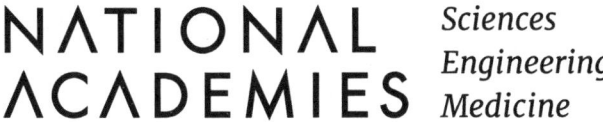

The Role of Seafood Consumption in Child Growth and Development

Committee on the Role of Seafood Consumption on Child Growth and Development

Food and Nutrition Board

Health and Medicine Division

Consensus Study Report

NATIONAL ACADEMIES PRESS 500 Fifth Street, NW Washington, DC 20001

This activity was supported by a contract between the National Academy of Sciences and the U.S. Department of Health and Human Services, U.S. Food and Drug Administration Grant No. 75F40122F19001, which includes funds from the National Oceanic and Atmospheric Administration, the U.S. Department of Agriculture, and the U.S. Environmental Protection Agency. Any opinions, findings, conclusions, or recommendations expressed in this publication do not necessarily reflect the views of any organization or agency that provided support for the project.

International Standard Book Number-13: 978-0-309-71698-7
International Standard Book Number-10: 0-309-71698-5
Digital Object Identifier: https://doi.org/10.17226/27623
Library of Congress Control Number: 2024937830

This publication is available from the National Academies Press, 500 Fifth Street, NW, Keck 360, Washington, DC 20001; (800) 624-6242 or (202) 334-3313; http://www.nap.edu.

Copyright 2024 by the National Academy of Sciences. National Academies of Sciences, Engineering, and Medicine and National Academies Press and the graphical logos for each are all trademarks of the National Academy of Sciences. All rights reserved.

Printed in the United States of America.

Suggested citation: National Academies of Sciences, Engineering, and Medicine. 2024. *The role of seafood consumption in child growth and development*. Washington, DC: The National Academies Press. https://doi.org/10.17226/27623.

The **National Academy of Sciences** was established in 1863 by an Act of Congress, signed by President Lincoln, as a private, nongovernmental institution to advise the nation on issues related to science and technology. Members are elected by their peers for outstanding contributions to research. Dr. Marcia McNutt is president.

The **National Academy of Engineering** was established in 1964 under the charter of the National Academy of Sciences to bring the practices of engineering to advising the nation. Members are elected by their peers for extraordinary contributions to engineering. Dr. John L. Anderson is president.

The **National Academy of Medicine** (formerly the Institute of Medicine) was established in 1970 under the charter of the National Academy of Sciences to advise the nation on medical and health issues. Members are elected by their peers for distinguished contributions to medicine and health. Dr. Victor J. Dzau is president.

The three Academies work together as the **National Academies of Sciences, Engineering, and Medicine** to provide independent, objective analysis and advice to the nation and conduct other activities to solve complex problems and inform public policy decisions. The National Academies also encourage education and research, recognize outstanding contributions to knowledge, and increase public understanding in matters of science, engineering, and medicine.

Learn more about the National Academies of Sciences, Engineering, and Medicine at **www.nationalacademies.org**.

Consensus Study Reports published by the National Academies of Sciences, Engineering, and Medicine document the evidence-based consensus on the study's statement of task by an authoring committee of experts. Reports typically include findings, conclusions, and recommendations based on information gathered by the committee and the committee's deliberations. Each report has been subjected to a rigorous and independent peer-review process, and it represents the position of the National Academies on the statement of task.

Proceedings published by the National Academies of Sciences, Engineering, and Medicine chronicle the presentations and discussions at a workshop, symposium, or other event convened by the National Academies. The statements and opinions contained in proceedings are those of the participants and are not endorsed by other participants, the planning committee, or the National Academies.

Rapid Expert Consultations published by the National Academies of Sciences, Engineering, and Medicine are authored by subject-matter experts on narrowly focused topics that can be supported by a body of evidence. The discussions contained in rapid expert consultations are considered those of the authors and do not contain policy recommendations. Rapid expert consultations are reviewed by the institution before release.

For information about other products and activities of the National Academies, please visit www.nationalacademies.org/about/whatwedo.

COMMITTEE ON THE ROLE OF
SEAFOOD CONSUMPTION IN CHILD GROWTH AND DEVELOPMENT

VIRGINIA A. STALLINGS (*Chair*), Professor of Pediatrics, Division of Gastroenterology, Hepatology, and Nutrition, The Children's Hospital of Philadelphia, University of Pennsylvania

LAURIE HING MAN CHAN, Canada Research Chair in Toxicology and Environmental Health, Department of Biology, University of Ottawa, Canada

ELAINE M. FAUSTMAN, Professor, Department of Environmental & Occupational Health Sciences and Director, Institute of Risk Analysis and Risk Communication, School of Public Health and Community Medicine, University of Washington

CLAUDE EARL FOX, Professor Emeritus, Department of Epidemiology, School of Public Health Sciences, University of Miami Miller School of Medicine

DELBERT M. GATLIN III, Regents Professor, Texas A&M AgriLife Research Senior Faculty Fellow, Department of Ecology and Conservation Biology, Texas A&M University

JULIE HERBSTMAN, Professor, Environmental Health Sciences, Director, Columbia Center for Children's Environmental Health, Columbia University, New York

MARGARET R. KARAGAS, James W. Squires Professor and Chair, Department of Epidemiology, Geisel School of Medicine, Dartmouth College, New Hampshire

SIBYLLE KRANZ, Associate Professor, Department of Kinesiology, Adjunct Associate Professor, Public Health Sciences, University of Virginia

MAUREEN LICHTVELD, Dean, Graduate School of Public Health, Jonas Salk Professor of Population Health, Professor of Environmental and Occupational Health, University of Pittsburgh

CHARLES A. NELSON, Professor of Pediatrics and Neuroscience, Richard David Scott Chair in Pediatric Developmental Medicine Research, Harvard Medical School, Boston Children's Hospital

EMILY OKEN, Alice Hamilton Professor and Vice Chair, Department of Population Medicine, Harvard Medical School and Harvard Pilgrim Health Care Institute

IAN J. SALDANHA, Associate Professor, Department of Epidemiology, Johns Hopkins Bloomberg School of Public Health, Johns Hopkins University, Baltimore

Consultants

JULEEN LAM, Assistant Professor, Department of Public Health, California State University East Bay

ALICE H. LICHTENSTEIN, Gershoff Professor of Nutrition Science, Jean Mayer USDA Human Nutrition Research Center on Aging at Tufts University, Massachusetts (*until March 2023*)

BARBARA O. SCHNEEMAN, Professor Emerita, University of California, Davis

ALICIA TIMME-LARAGY, Professor, School of Public Health & Health Sciences, University of Massachusetts Amherst

AMANDA MACFARLANE, Director, Texas A&M Agriculture, Food, and Nutrition Evidence Center

MAUREEN SPILL, Program Lead, Nutrition & Health, Texas A&M Agriculture, Food, and Nutrition Evidence Center

DAVID LOVE, Senior Scientist, Seafood, Public Health & Food Systems Project, Johns Hopkins Center for a Livable Future at the Bloomberg School of Public Health

ANDREW THORNE-LYMAN, Associate Research Professor, Department of International Health, Johns Hopkins Center for a Livable Future at the Bloomberg School of Public Health

Study Staff

ELIZABETTE ANDRADE, Study Director
KATHRYN GUYTON, Senior Program Officer (*until May 2023*)
ALICE VOROSMARTI, Associate Program Officer
JENNIFER STEPHENSON, Research Associate
JENNIFER MOUSER, Senior Program Assistant
THOMASINA LYLES, Senior Program Assistant (*until April 2023*)
REBECCA MORGAN, Senior Librarian
ANN L. YAKTINE, Director, Food and Nutrition Board

Reviewers

This Consensus Study Report was reviewed in draft form by individuals chosen for their diverse perspectives and technical expertise. The purpose of this independent review is to provide candid and critical comments that will assist the National Academies of Sciences, Engineering, and Medicine in making each published report as sound as possible and to ensure that it meets the institutional standards for quality, objectivity, evidence, and responsiveness to the charge. The review comments and draft manuscript remain confidential to protect the integrity of the process.

We thank the following individuals for their review of this report:

P. MICHAEL BOLGER, U.S. Food and Drug Administration (*retired*)
SUSAN E. CARLSON, University of Kansas Medical Center
PHILIPPE GRANDJEAN, University of Rhode Island
LORA IANNOTTI, Washington University in St. Louis
SHARON KIRKPATRICK, University of Waterloo
JIM RIVIERE, North Carolina State University
CATHERINE ROSS, Texas A&M University
MARCELA TAMAYO-ORTIZ, Columbia University
XIAOBIN WANG, Johns Hopkins Bloomberg School of Public Health
DANIELE WIKOFF, ToxStrategies

Although the reviewers listed above provided many constructive comments and suggestions, they were not asked to endorse the content of the report nor did they see the final draft before its release. The review of this report was overseen by **JACK EBELER,** Health Policy Alternatives, Inc., and **SUZANNE P. MURPHY,** University of Hawaii at Manoa. They were responsible for making certain that an independent examination of this report was carried out in accordance with standards of the National Academies and that all review comments were carefully considered. Responsibility for the final content rests entirely with the authoring committee and the National Academies.

Contents

ACRONYMS AND ABBREVIATIONS   xi

PREFACE   xv

SUMMARY   1

1 INTRODUCTION   13
Background for the Study, 13
Committee's Task and Approach, 14
Organization of the Report, 16
References, 16

2 METHODOLOGICAL APPROACH TO THE TASK   17
Systematic Reviews, 17
Supplementary Review of Systematic Reviews, 19
Seafood Intake Analyses, 21
Conceptual Framework, 22
References, 23

3 SEAFOOD CONSUMPTION PATTERNS IN THE UNITED STATES AND CANADA   25
Sources of Seafood, 25
Trends in Consumption of Fish and Seafood, 29
Survey Data on Seafood Consumption by Age and Sex Group, 31
Factors Influencing Seafood Consumption, 40
Seafood Consumption by Setting, 44
Findings and Conclusions, 52
Recommendations, 52
Research Gaps, 53
References, 53

4	**DIETARY INTAKE AND NUTRIENT COMPOSITION OF SEAFOOD**	57

Nutrient Composition of Seafood, 57
Dietary Patterns and Seafood Consumption, 67
Findings and Conclusion, 81
Research Gaps, 81
References, 81

5	**EXPOSURE TO CONTAMINANTS ASSOCIATED WITH CONSUMPTION OF SEAFOOD**	85

Toxins and Toxicants of Concern in Seafood, 85
Contaminants Resulting in Chronic Exposures, 86
Contaminants Resulting in Acute or Episodic Exposure, 93
Human Biomarkers of Toxicant Exposure Associated with Seafood Consumption, 96
Findings and Conclusions, 100
Research Gaps, 101
References, 102

6	**HEALTH OUTCOMES ASSOCIATED WITH SEAFOOD CONSUMPTION**	109

Seafood Consumption and Health Outcomes in Children and Adolescents, 109
Exposure to Toxicants in Seafood and Child Growth and Development, 114
Common Mechanisms of Action of Contaminants Commonly Found in Seafood, 121
Findings and Conclusions, 123
Research Gaps, 124
References, 124

7	**RISK–BENEFIT ANALYSIS**	129

Approach to Reviewing Evidence on Conducting a Risk–Benefit Analysis, 129
Assessment of the State of the Science on Risk–Benefit Analysis, 129
Methodologies and Frameworks Used to Conduct Risk–Benefit Analyses, 130
Modeling Benefits and Risks of Fish Consumption, 133
Developing a Framework for Conducting a Risk–Benefit Analysis, 135
Scientific Principles Underpinning a Risk–Benefit Analysis, 137
Approach to Conducting a Risk–Benefit Analysis, 138
Steps in Evaluating When or When Not to Conduct a Risk–Benefit Analysis, 139
A Basis for Decision Making, 140
Community Resilience and Access to Health Care, 141
Findings and Conclusions, 144
Recommendations, 145
Research Gaps, 145
References, 145

APPENDIXES[1]

A	**COMMITTEE MEMBER BIOSKETCHES**	147
B	**OPEN SESSION AGENDAS**	153
C	**COMMISSIONED SYSTEMATIC REVIEWS**	157
D	**SUPPLEMENTAL REVIEW OF SYSTEMATIC REVIEWS**	169
E	**NHANES DATA ANALYSIS METHODOLOGY**	185

---

[1] Three additional appendixes can be found at https://nap.nationalacademies.org/catalog/27623: Appendix F (Literature Searches Conducted for Systematic Reviews); Appendix G (Supplemental Literature Searches); and Appendix H (Commissioned Systematic Reviews: Final Report).

Acronyms and Abbreviations

ADHD	attention deficit hyperactivity disorder
ALA	alpha-linolenic acid
AMSTAR	A Measurement Tool to Assess Systematic Reviews
ASD	autism spectrum disorder
ATP	adenosine triphosphate
ATSDR	Agency for Toxic Substances and Disease Registry
BOND	biomarkers of nutrition for development
CCHS	Canadian Community Health Survey
CHD	coronary heart disease
CI	confidence interval
CSFII	Continuing Survey of Food Intakes by Individuals
CVD	cardiovascular disease
DALY	disability-adjusted life year
DEXA	dual x-ray absorptiometry
DGA	*Dietary Guidelines for Americans 2020–2025*
DHA	docosahexaenoic acid
DMA	dimethylarsinate
DNA	deoxyribonucleic acid
DXA	dual x-ray absorptiometry
EFSA	European Food Safety Authority
EPA	eicosapentaenoic acid
EPA	U.S. Environmental Protection Agency
ERS	Economic Research Service
EU	European Union

FADS	Food Availability Data System
FAO	Food and Agriculture Organization of the United Nations
FDA	U.S. Food and Drug Administration
FN	First Nations
FPED	Food Patterns Equivalent Database
g	gram
GRADE	Grading of Recommendations, Assessment, Development and Evaluation
HCL	hydrochloric acid
HDL	high-density lipoprotein
HEI	Healthy Eating Index
Hg	mercury
IF	intrinsic factor
IOM	Institute of Medicine
IQ	intelligence quotient
IU	international units
kcal	kilocalorie
LCPUFA	long-chain, polyunsaturated fatty acid
LDL	low-density lipoprotein
µg	microgram
MeHg	methylmercury
MeSH	Medical Subject Heading
mg	milligram
NHANES	National Health and Nutrition Examination Survey
NOAA	National Oceanic and Atmospheric Administration
NSLP	National School Lunch Program
PBDE	polybrominated diphenyl ether
PCB	polychlorinated biphenyl
PECOD	populations, exposures, comparators, outcomes, study design
PFAS	per- and polyfluoroalkyl substances
PFC	perfluorinated compounds
PIF	potential impact fraction
POP	persistent organic pollutant
PUFA	polyunsaturated fatty acids
QALY	quality-adjusted life year
RBA	risk–benefit analysis
RCT	randomized controlled trial

ACRONYMS AND ABBREVIATIONS

T3	tri-iodothyronine
T4	thyroglobulintetraiodothyronine or thyroxin
TrxR	thioredoxin reductase
TWI	tolerable weekly intake
UFCR	usual fish consumption rate
UK	United Kingdom
UL	Tolerable Upper Intake Level
USDA	U.S. Department of Agriculture
WCBA	women of childbearing age
WHO	World Health Organization

Preface

My childhood memories include the cultural and festive role of fish. Because my hometown is at the convergence of two rivers, many people fished for food and some for sport. With my grandfather, I learned of trotlines for huge catfish and the fun of catching sunfish and perch with a cane pole. A backyard fish fry was part of family reunions and parties, and our vacation to the Gulf involved shrimp and flounder for kids and crabs and oysters for adults. At those times, the safety of this freshwater and marine bounty was of no concern, nor was consumption of these foods considered to have health advantages.

At present, however, both the safety and the health advantages of fish and other seafood consumption are of high interest. The Committee on the Role of Seafood Consumption in Child Growth and Development of the National Academies of Sciences, Engineering, and Medicine was convened to understand the evidence of risks and benefits of seafood (including freshwater and marine) consumption in the United States. The committee was asked to examine seafood consumption and dietary intake by pregnant and lactating women, and by children, and its associations with growth, developmental, and health outcomes in children and adolescents. In addition, the committee evaluated the potential usefulness of the formal risk–benefit analysis methodology to inform public health recommendations issued by federal agencies, such as the U.S. Department of Agriculture, U.S. Food and Drug Administration, U.S. Environmental Protection Agency, and National Oceanic and Atmospheric Administration, and to make recommendations for seafood consumption in these two populations. It was also the committee's charge to consider racial and ethnic subgroups, as well as subsistence and sport fishers, in order to support a diverse, inclusive, and equitable approach to the task, to the extent possible.

Understanding the safety of seafood is a complicated process requiring information about each potential toxicant for each commonly consumed species. Information is then needed on the amount of each species consumed by the various life-stage groups (birth to 18 years, pregnant or lactating women, etc.). The search for this key information revealed limited high-quality evidence that was sometimes inconsistent.

One of the surprising findings for me was how little seafood is consumed by children and pregnant women, with few women and children meeting the recommendations in the *Dietary Guidelines for Americans* that call for two servings of seafood per week. Pregnant and lactating women merit special attention because of the potential for seafood consumption to result in both adverse and beneficial health effects on the fetus and infant; these issues are well covered in the report. Opportunity exists to increase consumption of seafood—a source of high-quality protein, healthful fatty acids, and several micronutrients—across all life stages evaluated.

Committee members were well suited to the report's tasks based on their scientific expertise and their experience in evaluating the quality of the evidence. After serving on this project for 20 months, the committee detailed its findings, conclusions, and recommendations. Among the recommendations are to collect additional, specific data to ensure that policy makers and other stakeholders have sufficient information for public health decision making, including promoting healthful dietary patterns while addressing safety concerns.

A technical expert panel (TEP) provided significant contributions that helped guide this report. In collaboration with the committee, TEP consultants Juleen Lam, Barbara Schneeman, Alicia Timme-Laragy, and Alice Lichtenstein worked with committee member Ian Saldanha to develop the conceptual framework to inform our approach to data gathering, review, and synthesis.[1] I also want to acknowledge the scientists at the Johns Hopkins Center for a Livable Future at the Bloomberg School of Public Health, David Love and Andrew Thorne-Lyman, as well as the team at Texas A&M University, Amanda McFarland and Maureen Spill, for their work to ensure the committee had the most current and comprehensive data for its analysis and deliberations.

As chair, I express my sincere appreciation to each committee member and to each member of our National Academies staff, including Ann Yaktine, Elizabette Andrade, Kate Guyton, Alice Vorosmarti, Jennifer Stephenson, Jennifer Mouser, Thomasina Lyles, and Rebecca Morgan, for your shared commitment to this project.

Virginia A. Stallings, *Chair*
Committee on the Role of Seafood in Child Growth and Development

---

[1] Alice Lichtenstein served on the TEP until March 2023.

Summary

BACKGROUND

Seafood, including marine and freshwater fish, mollusks, and crustaceans, is a protein food that is also a rich source of the nutrients needed in pregnancy and lactation as well as those vital to support growth and development from infancy through adolescence. The *Dietary Guidelines for Americans 2020–2025 (DGA)* includes an overarching recommendation that all U.S. adults aim to consume at least 8 ounces (two servings) of seafood per week.[1] For children, the *DGA* recommends two servings per week in amounts corresponding to an individual's total daily caloric intake. The *DGA* also includes a recommendation to introduce seafood to children when they are around 6 months of age.

Although seafood is an important source of key nutrients, it can also be a source of exposure to contaminants such as methylmercury, persistent pollutants including per- and polyfluoroalkyl substances, dioxins, polychlorinated biphenyls, and microbiological hazards that may be detrimental to the growth and development of children. The Closer to Zero action plan, launched by the U.S. Food and Drug Administration (FDA) in April 2021, proposed an approach to reduce exposure through food, including seafood, to four metals—arsenic, lead, cadmium, and mercury—that can have adverse effects on child development, particularly neurodevelopment, with the goal of reducing blood-level concentrations of these contaminants in infants and children by decreasing exposure from foods that contain them. The recommendations in the action plan serve as a foundation for *DGA* recommendations about consuming seafood.

The juxtaposition of nutritional benefits and toxicological risks associated with the consumption of seafood led FDA, in collaboration with the U.S. Environmental Protection Agency (EPA), the U.S. Department of Agriculture (USDA), and the National Oceanic and Atmospheric Administration (NOAA) to ask the National Academies of Sciences, Engineering, and Medicine (the National Academies) to convene a committee to review the role of seafood in the diets of pregnant and lactating women and children, including adolescents—with consideration of the components found in seafood that are potentially detrimental as well as those that are beneficial—to evaluate their respective, interacting, and complex roles in child development and lifelong health. Additionally, these federal sponsoring agencies asked the committee to evaluate when or when not to conduct a formal risk–benefit analysis (RBA) relative to risk–benefit factors including how to assess the quality and uncertainty of an RBA

---

[1] Throughout the report, seafood consumption guidelines refer to the recommendations in the Dietary Guidelines for Americans. This clarification was added after release of the report to the study sponsor.

and to provide scientific information and principles that can serve as a foundation to evaluate confidence in the potential conclusions of an RBA. The committee was further asked to identify and comment on additional context, including equity, diversity, inclusion, and access to health care, that may be additive to the findings of an RBA approach to the task.

The committee approached its task by evaluating evidence submitted by the study sponsors, supplemented with additional searches of existing databases and published literature. The committee contracted with the Texas A&M University Agriculture, Food, and Nutrition Evidence Center to conduct an update of two systematic reviews from the USDA Nutrition Evidence Systematic Review—one on seafood consumption during childhood and adolescence and neurocognitive development and the other on seafood consumption during pregnancy and lactation and neurocognitive development in the child. In addition, the committee requested the Evidence Center conduct a *de novo* systematic review on toxicants in seafood and neurocognitive development in children and adolescents. The committee also commissioned two scientists from the Johns Hopkins Center for a Livable Future at the Bloomberg School of Public Health to perform analyses using National Health and Nutrition Examination Survey (NHANES) cross-sectional data on seafood consumption and factors that affect decision making and dietary patterns. To provide deeper context for both nutrient intake and exposure to contaminants, particularly among at-risk groups, the committee's review of evidence included the assessment of data from the United States and from Canadian populations, including Native and Indigenous peoples. While this evidence was considered, the committee's recommendations apply only to U.S. populations.

As part of its task, the committee was asked to develop and implement an approach to integrating scientific evidence in a transparent way and draw conclusions on questions related to seafood and child development outcomes. To facilitate this, the committee developed a conceptual framework (Figure S-1). The conceptual framework indicates the relationships of sources of nutrient, contaminant, and micro-organism exposures in seafood with health outcomes. The framework also identifies relevant time periods over the life course of the population groups of interest. The framework was used to guide the committee's discussions, particularly on exposure and health outcomes through consumption of seafood by these population groups.

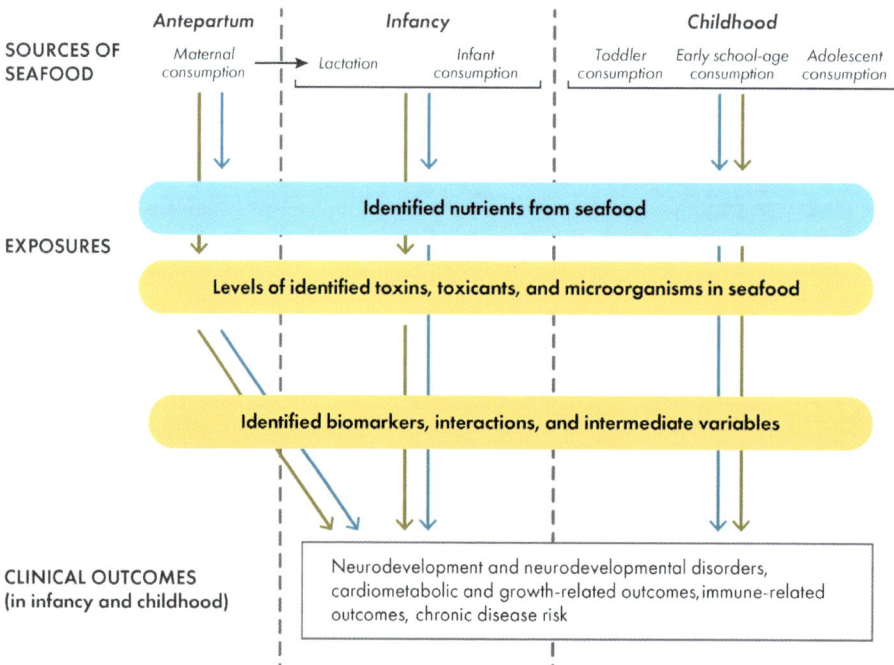

FIGURE S-1 Conceptual framework for mapping nutrient, contaminant, and micro-organism exposures to health outcomes.

FACTORS ASSOCIATED WITH CONSUMING SEAFOOD

Types and Amounts of Seafood Consumed

According to dietary intake data from 2018–2019, the 10 most consumed seafood species for the total U.S. population accounted for about three-quarters of the total seafood consumption. All of the 10 most consumed species in both the United States and Canada are rich in protein. Several of them, such as salmon and albacore tuna, are also rich in docosahexaenoic acid (DHA) and eicosapentaenoic acid (EPA), which are n-3 long-chain polyunsaturated fatty acids (LCPUFAs). The remaining most consumed seafood species are lower in total lipids, including n-3 LCPUFAs.

During the past century, overall consumption of seafood has increased and is attributable to a combination of increasing population and greater per capita consumption. Most of the increase has been in the consumption of fresh and frozen seafood, as consumption of canned seafood has remained generally stable and cured seafood (e.g., fermented, pickled, or smoked) has had a negligible contribution to overall seafood consumption. Most seafood consumed in the United States is imported.

Most of the seafood consumed by women of childbearing age and children comes from retail purchases (e.g., supermarket, grocery store, or convenience store) and is consumed at home as part of lunch or dinner meals and, less frequently, as restaurant meals. School and other institutional meals provide a negligible contribution to overall seafood intake.

Factors Influencing the Choice to Consume Seafood

Factors, including cultural background, income, and geographic locations, influence the types and amounts of seafood consumed. Native and Indigenous peoples and recreational fishers are likely to consume seafood more frequently than other groups. Individuals with lower household incomes may tend to eat fish less frequently and consume fish that are less rich in n-3 LCPUFAs. With regard to the types of seafood, individuals identifying as non-Hispanic Asian and non-Hispanic Black most commonly consume shrimp, salmon, other fish, and other unknown fish or catfish, whereas those who identify as Hispanic, non-Hispanic White, and those of other racial and ethnic identities consume more shrimp, tuna, salmon, and crab.

Residence in a geographic area near the Atlantic, Pacific, or Gulf of Mexico coasts, or the Great Lakes, is associated with greater average seafood consumption, although few children or women in these areas consume the recommended two servings of seafood per week.

Limited information is available regarding the awareness of fish consumption guidelines for women of childbearing age and children. Longitudinal data from over a decade ago suggest that there was consumer awareness about prior guidelines. However, consumer awareness was not a factor in amounts of seafood consumed.

Nutrient Intake from Seafood Consumption

Seafood is a source of protein that is high in biological value (i.e., contains all the essential amino acids and has high absorption rates); therefore, the *DGA* includes seafood as a subgroup of dietary protein that also includes the subgroup of meat, poultry, and eggs.[2] Some types of seafood contain EPA and DHA, which are necessary for fetal development as they form key components of cell membranes; they are also precursors of several metabolites that are potential lipid mediators. Although EPA and DHA can be synthesized from alpha-linolenic acid (an essential short-chain n-3 fatty acid), the conversion rate is less than 10 percent in humans.

NHANES data for adults indicate that, compared with women 25 years of age or older, younger women consume lower amounts of micronutrients from seafood, except for vitamin B12. No large differences in the average intakes of any nutrients were observed by racial and ethnic identity. Higher income is associated with higher intake

---

[2] Available at https://health.gov/our-work/nutrition-physical-activity/dietary-guidelines/previous-dietary-guidelines/2015/advisory-report/appendix-e-3/appendix-e-31a1 (accessed February 13, 2024).

from seafood for all nutrients, except vitamin D, which was the same in women from middle- and high-income households. Differences in nutrient intake between seafood consumers and nonconsumers are small.

NHANES data for children indicate that a small proportion of daily protein intake is from seafood and that average protein intake from seafood high in n-3 LCPUFA is less than 2 grams per day. Those in the highest percentile of protein intake from seafood that is also high in n-3 LCPUFAs consume only about 27 grams of protein per day, which contributes approximately 25 percent of their daily total protein intake. Boys showed a higher protein intake from seafood compared with girls; however, the proportion of total protein intake from seafood was below 25 percent in all age groups. Non-Hispanic Asian children had higher intakes of n-3 LCPUFAs compared with all other children, and Hispanic children had the second-highest intakes of n-3 LCPUFAs.

Primary Findings and Conclusions

Findings

1. Despite population-level increases in seafood disappearance during the past decade, seafood consumption among women of childbearing age and children and adolescents is generally low and has remained similar to that reported in *Seafood Choices: Balancing Benefits and Risks* (IOM, 2007).
2. Limited evidence is available to suggest that the public is knowledgeable about both the types and amounts of seafood that are recommended for consumption by women of childbearing age and children and adolescents.
3. Most of the seafood consumed by both women of childbearing age and children and adolescents comes from retail purchases and is consumed at home as part of lunch or dinner meals. School lunch is a negligible contributor of seafood to children's diets.
4. Limited evidence is available on the types and preparation methods of seafood consumed by pregnant and lactating women and children and adolescents in the general population.
5. Although few women of childbearing age and children and adolescents in the general population meet the recommended intake of two servings of seafood per week, some from certain ethnic or cultural backgrounds—such as those of Asian or Native American heritage, Indigenous peoples, and sport and subsistence fishers and their families—consume greater than average amounts of seafood.
6. Multiple factors influence patterns of seafood consumption, including residence in coastal areas or near bodies of water such as the Great Lakes, familiarity with fish preparation methods, and cultural and traditional practices.
7. Current evidence on the nutrient content of seafood indicates that seafood is a rich source of multiple nutrients, including vitamin D, calcium, potassium, and iron, which are identified as nutrients of public health concern by the *Dietary Guidelines for Americans* and play roles in supporting pregnancy and lactation as well as growth and development.
8. Seafood is an important source of n-3 LCPUFAs, which are key nutrients for the prenatal period, during lactation, and throughout childhood. Choline, iodine, and magnesium are additional nutrients that are provided by seafood and have important functions throughout childhood and adolescence.
9. Individuals who do not consume seafood likely have intakes of n-3 LCPUFAs below recommended amounts.
10. Seafood is one component of healthful dietary patterns described in the *Dietary Guidelines for Americans*. The majority of the U.S. and Canadian population has lower-than-recommended intakes of n-3 LCPUFAs from seafood. Intakes are highest among high-income women and children, but income status, however, is not consistently associated with intake levels of other nutrients.
11. Among Native and Indigenous populations who are transitioning away from traditional diets, limiting seafood consumption increases the risk of not achieving optimal intake of a range of nutrients, including n-3 LCPUFAs. Low seafood consumption may also contribute to inadequate nutrient intakes among other at-risk populations who are low consumers, such as non-Hispanic Black and Hispanic Americans, and especially among those with lower incomes or experiencing food insecurity.

Conclusions

1. *Most women of childbearing age and children and adolescents do not consume the recommended amounts and types of seafood. Strategies to support increasing consumption toward meeting recommendations are needed.*
2. *Identification of strategies to overcome barriers to seafood consumption are needed so (1) individuals who consume some seafood will increase their intake toward recommended amounts, and (2) nonconsumers will begin consuming seafood with the goal of meeting recommended amounts.*
3. *Insufficient evidence exists to suggest a need to revise seafood consumption guidelines, but a need does exist to identify strategies to help individuals meet current guidelines.*
4. *Taken together, the committee concludes that nutrient intakes from seafood by women of childbearing age and children are low.*

RECOMMENDATIONS

Recommendation 1: The Centers for Disease Control and Prevention should identify strategies to address gaps in the current National Health and Nutrition Examination Survey monitoring to better assess the sources, types, amounts, and preparation methods of seafood consumed by women of childbearing age, pregnant and lactating women, and children and adolescents up to 18 years of age.

Recommendation 2: The U.S. Department of Agriculture should reevaluate its federal nutrition programs, especially school meals, to support greater inclusion of seafood in meal patterns.

RESEARCH GAPS

- Research is needed to characterize the knowledge of, and responses to, current seafood consumption guidelines among women of childbearing age and children and adolescents. This should include research of seafood consumption by children, particularly in school settings and other meals consumed outside the home.
- Further research is needed to assess the types, amounts, and patterns of seafood consumed during pregnancy and lactation.
- Additional research is needed to assess the barriers to providing seafood as a component of meals served in schools and other settings frequented by children.
- Data are needed on levels of nutrient intake by seafood consumers who meet current seafood intake recommendations compared to nonconsumers and low consumers of seafood.
- Additional data are needed on the nutrient composition of types of seafood frequently consumed in different geographic regions in the United States and Canada.

HEALTH OUTCOMES ASSOCIATED WITH EXPOSURE TO CONTAMINANTS IN SEAFOOD

Exposure to Contaminants in Seafood

Estimates of exposure to contaminants of concern through consumption of seafood depend principally on two factors: the amount of seafood consumed and the amount of the contaminant in seafood. Using the reported consumption rates from national surveys such as NHANES and the Canadian Community Health Survey, it is possible to quantitatively estimate the exposure of different contaminants from seafood consumption among women of childbearing age, children, and adolescents. The concentration of contaminants in seafood depends on many factors including the species, age of the fish, its geographic origin, how it is prepared, and which part of the fish is consumed.

Seafood can contain a broad range of contaminants, including microbial contaminants. Concentrations of contaminants such as metals, metalloids, and other trace elements along with organic compounds such as polychlorinated biphenyls (PCBs), polybrominated diphenyl ethers (PBDEs), and per- and polyfluoroalkyl substances (PFAS) vary widely among species and geographic region, by the size and age of the organism, and according to whether they are wild caught or cultivated, among other factors. Mercury is the most studied contaminant in seafood, but because seafood consumption is generally below recommendations and the concentrations of mercury for commonly consumed seafood (except for tuna) tend to be relatively low, exposure will likely not exceed guideline values for most people. Certain subgroups of the population, including Native and Indigenous peoples and subsistence or sport fishers could be at greater risk from exposure to seafood toxicants because of their pattern of seafood intake or source of seafood.

Exposures to pathogens and microbial toxins occur episodically as "outbreaks" at a specific time and location, or as food poisoning cases among individuals who consume contaminated seafoods. These risks are often mitigated by the closing of the harvest at specific times or locations or by removing contaminated seafood from the market before it is sold.

FDA oversees the inspection of both domestic and imported seafood to ensure its safety to consumers. Products are assessed for various adulterations including the presence of contaminants and pathogens as well as mislabeling and unsanitary manufacturing, processing, or packing. An Institute of Medicine (IOM) report indicates that most of the seafood sold in the United States is wholesome and unlikely to cause illness. Potential differences in contaminants and pathogens from imported and domestic products are difficult to assess owing to the great variety of seafood products and processing methods.

Biomarkers of Exposure to Toxicants Associated with Seafood Consumption

Epidemiological studies relating seafood intake during pregnancy to biomarkers of contaminant exposure have largely focused on mercury, with findings of higher blood, hair, and toenail mercury concentrations among those who consumed more seafood. Evidence from NHANES indicates that higher seafood intake is positively correlated with blood levels of mercury and urinary concentrations of total arsenic, domoic acid, and arsenobetaine, among both women of childbearing age and children. Studies of the biomarker concentrations of other contaminants associated with seafood consumption are relatively scarce, and for all contaminants very little data exist on biomarker associations with seafood intake specifically during lactation, infancy, and childhood.

Health Outcomes

Higher fish consumption by women of childbearing age, including women who are pregnant and lactating, and by children is either generally associated with a lower risk of adverse health outcomes or no association with health outcomes is found. An exception is higher exposures among certain population subgroups such as consumers of sport-caught species or groups dependent on subsistence fishing. Moreover, there is evidence that greater fish consumption by women during pregnancy is likely associated with several health benefits, including improved birth outcomes. Taken as a whole, the evidence reviewed by the committee indicates that higher fish consumption is associated with lower risk of adverse health outcomes or no association with health outcomes. The evidence for increased risk of adverse health outcomes associated with seafood consumption was insufficient to draw a conclusion.

Mechanisms of Action

Some experimental evidence supports that the toxicity of mercury and PCBs can be modified by other factors (i.e., in antioxidant response pathways). This literature is complex, and the committee was not able to identify supportive evidence in humans.

Primary Findings and Conclusions

Findings on Contaminants of Concern and Exposure Through Seafood

1. Toxins, toxicants, and microbes, including persistent bioaccumulative chemicals, metals and metalloids, infectious organisms, microplastics, and micro-organisms, may be present in seafood at levels hazardous to consumers. The concentration of these various contaminants in seafood depends on many factors, including species, trophic position, size, age, geographic location, and origin—wild caught or farm raised.
2. With the exception of some types of tuna, the most commonly consumed seafood species in the United States and Canada contain relatively low concentrations of methylmercury, and concentrations of other metals and metalloids tend to be limited to certain species and geographic areas.[3]
3. Among adults and children, seafood consumption is associated with higher blood, hair, and toenail levels of mercury, and urinary concentrations of certain forms of arsenic, particularly those common to seafood such as arsenobetaine.
4. Average intake levels of methylmercury from seafood are below the FDA "Closer to Zero" recommended limits among women of childbearing age, infants, and children, except for those who frequently consume tuna.[4]
5. PCBs and mercury are the key drivers for fish consumption advisories and PCBs are particularly relevant in the Great Lakes region.
6. Certain population groups, in particular Native Americans and Indigenous peoples, as well as subsistence and sport fishers and their families, may consume more seafood species or seafood components from geographic locations that could have high concentrations of mercury and PCBs than individuals in the general population, thereby exceeding recommended limits.[5]

Findings on Health Outcomes

1. Many of the studies reviewed by the committee reported outcomes correlated with seafood consumption generally and without differentiation as to species. One commonly accepted assumption has been that omega-3 long-chain fatty acids in seafood, particularly DHA, contribute benefits, possibly in combination with other nutrients.
2. The evidence reviewed indicates that some gains in neurodevelopment may be achieved during childhood and are apparent in the children of women who consume greater quantities of seafood during pregnancy compared to those who consume lower quantities or no seafood.
3. Seafood consumption by women during pregnancy may also have a protective effect against adverse neurocognitive outcomes in their children that is linked to the nutrients in seafood, particularly the n-3 long-chain polyunsaturated fatty acids that are essential to brain development. Associations of health outcomes with seafood intake differ between the general populations and recreational and subsistence fishers.

Conclusions

1. *The committee found insufficient evidence to assess exposure to most consumers associated with emerging contaminants in seafood, including PFAS, microplastics, and domoic acids.*
2. *PBDE exposure is not due primarily to seafood consumption; however, as PBDEs migrate into aquatic environments, risk of increased exposure through seafood may emerge.*
3. *Although seafood consumption is generally low across population groups, it continues to be an important predictor of methylmercury, arsenic, and PCB exposure and may be important for assessing PFAS exposure,*

---

[3] The sentence was revised after release of the report to the study sponsor to clarify that concentrations of methylmercury vary in different types of tuna after release of the report to the study sponsor.

[4] This sentence was modified after release of the report to the study sponsor to clarify that recommended limits of contaminant exposure are based on the Closer to Zero Action Plan.

[5] This section was modified after release of the report to the sponsor to reference recommended limits rather than acceptable risk levels.

where evidence is beginning to emerge. Therefore, if fish intake were to increase to DGA-recommended levels, then exposures would likely increase.
4. *The results of the studies identified through the committee's evidence reviews did not support a beneficial association of seafood consumption during childhood and adolescence and reduced risk of cardiovascular disease.*
5. *No evidence was identified to determine whether seafood consumption among children or adolescents is associated with benefits to reducing risk of other diseases such as immune disease.*
6. *The evidence reviewed on health outcomes associated with seafood consumption for women of childbearing age, children, and adolescents is not adequate to support an accurate assessment of the health benefits and risks associated with meeting the recommended intakes of seafood for this population group.*

Research Gaps

- Additional research is needed to assess geographic and temporal trend data for levels of methylmercury, mercury, and other contaminants in seafood, and to monitor intake levels of these contaminants among women of childbearing age, infants, and children. Special attention should be given to at-risk population groups such as Native Americans and Indigenous peoples, and to other at-risk groups, such as subsistence and sport fishers and their families.
- Research is needed for specific studies that examine arsenic and selenium in fish. Additional research is needed to assess the potential protective role of nutrients and other factors, such as selenoneine effects on mercury (Hg) toxicity.
- More quantitative characterization is needed to assess the risk of chronic exposure to less studied contaminants such as PFAS, arsenic species, microplastics, and domoic acid to assess bioaccumulation in food chains at the levels of exposure and toxicity.
- Research is needed to characterize biomarkers of exposure to contaminants in seafood among women of childbearing age, infants, children, and adolescents. This research is needed to identify and characterize dose–response relationships between contaminants and contaminant mixtures in seafood and adverse outcomes among the children of women exposed during pregnancy and lactation.
- Additional research is needed to assess childhood health outcomes related to seafood consumption by children. This should include not only amounts and types consumed but also the age of introduction of seafood to infants and children.
- Additional research is needed to determine whether there are sensitive periods in child development during which seafood consumption or exposure to contaminants in seafood might have different effects on child health.
- Population studies that examine the effects of maternal and child seafood consumption on child health outcomes need to better characterize the seafood species (e.g., type of fish, source, and location) as well as nutrient composition and contaminant concentrations in the seafood consumed.
- Additional research is needed on the health effects of contaminant mixtures and varied exposure levels to determine applicability for these observations in seafood-consuming populations in the United States and Canada.
- Additional research is needed to assess how to effectively communicate seafood consumption recommendations to women of childbearing age, children, and adolescents.

RISK–BENEFIT ANALYSIS

The assessment of risks and benefits to human health associated with seafood consumed as a food product as well as a part of a dietary pattern can be either quantitative or semiquantitative. The four steps in the risk assessment process are (1) identification of chemical and/or microbiological hazards, (2) assessment of intake response, (3) assessment of the nature of the risk, and (4) characterization of health outcomes. The balance of positive and negative health outcomes identified in the risk assessment is used to inform policy decisions and develop guidelines for public health practitioners.

Approaches to Conducting Risk–Benefit Analyses

An evidence scan, provided by the study sponsors, identified three tiers of risk–benefit analyses (RBAs). These are:

- Tier 1: Initial—a qualitative RBA that determines whether the health risks clearly outweigh the health benefits or vice versa.
- Tier 2: Refined—a semi-quantitative or quantitative estimate of risks and benefits at relevant (toxicant, essential nutrient) exposure levels.
- Tier 3: Composite metric—a quantitative RBA that compares risks and benefits as a single net health effect value, such as disability-adjusted life year (DALY) or quality-adjusted life years (QALY).

Across the body of epidemiological evidence, the evidence scan identified differences in exposure levels and in exposure and outcome measurements and windows, questionable population representation, and generalizability of diverse and specialized study samples. From a biostatistical perspective, variation existed in the covariates, confounders, and effect modifiers that were considered. The findings from the evidence scan show the importance of sufficient planning, preparation, discussion, consensus building, and further innovation when applying evolving review methodologies, incorporating emerging findings from new studies, and exploring approaches for integrating and synthesizing evidence.

The European Food Safety Authority (EFSA) scientific commission recommended that risk assessors consider the risks and benefits independently and compare health outcomes to determine whether the benefits outweigh the risks or vice versa. Step 1 of the EFSA model indicates the sources of evidence used to evaluate whether the evidence is of sufficient quality and quantity to justify an RBA. Step 2 indicates the methodologies and framework for comparing risks and benefits as a single net health effect value. Step 3 identifies the factors that influence the decision of whether to conduct an RBA. Step 4 considers factors that the committee considered in developing a process for evaluating confidence and conclusions in the evaluation process. If the results demonstrate that neither a substantial risk nor benefit exists, the assessment is terminated.

A Decision Tree for Evaluating When to Conduct a Risk–Benefit Analysis

Figure S-2 shows the committee's steps for evaluating when or when not to conduct a formal risk–benefit analysis. The committee based its steps for refining risk–benefit decision making on the EFSA model.

The committee considered a range of contextual factors—such as access to health care, access to food, community resilience, and stress—that modify the risk–benefit decision process. Specifically, higher perceived stress levels have been associated with lower adherence to a healthful dietary pattern. Social environments (family and peer influence), physical environments (schools and restaurants), and economic factors (income and socioeconomic status) also have an effect on food choice behaviors. Factors related to diversity, equity, and inclusion such as ethnicity, culture, and identity can affect food choice as well as availability.

Primary Findings and Conclusions

Findings

1. The integration of diverse data sources and the heterogeneous nature of information available about risks and benefits presents a challenge when selecting metrics to adequately evaluate and compare these risks and benefits in a formal RBA. To date, many formal RBAs have focused on methylmercury (MeHg) as the contaminant and have not assessed contaminant mixtures and toxins. Many other contaminants present in mixtures showed gaps in evidence and hence were less suitable to conduct a formal RBA. Key factors influencing the conduct of RBAs include the social determinants of health at the individual level, such as poverty and health disparities, and cultural traditions and vulnerability at the community level.

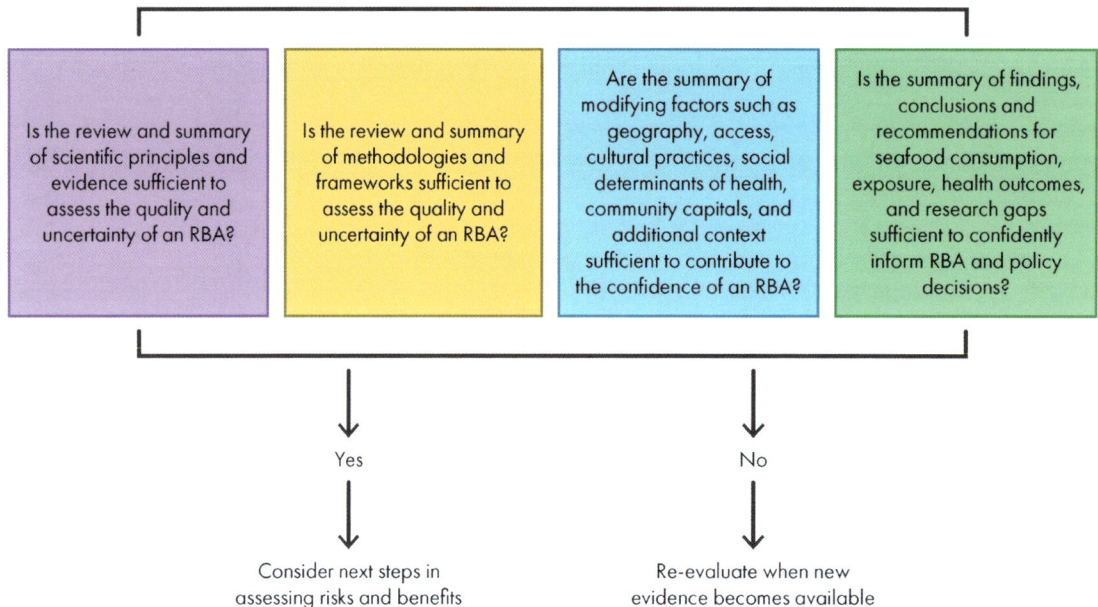

FIGURE S-2 Steps in evaluating when or when not to conduct a formal risk–benefit analysis.
NOTE: RBA = risk–benefit analysis.

2. All 50 U.S. states issue voluntary fish consumption advisories on potential contaminant exposure from consuming local fish. Advisories often include specific information about contaminants found in distinct fish species and waters. The evidence available showed variability in the information included in fish advisories for how these hazards are described, and even more variability in what (or if) nutritional information is included in these advisories, yet they are an information source for consumers. A key focus was observed on risks associated with the consumption of MeHg-contaminated fish by pregnant women. Most advisories do not adequately address the risk for specific vulnerable populations, especially subsistence fishers. The committee finds that this irregularity across advisories makes comparison of risks and benefits difficult for most consumers.

Conclusions

1. *A risk–benefit analysis can be an excellent tool to analyze, in a transparent matter, factors that affect both benefits and risks in an integrated approach, rather than as independent domains. This integrated approach toward assessing benefits and risks positions an RBA to effectively support decision-making processes regarding fish consumption. This tool can be applied at the population and individual levels and its scope extended beyond health concerns by including costs, environmental sustainability, and ethics.*
2. *The process for evaluating when or when not to conduct a formal risk–benefit analysis requires assessing the following four key areas: the state of evidence aided by systematic reviews of existing literature, the existence of validated approaches and metrics, an analysis of contextual factors affecting benefits or risk tailored to specific target populations, and the quality and uncertainty of the overall RBA evaluation.*
3. *Formal risk–benefit analyses of fish consumption are seldom conducted because no comprehensive source exists that provides necessary, available data on consumption, contextualization factors, and contamination.*
4. *Maximizing the usefulness of a risk–benefit analysis requires the integration of datasets addressing life stages, consumption patterns, information on nutrient status, exposure to contaminants, health outcomes, and contextual factors.*

5. *Communication about potential health benefits conferred by specific nutrients in seafood is varied. The advisories reviewed by the committee were voluntary and not subject to regulation.*
6. *Strengthening the links between a formal risk–benefit analysis, management decisions, and dietary recommendations communicated to the public can improve transparency and advance public health outcomes by ensuring that the best science informs management decisions.*

RECOMMENDATIONS

Recommendation 3: The U.S. Food and Drug Administration should consider conducting a risk–benefit analysis of maternal and child seafood intake and child growth and development, and, in doing so, routinely monitor data and scientific discoveries related to the underlying model and assumptions to ensure the assessment reflects the best available science.

Recommendation 4: In conducting a risk–benefit analysis, the U.S. Food and Drug Administration and the U.S. Environmental Protection Agency should include reviews of current evidence scans, systematic and supplemental reviews, approaches and metrics, benefit–harm characterization, and quality and assurance in evaluating the confidence in a risk–benefit analysis for policy decision making.

Recommendation 5: The U.S. Food and Drug Administration, in collaboration with the U.S. Environmental Protection Agency, should create an integrated database to support risk–benefit analyses for fish consumption, thoroughly considering implications of using a metric that reflects transparency and conflicts of interest for both risk and benefit.

Recommendation 6: To maximize the use of a formal risk–benefit analysis, the U.S. Food and Drug Administration in collaboration with the U.S. Environmental Protection Agency should present conclusions of a risk–benefit analysis, including a risk estimate, in a readily understandable and useful form to risk managers and be made available to other risk assessors and interested parties.

RESEARCH GAPS

- Research is needed to inform the use of emerging technologies, such as artificial intelligence and machine learning, to develop a comprehensive data integration framework to support the conduct of risk–benefit analyses.
- Research is needed to determine both the individual effect as well as the potential cumulative effects of factors that influence the conduct of a risk–benefit analysis.
- The science undergirding the conduct of a risk–benefit analysis should be periodically reviewed, such as every 3–5 years, and updated when needed.

1

Introduction

BACKGROUND FOR THE STUDY

Seafood is considered a healthful food choice—it is a source of high-quality protein, long-chain polyunsaturated fats, and essential micronutrients such as vitamin D, selenium, and iodine. In this report, seafood includes marine and freshwater fish, mollusks, and crustaceans. The *Dietary Guidelines for Americans 2020–2025 (DGA[1])* recommends that U.S. adults eat at least 8 ounces (oz) of seafood per week, with lower total amounts for children in proportion to their overall energy intake. Individuals who are pregnant or breastfeeding are advised to consume 8–12 oz of seafood per week, and to choose options lower in mercury. The *DGA* also includes a recommendation to introduce seafood to children when they are around 6 months of age. Seafood is also a potential source of exposure to contaminants that may be harmful to the growth and development of children. Contaminants of particular concern include methylmercury (MeHg), persistent pollutants, such as per- and polyfluoroalkyl substances (PFAS), dioxins, polychlorinated biphenyls (PCBs), and microbiological hazards.

The U.S. Food and Drug Administration (FDA) and U.S. Environmental Protection Agency (EPA) published "Advice About Eating Fish: For Those Who Might Become or Are Pregnant or Breastfeeding and Children Ages 1–11 Years" (also known as the FDA/EPA Fish Advice) (FDA, 2021). This advice is intended to help those who might become or are pregnant or breastfeeding as well as parents and caregivers who are feeding children to make informed choices about the types of fish that are nutritious and safe to eat. In the advice, "fish" refers to both finfish and shellfish from both marine and fresh water sources. The FDA and EPA recommendations serve as the foundation for the *DGA* advice. Health Canada maintains a website, "Mercury in Fish—Questions and Answers," that provides consumption advise to the population. The advice is centered around MeHg in various species of tuna and other fish commonly consumed by Canadians.[2] FDA, EPA, and the National Oceanic and Atmospheric Administration (NOAA) requested a more holistic review of the role of seafood in the diet—with consideration of components found in seafood that are potentially detrimental (e.g., MeHg, PFAS, dioxins, and PCBs) as well as those that are beneficial (e.g., essential nutrients)—to evaluate their respective, interacting, and complex roles in child development and lifelong health. The goals are to have

---

[1] Throughout the report, seafood consumption guidelines refer to the recommendations in the Dietary Guidelines for Americans. This clarification was added after release of the report to the study sponsor.

[2] Available at: https://www.canada.ca/en/health-canada/services/food-nutrition/food-safety/chemical-contaminants/environmental-contaminants/mercury/mercury-fish-questions-answers.html (accessed October 14, 2023).

an up-to-date understanding of the relationships between fish consumption in a total diet context and children's health, and to determine if and how to calibrate the FDA/EPA Fish Advice in the future.

In addition, the Closer to Zero Action Plan, launched by FDA in April 2021, sets forth FDA's approach to reduce exposure through food to four metals (arsenic, lead, cadmium, and mercury) that can have adverse effects on child development, particularly neurodevelopment (FDA, 2023). The agency's goal is to work with other federal partners to help reduce the concentrations of toxic elements in the blood of infants and children by decreasing exposure from foods containing them (Mayne, 2023).

In 2004, NOAA, in collaboration with FDA and EPA, asked the Institute of Medicine (IOM) to examine the relationships between risks and benefits associated with seafood consumption through a consensus study to help consumers make informed choices. The findings were published in *Seafood Choices: Balancing the Benefits and Risks* (IOM, 2007). That report concluded that the ability to quantify benefits and risks and benefit–risk interactions at that time was limited. The report articulated an approach to balance the benefits and risks of seafood consumption whereby expert judgment was used to produce a qualitative scientific benefit–risk analysis. The analysis relied on the health benefits of omega-3 fatty acids alongside the health risks of toxic contaminants, with the latter based on some available data for MeHg and very little on persistent pollutants.

When the IOM (2007) study was conducted, the systematic review methodology that is relied on today as a gold standard in evidence review was not as commonly used as it is now. Recent systematic reviews use rigorous and transparent methods to search for, evaluate, analyze, and synthesize all relevant research studies to answer specific scientific questions. Given that more than 15 years have passed since the National Academies' last scientific review on seafood and health, scientific evidence has grown substantially, and robust systematic review methodologies now exist, the time is right for an updated evaluation of the totality of evidence on seafood and its relationship to health.

COMMITTEE'S TASK AND APPROACH

The U.S. Department of Agriculture (USDA), FDA, EPA, and NOAA asked the National Academies to review the role of fish and seafood in the diet, considering components that are potentially detrimental (e.g., MeHg, PFAS, dioxins, and PCBs), as well as those that are likely beneficial (e.g., essential nutrients) and evaluate their respective, interacting, and complex roles in child development and lifelong health. Specifically, the National Academies was asked to convene a committee of scientific experts in the disciplines of nutrition, toxicology, and evidence synthesis to study the associations between seafood intake (maternal and child) and child growth and development. The committee's task includes:

- evaluating dietary intake and seafood composition data provided by the co-sponsors,
- conducting systematic reviews of the scientific literature covering the areas of seafood nutrition and toxicology,
- reviewing existing sources of evidence on seafood consumption and child growth and development, and
- integrating the available evidence using existing, adapted, or new evidence synthesis methodologies, where warranted.

The committee's findings will be used to inform the federal government on the state of scientific evidence on types (e.g., based on species/variety and nutrient and contaminant composition) and amounts of seafood to consume to support healthy growth and allow children to attain their full development. The committee's statement of task is shown in Box 1-1. In response to the request from FDA, USDA, EPA, and NOAA, an expert committee was appointed to review the evidence, conduct systematic reviews, and recommend amounts of seafood to consume to support healthy child growth and development.

Interpretation of the Task

As the committee reviewed, discussed, and interpreted its task, it determined that including data from Canada in addition to the data from the United States would be useful to understand the context of seafood consumption in the target population groups. Additionally, because the United States and Canada are important trading partners

> **BOX 1-1**
> **Statement of Task**
>
> An ad hoc committee of the National Academies of Sciences, Engineering, and Medicine will be convened to examine associations between seafood intake (maternal and child) and child growth and development. Specifically, the committee will:
>
> - Evaluate dietary intake and seafood composition data provided by the sponsors.
> - Conduct systematic reviews of the scientific literature covering the areas of seafood nutrition and toxicology associated with seafood consumption and child growth and development.
> - Review existing sources of evidence on maternal and child seafood consumption and child growth and development.
> - Develop an approach to synthesize the scientific evidence and use that strategy to develop findings and conclusions (quantitative and/or qualitative) about associations between seafood consumption and child growth and development. The committee's approach to evidence synthesis will be described in its report.
>
> The committee will evaluate when to or not to conduct a formal risk–benefit analysis (RBA), relative to risk–benefit factors including how to assess the quality and uncertainty of an RBA; provide scientific information and principles that can serve as a foundation to evaluate confidence in the potential conclusions of an RBA relative to these factors; and identify and comment on additional context, including equity, diversity, inclusion, and access to health care that is additive to the findings of an RBA and any implications/applications capable of informing policy decisions by decision makers.
>
> The committee will produce a report of its findings, conclusions, and recommendations, including research recommendations to inform the federal sponsors on the state of scientific evidence on types (e.g., based on species/variety and nutrient and contaminant composition) and recommended amounts of seafood to consume to support healthy growth and allow children to attain their full development.

for seafood, knowledge and understanding of consumption patterns and availability of seafood across both populations is important.

This approach allowed the committee to consider a broader range of data on otherwise relatively small populations. In addition, the committee determined there was a specific need for evidence on at-risk population groups, principally Indigenous peoples and subsistence fishers. Many of these groups share waterways between the United States and Canada as well as common heritage and backgrounds, particularly between Alaska and the Northern Territories. Thus, the committee sought to be inclusive of populations in both countries to better understand their relationships with fish and seafood as a common dietary resource. The committee's task, however, did not specify inclusion of Canadian populations and therefore these populations were not included in the recommendations.

The committee determined that in this report the term "fish" refers to both finfish and shellfish (e.g., pelagic, demersal, freshwater), mollusks (including cephalopods), and crustaceans from both marine and freshwater sources. Similarly, the term "seafood" is used in the same context, consistent with its use in the *DGA* (USDA and HHS, 2020). The committee did not consider sea mammals and seaweed to be included in its task.

Approach to the Task

The committee evaluated data and evidence submitted by the study sponsors, supplemented with additional searches of existing databases and published literature. The committee contracted with Texas A&M University to conduct an update of two previously published systematic reviews provided by the sponsor: one on seafood consumption during childhood and adolescence and neurocognitive development, and the second on seafood consumption during pregnancy and lactation and neurocognitive development in the child. In addition, consultants to the committee with expertise in systematic reviews developed a protocol that was carried out by Texas A&M

University for a *de novo* systematic review on toxicants in seafood and neurocognitive development in children and adolescents. The protocols for the systematic reviews are in Appendix C.

The committee also gathered information from publicly available data sources, including both original research and systematic reviews from the published peer-reviewed literature. The committee commissioned analyses from the Johns Hopkins Center for a Livable Future at the Bloomberg School of Public Health of seafood consumption and nutrient intake in the target population groups using data from the U.S. National Health and Nutrition Examination Survey (NHANES). The committee also assessed data from the Canadian Community Health Survey. The committee also held two public workshops to obtain additional information relevant to its task.

ORGANIZATION OF THE REPORT

The report is organized into seven chapters. In this chapter, the background for the study, the statement of task and the study strategy are described. In Chapter 2, the committee elaborates on its methodological approach to the task. Chapter 3 describes data on seafood consumption patterns in the United States and Canada. Chapter 4 reports the committee's analysis of dietary intake and nutrient composition of seafood. Chapter 5 discusses exposure to contaminants associated with consumption of seafood. Chapter 6 discusses relationships between seafood consumption and health outcomes. Chapter 7 presents the committee's guidance on the use of risk–benefit analyses to guide the sponsor's decision making about public guidance on seafood consumption. Biographical sketches of the committee members are provided in Appendix A. Workshop agendas are presented in Appendix B. Appendix C presents details of the commissioned systematic reviews. Information on the supplemental reviews of systematic reviews is given in Appendix D, and Appendix E presents the methodology for the NHANES data analysis. Three additional appendixes are available online.[3] Online Appendix F contains the search terms and results for the literature searches conducted for the commissioned systematic reviews. Online Appendix G provides the search terms and results for the supplemental literature searches. The final report from Texas A&M University on the commissioned systematic reviews is found in Online Appendix H.

REFERENCES

FDA (U.S. Food and Drug Administration). 2021. *Advice about eating fish: For those who might become or are pregnant or breastfeeding and children ages 1–11 years.* https://www.fda.gov/food/consumers/advice-about-eating-fish (accessed October 30, 2023).

FDA. 2023. *Closer to Zero: Reducing childhood exposure to contaminants from foods.* https://www.fda.gov/food/environmental-contaminants-food/closer-zero-reducing-childhood-exposure-contaminants-foods (accessed October 30, 2023).

IOM (Institute of Medicine). 2007. *Seafood choices: Balancing benefits and risks.* Washington, DC: The National Academies Press.

Mayne, S. T. 2023. The FDA's action plan to reduce dietary exposure to arsenic, lead, cadmium, and mercury for infants and young children. *American Journal of Clinical Nutrition* 117(4):647-648. https://doi.org/10.1016/j.ajcnut.2023.02.004 (accessed August 23, 2023).

USDA and HHS (U.S. Department of Agriculture and U.S. Department of Health and Human Services). 2020. *Dietary Guidelines for Americans, 2020–2025.* https://www.dietaryguidelines.gov/sites/default/files/2021-03/Dietary_Guidelines_for_Americans-2020-2025.pdf (accessed September 19, 2023).

---

[3] The online appendixes can be found at https://nap.nationalacademies.org/catalog/27623.

2

Methodological Approach to the Task

The committee developed a systematic approach to support its synthesis of the evidence on relationships between seafood consumption and health outcomes (including behavioral outcomes), both advantageous and harmful. As part of its evidence-gathering approach, the committee commissioned an update of two systematic reviews of the literature and a *de novo* systematic review. The committee also gathered and reviewed publicly available information, including both original research and systematic reviews from the published peer-reviewed literature, that has become available since the previous study on these topics, *Seafood Choices: Balancing Benefits and Risks* (IOM, 2007). Finally, the committee commissioned analyses of seafood consumption and nutrient intake using data from the National Health and Nutrition Examination Survey (NHANES) and the Canadian Community Health Survey.

The committee's approach to integrate scientific evidence from a range of sources to inform conclusions helped support a key goal of the study, which is to produce the most up-to-date understanding of the science on fish consumption in a whole diet context to determine whether the U.S. Food and Drug Administration (FDA) and the Environmental Protection Agency's current fish consumption advice (FDA, 2021) should be updated. As discussed in Chapter 1, the committee's scientific review will also help inform FDA in its efforts through the Closer to Zero Action Plan (FDA, 2023), which launched in April 2021 and sets forth the agency's approach to reduce the public's dietary exposure to contaminants to as low as possible.[1]

SYSTEMATIC REVIEWS

The sponsors provided the committee two existing systematic reviews conducted to support the Scientific Advisory Committee for the *Dietary Guidelines for Americans 2020–2025 (DGA)*. These reviews covered (1) the relationship between seafood consumption during childhood and adolescence and neurocognitive development (up to 18 years of age) (Snetselaar et al., 2020a) and (2) the relationship between seafood consumption during pregnancy and lactation and neurocognitive development in children up to 18 years of age (Snetselaar et al., 2020b). The committee was asked to update these existing systematic reviews (referred to in this report as the "nutrition reviews") and to also conduct a *de novo* systematic review of the relationship of toxins, toxicants, and microorganisms in seafood with health outcomes in children and adolescents (the "toxicology review").

---

[1] This section was modified after release of the report to the study sponsor to accurately reflect the study scope.

Scoping Reviews

Prior to conducting systematic reviews on toxicants from seafood consumed during pregnancy, lactation, childhood, or adolescence and child development and health outcomes, the Texas A&M Agriculture Food and Nutrition Evidence Center (Evidence Center) conducted a scoping review to identify toxicant exposures with sufficient evidence to warrant a systematic review, as well as gaps in the evidence. The scoping review protocol is described in Appendix C. The committee prioritized the list of outcomes to narrow the scope and inform decisions about which exposure–outcome pairs would have sufficient evidence to warrant a systematic review.

Protocols for Updated Existing and Conducting *De Novo* Systematic Reviews

The committee appointed a technical expert panel (TEP) composed of three consultants to develop a protocol to update the two existing systematic reviews with articles published from January 1, 2019, through May 15, 2023. The committee also asked the TEP to design a protocol for a *de novo* systematic review on toxins, toxicants, and micro-organisms in seafood. For consistency and to facilitate comparison between the updated nutrition systematic reviews and the new toxicology systematic review, the toxicology review protocol was generally aligned with the search strategy used in the nutrition reviews (see Appendix C). It was based on two overarching questions provided by the sponsors:

1. What is the relationship between maternal seafood consumption in the United States and Canada and child growth and development?
2. What is the relationship between seafood consumption in the United States and Canada during childhood and adolescence and neurocognitive development?"

The specific subquestions relevant to the toxin/toxicant systematic review are as follows:

1. What are the exposures to toxins and toxicants from seafood in the perinatal period, including lactation, and childhood?
2. What are the associations between seafood toxins and toxicant exposure during pregnancy, lactation, and childhood and child growth and development?
3. What are the biological mechanisms of action (single actions, interactions, compound effects, and/or synergistic effects) through which toxins and toxicants from seafood potentially affect child growth and development?

For each of these three subquestions, the committee identified two additional subquestions:

a) What are the differences by social, economic, and/or environmental factors (e.g., race/ethnicity, income, cumulative exposure to nonchemical stressors such as psychosocial stress and depression, cumulative exposure to environmental stressors)?
b) What are the differences by preexisting disease burden in the mother or child (e.g., asthma, allergy, neurodevelopmental disorders, other developmental disorders, cardiovascular disease, growth disorders, psychomotor performance)?

To assist the committee in understanding the state of the published literature and to afford a basis for structuring the systematic reviews the sponsors provided three evidence scans: (1) epidemiology, (2) mechanisms of action, and (3) risk–benefit analysis. The first scan focused on studies of exposures from seafood and all available outcomes in all populations. The second scan reviewed the available evidence on how the composition of the seafood matrix may function as exposures within the body that have various mechanisms of action and interplay. The third scan reviewed existing risk–benefit analyses and methodologies within the published literature.

The committee asked the National Academies' Research Center to carry out the literature search for the updated and the *de novo* systematic reviews. National Academies staff, working with the committee's consultants, created initial lists of relevant controlled vocabulary terms (Medical Subject Heading [MeSH] terms for Medline and Emtree terms for Embase). The committee then reviewed the lists and suggested additional terms. The search was carried out in Medline using PubMed, Embase, and the Cochrane Central Register of Controlled Trials, using Ovid for the latter two databases. Reports published in English between January 2019 and May 2023 for the nutrition updates and between January 2000 and July 2023 for the *de novo* toxicology review were included. Appendix C describes additional eligibility criteria for the two nutrition reviews and the toxicology review. The eligibility criteria follow the populations, exposures, comparators, outcomes, and study design (PECOD) formulation. The complete series of commissioned systematic reviews is available online in Appendix H.[2] The protocols for the systematic reviews were prospectively registered in PROSPERO (CRD42023432844),[3] an international prospective register of systematic reviews.

The committee developed an internal check to ensure that the search strategy was capturing known relevant studies. Individual committee members suggested five to six key articles that they expected to find in the search results. Research Center staff checked whether the search had identified the submitted articles. Audit results were consistent with expected outcomes; therefore, no further refinements were made to the literature search and the search syntax was finalized. The search strategy is available online in Appendix F.[4]

The committee then commissioned the Evidence Center to perform the updates to the two existing nutrition reviews and the new toxicology review. As noted above, the committee provided the PECOD formulation, inclusion/exclusion criteria, and search strategy for each of the systematic reviews to the Evidence Center. The Evidence Center then carried out the screening, data extraction, and risk-of-bias assessment as described in Appendix C. The PRISMA flow charts for each review are shown in Figures 2-1 and 2-2.[5] For the nutrition reviews updates, there were 12 new articles related to maternal seafood consumption and 4 new articles related to seafood consumption during childhood since the time period covered by the existing systematic reviews.

The *de novo* systematic review on associations between contaminants in seafood and health outcomes found 73 included articles. Prior to full data extraction, the Evidence Center conducted a scoping review and extracted high-level data from each included article (see description above). These data were used to inform committee decisions on prioritizing toxicant and outcomes relationships for further systematic review. Based on these decisions, two toxicant exposure pairs were identified for full systematic review: polychlorinated biphenyls (PCBs) and growth and body composition, and lead and developmental domains. Four articles on PCBs and three on lead were included for data extraction (see Appendix H online for full details).[6]

SUPPLEMENTARY REVIEW OF SYSTEMATIC REVIEWS

In response to the two overarching questions and specific subquestions submitted by the sponsor, the committee was interested in identifying additional health outcomes, toxic elements, and micro-organisms. Those terms not included in the commissioned systematic reviews were searched in a supplementary review of systematic reviews in the published literature. The supplementary reviews included seafood consumption and cardiometabolic, immune-related, and cancer outcomes.

To execute the supplementary reviews, the committee followed a similar process as described for the systematic reviews. The committee identified key topics relevant to its statement of task that were not included in the systematic reviews. The committee then defined search terms and eligibility criteria (Appendix D) and conducted literature searches in PubMed, Web of Science, and Embase for articles published from 2010 to 2023. The search results were uploaded to a systematic review management program (Pico Portal) for screening. Two staff independently screened each article title and abstract. Any conflicting results were discussed by the staff reviewers and

---

[2] Appendix H can be found online at https://nap.nationalacademies.org/catalog/27623.
[3] See https://www.crd.york.ac.uk/prospero/display_record.php?RecordID=448200; https://www.crd.york.ac.uk/prospero/display_record.php?RecordID=432844 (both accessed April 10, 2024).
[4] Appendix F can be found online at https://nap.nationalacademies.org/catalog/27623.
[5] The Preferred Reporting Items for Systematic Reviews and Meta-Analyses (PRISMA) flow chart depicts the flow of information through the different phases of a systematic review. For more information on PRISMA, see http://prisma-statement.org/ (accessed February 13, 2024).
[6] Appendix H can be found online at https://nap.nationalacademies.org/catalog/27623.

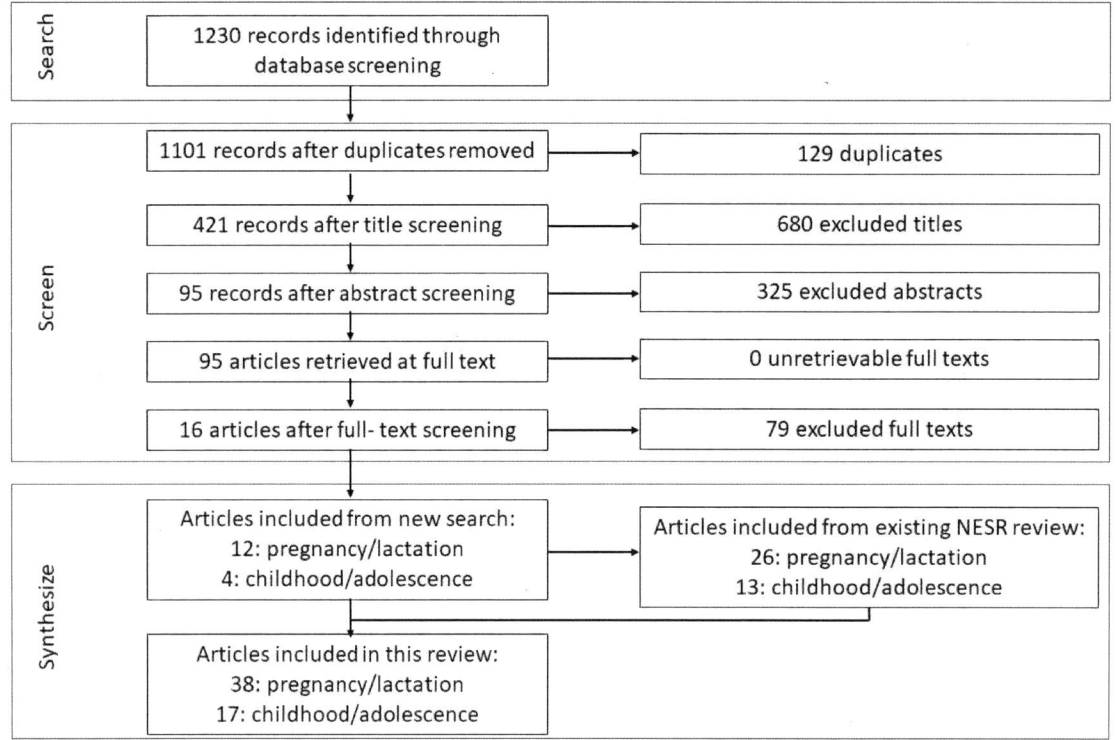

FIGURE 2-1 PRISMA flow chart for updated systematic reviews on seafood consumption during pregnancy and lactation and childhood and adolescence and neurocognitive development in the child. The diagram shows the number of articles included after electronic searching and each step of screening. The literature search dates included articles published from January 1, 2019, to May 15, 2023.
NOTE: NESR = Nutrition Evidence Systematic Review.
SOURCE: Texas A&M Agriculture, Food, & Nutrition Evidence Center.

resolved by consensus. The final full-text screening was conducted independently by a committee member and consultant team with a similar conflict resolution process as described above. Following extraction, data synthesis was conducted independently for each of the key topics.

The committee did not conduct meta-analyses or other reanalyses of data. Risk-of-bias analyses and AMSTAR 2[7] (or equivalent) certainty-of-evidence conclusions were considered as reported within the existing publications. In addition, the methodological quality of each systematic review identified in the supplementary review of systematic reviews was evaluated using the A Measurement Tool to Access Systematic Reviews (AMSTAR 2) quality-assessment tool (Appendix D). The AMSTAR 2 questions were answered for each article and given an overall assessment of the quality of each review. Extracted data for the supplemental systematic reviews is in Appendix D. The complete search strategy is described in online Appendix G.[8]

The committee was also interested in examining the association between mercury and child health outcomes using studies that did not explicitly report fish or seafood consumption. The search was focused on relevant, timely, and high-quality systematic reviews on mercury exposure during pregnancy, lactation, childhood, or adolescence on child health and development outcomes. Two reviewers screened all search results at the full-text level, and conflicts were resolved by a third reviewer. Each reviewer conducted independent assessments for each systematic

---

[7] The sentence was edited after release of the report to the study sponsor in order to correctly identify the method used for assessing systematic review quality.

[8] Appendix G can be found online at https://nap.nationalacademies.org/catalog/27623.

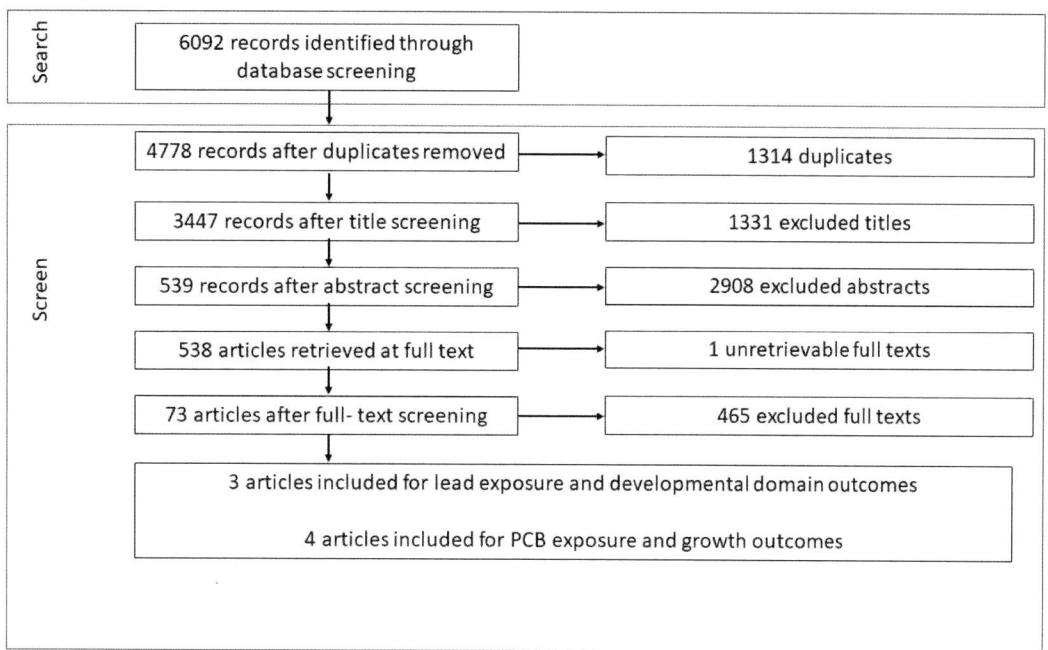

FIGURE 2-2 PRISMA flow chart for *de novo* systematic review on toxicant exposure from seafood consumed by pregnant and lactating women, children, and adolescents. The diagram shows the number of articles included after electronic searching and each step of screening. The literature search dates include articles published from January 1, 2000, to July 12, 2023.
NOTE: PCB = polychlorinated biphenyl.
SOURCE: Texas A&M Agriculture, Food, & Nutrition Evidence Center.

review that met inclusion criteria. Conflicts were discussed and resolved by the two reviewers. The AMSTAR 2 quality-assessment tool was used to assess the quality of included systematic reviews (Appendix D). A total of 53 articles were identified in the search for existing systematic reviews related to the association between mercury exposure during pregnancy, lactation, or childhood and child outcomes. Existing systematic reviews were identified for all but two prioritized outcomes. No articles were identified in the search related to blood pressure; however, a review from 2019 was identified through manual searching and included.

SEAFOOD INTAKE ANALYSES

The committee also commissioned analyses of seafood intake data from the NHANES, a nationally representative sample of the U.S. population. Data from survey cycles 2011–2012 to 2017–March 2020 were analyzed for the following age/sex subgroups of the exposed population:

- Female individuals of childbearing age (16–50 years)
- Male and female children ages 12–24 months, and 2–5, 6–11, and 12–19 years.

Usual intake of seafood was estimated using modeling approaches based on 24-hour recalls from 2 nonconsecutive days for children (2–19 years old, $n = 13,171$) and women of childbearing age (16–50 years old, $n = 7,355$) in year cycles 2011–2012 to 2017–March 2020. As seafood is known to be episodically consumed, special modeling methods are required to estimate usual intake and intake distributions from 24-hour recall data. The National Cancer Institute approach was used for such estimates (Appendix E). Analyses adjusted for complex sampling design and the contributions of multiple NHANES cycle years to the dataset. Mean usual intake and usual intake distributions were estimated for total seafood, seafood groups high and low in long-chain n-3 polyunsaturated fatty acids, total protein foods (e.g., red meat, processed meat, poultry, eggs, nuts and seeds, legumes, soy), seafood species, fatty acids, and micronutrients for demographic groups above, and stratified estimates generated by age, sex, race/ethnicity, and income.

To understand consumption of common seafood species the committee used the NHANES 30-day food frequency questionnaire (FFQ), which includes questions about consumption of meals containing 31 different species (but not amounts). The frequency of seafood intake by food source (retail, restaurant, etc.), meal type (breakfast, lunch, dinner), and by the top 10 most commonly consumed species (shrimp, tuna, salmon, etc.) was analyzed by age, sex, race/ethnicity and income groups. Frequencies of the top 10 species were developed using the 30-day FFQ counts multiplied by the average seafood meal size weighted by meal type (breakfast, lunch, dinner). Average seafood meals sizes were estimated for age-sex group. A separate analysis was conducted of infants and children ($n = 1,750$) 6 months to 2 years of age for the same time period to examine patterns related to the timing of introduction of seafood. See Appendix E for the full methodology report.

CONCEPTUAL FRAMEWORK

The committee was asked to develop and implement an approach to integrate scientific evidence in a transparent way and to draw conclusions (quantitative and/or qualitative) on questions related to seafood and child development outcomes. To facilitate this task, the committee developed the conceptual framework shown in Figure 2-3. The committee used iterative discussions to achieve consensus regarding the framework. The framework is organized such that relationships between sources of nutrient, toxin, toxicant, and micro-organism exposures in seafood and their relationships with clinical outcomes are depicted along the vertical direction (from top to bottom). The horizontal direction of the framework (from left to right) follows the relevant time periods of the life course of the exposed population and the outcome population. The framework was used to guide the committee's discussions, particularly on health outcomes related to nutrient and toxicant exposures through seafood (see Chapter 6).

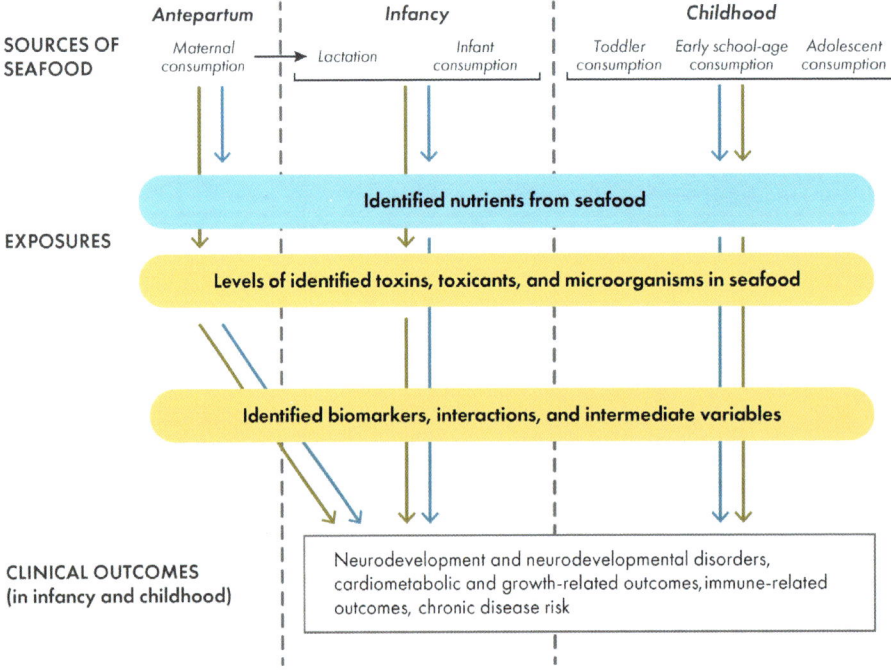

FIGURE 2-3 Conceptual framework for mapping nutrient, toxin, toxicant, and micro-organism exposures to clinical outcomes.
NOTE: Interactions refer to possible nutrient–toxin interactions.

REFERENCES

FDA (U.S. Food and Drug Administration). 2021. *Advice about eating fish: For those who might become or are pregnant or breastfeeding and children ages 1–11 years.* https://www.fda.gov/food/consumers/advice-about-eating-fish (accessed October 30, 2023).

FDA. 2023. *Closer to Zero: Reducing childhood exposure to contaminants from foods.* https://www.fda.gov/food/environmental-contaminants-food/closer-zero-reducing-childhood-exposure-contaminants-foods (accessed October 30, 2023).

IOM (Institute of Medicine). 2007. *Seafood choices: Balancing benefits and risks.* Washington, DC: The National Academies Press.

Snetselaar, L., R. Bailey, J. Sabaté, L. Van Horn, B. Schneeman, J. Spahn, J. H. Kim, C. Bahnfleth, G. Butera, N. Terry, and J. Obbagy. 2020a. *Seafood consumption during childhood and adolescence and neurocognitive development: A systematic review.* USDA Food and Nutrition Service, Center for Nutrition Policy and Promotion, Nutrition Evidence Systematic Review. https://doi.org/10.52570/NESR.DGAC2020.SR0503 (accessed January 30, 2023).

Snetselaar, L., R. Bailey, J. Sabaté, L. Van Horn, B. Schneeman, J. Spahn, J. H. Kim, C. Bahnfleth, G. Butera, N. Terry, and J. Obbagy. 2020b. *Seafood consumption during pregnancy and lactation and neurocognitive development in the child: A systematic review.* USDA Food and Nutrition Service, Center for Nutrition Policy and Promotion, Nutrition Evidence Systematic Review. https://doi.org/10.52570/NESR.DGAC2020.SR0502 (accessed January 30, 2023).

3

Seafood Consumption Patterns in the United States and Canada

This chapter provides an overview of evidence reviewed by the committee on the sources of seafood, the major types of seafood consumed, maternal and child seafood consumption in the United States and Canada—including trends over time, and factors that influence consumption. The committee also commissioned two scientists from the Johns Hopkins Center for a Livable Future at the Bloomberg School of Public Health to perform analyses using the National Health and Nutrition Examination Survey (NHANES) data from 2011 to March 2020 on seafood consumption and factors that are associated with dietary patterns. Consideration is given to special population subgroups, including racial and ethnic groups, Indigenous populations, and subsistence and sport fishers, as well as geographic area.

SOURCES OF SEAFOOD

The Role of Aquaculture in Fish and Seafood Supplies

Aquaculture continues to play an increasingly important role in providing seafood to the world's expanding population. Of the 214 million metric tons of seafood harvested globally in 2020, aquaculture contributed a record 122.6 million metric tons, with aquatic animals accounting for 87.5 million metric tons and algae (principally various species of macroalgae or seaweed) accounting for 35.1 million metric tons (FAO, 2022). Considering the portion of fish from capture fisheries that is processed for nonhuman use (e.g., rendered into fishmeal and fish oil) and excluding algae production, world aquaculture has continued to increase its contribution of seafood destined for human consumption to the present figure of more than 50 percent (FAO, 2022).

In 2020, global aquaculture production had grown by 6 percent from 2018 levels and 2.7 percent from 2019 levels. This expansion in production was marked by increases in all regions, except Africa, which recorded a decrease owing to reduced production from Egypt and Nigeria, the two major producing countries in that region (FAO, 2022). The remaining countries in Africa experienced 14.5 percent growth from 2019. Asian countries contributed 70 percent of the total production of aquatic animals in 2020, followed by the Americas, Europe, Africa, and Oceania. Chile, China, and Norway were the top producers in their regions. With 35 percent of the total, China continued to be the world's leading producer of aquatic animals and exports more aquatic animal products than any other country, although it also consumes a large quantity of domestically produced seafood. Other major exporting countries are Norway and Vietnam (FAO, 2022).

Seafood production for human consumption amounted to 20.2 kg per capita in 2022, slightly less than the all-time high of 20.5 kg in 2019 but more than double the average of 9.9 kg in the 1960s (FAO, 2022). Global consumption of seafood[1] has increased annually at an average rate of 3.0 percent since 1961, compared with a 1.6 percent population growth rate (FAO, 2022). The relative contribution of seafood from aquaculture is expected to continue to increase to meet the demands of the world's growing population; meanwhile, the global fishing fleet continues to decrease (a 10 percent reduction was estimated in 2020 compared with 2015). Moreover, most capture fisheries continue to decline in the amount of their catches because of factors such as overfishing, pollution, and poor management, although the number of landings from biologically sustainable stocks is reported to be on the rise (FAO, 2022). Overall, sustainable aquaculture development remains essential to supply the increasing demand for aquatic foods by an expanding global population. The Food and Agriculture Organization of the United Nations (FAO) projects that aquatic animal[2] production will increase 14 percent by 2030 (FAO, 2020).

The European Union is (collectively) the world's largest importing market for seafood; individual countries that import the most are the United States, China, and Japan (FAO, 2022). China imports large quantities of aquatic species for domestic consumption but also as raw material that is processed in China and reexported, at least since the year 2000 (Asche et al., 2022). Asche et al. (2022) proposed that Chinese domestic seafood demand is not a primary driver of its fish imports and that an estimated 74.9 percent of imported fish, such as imported Russian Alaskan pollock and Norwegian cod, are processed and reexported.

Data from the National Marine Fisheries Service's (NMFS's) *Fisheries of the United States* report indicate that aquaculture currently accounts for about 7 percent of the total U.S. domestic seafood production by weight (NMFS, 2022). From a cost perspective, aquaculture contributes approximately 24 percent of the value of domestic seafood products. For example, aquaculture production in the United States did not fluctuate between 2014 and 2019, but the value of sales of domestic aquaculture increased by an average of 2.3 percent per year within the same time frame (NMFS, 2022).

Domestic Seafood Supply

Seafood products available from domestic sources come from both capture fisheries and aquaculture. As the United States and Canada are bordered by the Atlantic and Pacific Oceans and the Gulf of Mexico is along the U.S. southern border, substantial quantities of seafood are obtained from commercial fishing from ports in those areas. A large diversity of aquatic species is harvested from the wild. The National Oceanic and Atmospheric Administration (NOAA) maintains yearly harvest records for several hundred fish, crustacean (e.g., crab, lobster, shrimp), and molluscan (e.g., abalone, clam, and oyster) species obtained from various U.S. regions, including the Great Lakes. Commercial harvest of aquatic species from U.S. inland waters is minor compared to that from marine waters (NMFS, 2020).

Commercial aquaculture in the United States also provides a diversity of seafood particularly for regional markets. For example, catfish aquaculture—the largest U.S. aquacultural—is primarily practiced in earthen ponds in Mississippi, Arkansas, Alabama, and Texas, whereas crayfish aquaculture principally occurs in Louisiana (USDA/FSIS, 2022). Aquaculture of rainbow trout occurs in flow-through raceway systems primarily in Idaho and North Carolina, where water and climatic conditions for this cold-water species are suitable and markets are well established (Hinshaw et al., 2004).

Production of Atlantic salmon occurs primarily in ocean net pens off the coast of Maine and both the east and west coasts of Canada, although aquaculture industries in Norway and Chile produce much larger quantities of Atlantic salmon (FAO, 2022). Oysters are produced in waters along the eastern, western, and southern coasts of the United States and are a primary domestic-origin product. Many other species of aquatic organisms (fish, crustaceans, and mollusks) are produced by aquaculture in various U.S. regions, but those species constitute a small percentage of the total seafood available to U.S. consumers compared with similar species produced by

---

[1] Aquatic food consumption data are expressed in live weight equivalents.

[2] Aquatic animals include finfish harvested from inland aquaculture as well as marine and coastal aquaculture, mollusks, crustaceans, marine invertebrates, aquatic turtles, and frogs.

aquaculture imported from other countries. They also make a minor contribution compared with various seafood species commercially harvested from the wild such as cod, Pacific salmon, pollock, and tuna (NMFS, 2020, 2022).

Canada produced 0.9 million tons of fish and seafood in 2020, with a value of $5.0 billion (CAD). Marine fisheries accounted for 750,000 tons, freshwater fisheries accounted for 22,000 tons, and aquaculture production accounted for 170,000 tons (Agriculture Canada, 2023).

The United States and Canada are important trading partners in fisheries. The United States is Canada's largest export market. The top three imported foods were lobsters, prepared/preserved salmon, and sockeye salmon (Agriculture Canada, 2023).

Imported Seafood Supply

It has been reported that 60–65 percent of the U.S. seafood supply is imported (Gephart et al., 2019; NMFS, 2022), primarily from Asia, and that 70–85 percent of that proportion is imported for consumption (NMFS, 2020). More than 170 countries export seafood to the United States, with Canada, Chile, China, India, Indonesia, and Vietnam being the top six in order, based on value (Love et al., 2021).

Many imported seafood products are produced by aquaculture including penaeid shrimp, pangasius catfish,[3] tilapia, and Atlantic salmon; these species constitute approximately half of U.S. seafood consumption (Shamshak et al., 2019), and the other half is composed of canned tuna, pollock, cod, crab, and clams (NFI, 2023).

Calculation of Seafood Consumption in the United States and Canada

NOAA compiles fisheries statistics from the previous year into an annual overview of the contribution of fishing to the U.S. food supply (NMFS, 2022).[4] This annual report provides information on the total catch for domestic commercial and recreational fisheries by species and provides data on the U.S. fishery processing industry, imports and exports of fishery-related products, domestic supply, and per capita consumption of fishery products (NMFS, 2022). These data allow for tracking important indicators, such as annual estimates of seafood consumption. To capture more typical consumption patterns, the committee selected data from the 2018–2019 report rather than data collected during years covering the COVID-19 pandemic.

Per capita consumption is calculated by NOAA fisheries and based on a "disappearance" model using data derived primarily from secondary sources. Specifically, the total supply of imports and landings is converted to edible weight by decreases in supply, including exports and industrial uses. To estimate per capita consumption, the remaining total is divided by the U.S. population size. Limitations in the model include changes in source data and invalid model assumptions, with potentially inaccurate or outdated conversion factors that may affect calculations (Pulver et al., 2020). There are additional limitations to this estimate, as geographic location (i.e., interior regions compared to coastal regions) could affect the level of seafood consumption. Furthermore, the model used to calculate consumption does not consider inventories of products on hand at the beginning and end of the year and it assumes that all production is consumed within the year it is produced (NMFS, 2022).

Using this model, the top 10 most consumed species among the U.S. population in 2018–2019 accounted for 74 percent of total seafood consumption (Table 3-1) and the remaining 26 percent came from other seafood products from various sources (NFI, 2023). Half of the species listed in Table 3-1 (including penaeid shrimp, pangasius catfish, tilapia, and Atlantic salmon) are produced by aquaculture and are largely imported in contrast to domestic catfish. The other half of the species in Table 3-1 includes canned tuna, pollock, cod, crab, and clams.

In Canada, data on types and amounts of seafood consumed are collected through the Canadian Community Health Survey (CCHS). The CCHS is a series of nationally representative cross-sectional surveys that collect information on health status, use of health care services, and the determinants of health for the Canadian population during each survey cycle (Hu and Chan, 2021). The 2015 survey included a 24-hour dietary recall that gathered information on foods and beverage consumption via a computer-assisted participant interview for the total sample

---

[3] Pangasius is a type of large catfish imported from South and Southeast Asia.
[4] Available at https://www.fisheries.noaa.gov/national/sustainable-fisheries/fisheries-united-states (accessed August 29, 2023).

TABLE 3-1 Seafood Species Most Frequently Consumed, U.S. Per Capita Consumption, 2019

United States	Per Capita Consumption, 2019, lb (g)
1. Shrimp	4.70 (2,131.9)
2. Salmon	3.10 (1,406.1)
3. Canned tuna	2.20 (997.9)
4. Alaska pollock	1.00 (453.6)
5. Tilapia	0.98 (444.5)
6. Cod	0.59 (267.6g)
7. Catfish	0.55 (249.5)
8. Crab	0.52 (235.9)
9. Pangasius	0.36 (163.3)
10. Clams	0.30 (136.1)

NOTE: Per capita consumption is calculated from disappearance data by type of seafood (see NMFS, 2022).
SOURCE: Table created from data in NMFS, 2022.

(day 1), and via a telephone interview for a subsample (day 2) of participants. Table 3-2 summarizes 1-day 24-hour recall data on the top 10 seafood species consumed per capita among consumers in Canada.

Direct comparison of Canadian and U.S. values cannot be made because they are based on different data collection methodologies (food disappearance data vs. self-reported 24-hour dietary recall data), but per capita fish consumption appears to be lower in Canada. The United States consumes more imported species such as tilapia and pangasius than Canada, and differences exist between the native species consumed in the two countries, as shown in Tables 3-1 and 3-2. All species on the top 10 lists in both countries are rich in protein, and several (including salmon and albacore tuna) are also rich in docosahexaenoic acid (DHA). The other top 10 consumed seafood species are lower in total lipids and thus lower in long-chain polyunsaturated fatty acids (n-2 LCPUFAs) (Love et al., 2022). In terms of contaminants, species produced from aquaculture are typically exposed to more regulated environments than wild species (NOAA, n.d.) and are less likely to be exposed to toxins and toxicants that tend to accumulate and/or become concentrated in marine organisms in the wild (Burridge et al., 2010).

TABLE 3-2 Seafood Species Most Frequently Consumed, Canada Per Capita Consumption, 2015

Canada	Per Capita Consumption, 2015, lb (g)
1. Sardine	0.24 (109.7)
2. Salmon	0.20 (92.4)
3. Herring	0.20 (91.3)
4. Trout	0.20 (89.6)
5. Cod	0.17 (74.9)
6. Tuna	0.14 (62.2)
7. Clams	0.09 (42.5)
8. Crab	0.09 (39.3)
9. Shrimp	0.08 (36.4)
10. Scallops	0.08 (34.8)

SOURCE: Hu and Chan, 2020.

Summary of Evidence on Sources of Seafood

The majority (70–85 percent) of seafood consumed in the United States is imported, and aquaculture accounts for about half of seafood consumed (NMFS, 2022). The top 10 most consumed species for the total U.S. population in 2018–2019 accounted for about three-quarters of the total seafood consumption (NFI, 2023). Compared to consumption during 2004 as reported in the *Seafood Choices: Balancing Benefits and Risks* report (IOM, 2007), shrimp remains the most consumed seafood, but salmon has now surpassed tuna and is the second most consumed seafood in both the United States and Canada. Because of different data sources and collection methods, it is not possible to directly compare absolute intake of seafood in the United States and Canada.

TRENDS IN CONSUMPTION OF FISH AND SEAFOOD

To understand current trends in seafood consumption, the committee accessed the U.S. Department of Agriculture (USDA) Economic Research Service (ERS) Food Availability (Per Capita) Data System (FADS).[5] This data source includes three data series on food and nutrient availability for consumption: (1) food availability data, (2) loss-adjusted food availability data, and (3) nutrient availability data. The FADS calculates the amount of food available for human consumption using the difference between available commodity supplies and nonfood use for each specific food item. The calculated data are a proxy for actual consumption of foods at the national level for consumers in the United States and Armed Forces overseas and for time-series data on food availability in the United States.

Figure 3-1 shows trends in seafood consumption from disappearance data over the past century in the United States. Overall, since 1909 consumption of cured seafood has decreased and remains low since 1930 while total intake increased to 16.1 lb (7.3 kg) per capita per year, a trend driven largely by intake of fresh and frozen seafood, which tripled since 1909. Canned seafood consumption has remained relatively stable at 2.6–3.5 lb (1.2–1.6 kg) per capita per year.

In Canada, there are no similar long-term trending data. From 1988 to 2022, the amount of seafood available for consumption per person per year ranged from 7.2 to 10.0 kg (15.9–22 lb) and there was no clear trend. In 2021, seafood consumption in Canada was 8.44 kg (18.6 lb)/per person per year and consisted of 6.6 kg (14.6 lb) of marine fish,[6] 0.89 kg (2 lb) of freshwater fish, and 0.95 kg (2.1 lb) of shellfish.

Table 3-3 shows trends in the past decade in U.S. per capita consumption of fresh and frozen, canned, and cured seafood collected by NMFS, Office of Science and Technology (NMFS, 2022). Data show that consumption of cured seafood has remained stable at 0.3 lb/per person per day while fresh and frozen as well as canned seafood intake has fluctuated, with an increasing trend starting in 2015. It is noteworthy to point out that in the same time frame, the population increased by approximately 7 percent. Consumption of fresh and frozen seafood increased more than canned seafood consumption, reflecting a change in food preference.

Summary of Evidence on Trends in Seafood Consumption

Over the past century, consumption of seafood has increased because of a combination of both increasing population and greater per capita consumption. Most of the increase in consumption relates to fresh and frozen seafood, whereas consumption of canned seafood has remained generally stable and cured seafood contributes negligibly to overall seafood consumption. Even during the past few decades, consumption of fresh and frozen seafood has continued to increase.

---

[5] Available at https://www.ers.usda.gov/data-products/food-availability-per-capita-data-system/ (accessed February 25, 2024).

[6] Available at https://www.statista.com/statistics/451558/volume-of-fish-products-available-for-consumption-per-person-canada/ (accessed February 25, 2024).

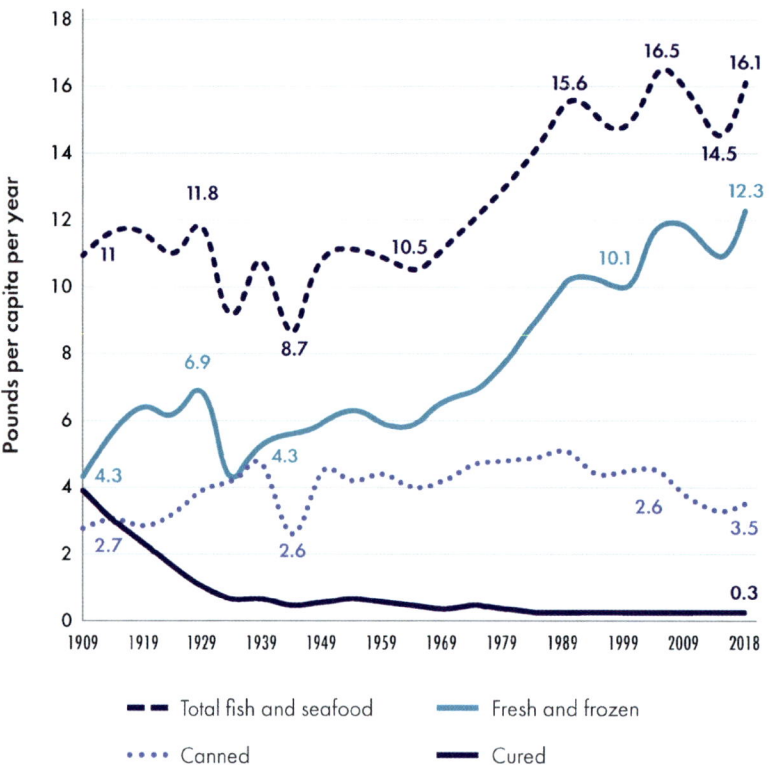

FIGURE 3-1 Trends in U.S. consumption of total fishery products (boneless, trimmed [edible] weight), by type in pounds per capita per year, 1909–2018. Based on edible raw fish and shellfish. Excludes edible offal, bones, and viscera for fishery products. Excludes animal consumption for fishery product. Calculated from data not rounded.
SOURCE: ERS, 2020.

TABLE 3-3 Annual Per Capita Consumption of Fish and Shellfish, United States, 2011–2020

Year	U.S. Civilian Resident Population (millions)	Per Capita Consumption in Pounds (grams)			
		Fresh and Frozen	Canned	Cured	Total
2011	310	13.4 (6,078)	4.0 (1,814)	0.3 (136)	17.8 (8,074)
2012	313	12.9 (5,851)	3.6 (1,633)	0.3 (136)	16.8 (7,620)
2013	315	13.8 (6,260)	3.8 (1,724)	0.3 (136)	17.9 (8,119)
2014	318	13.5 (6,124)	3.5 (1,588)	0.3 (136)	17.3 (7,847)
2015	320	14.6 (6,622)	4.0 (1,814)	0.3 (136)	18.8 (8,528)
2016	322	14.4 (6,532)	3.6 (16,323)	0.3 (136)	18.3 (8,301)
2017	325	15.1 (6,849)	3.8 (1,724)	0.3 (136)	19.1 (8,664)
2018	326	15.0 (6,804)	3.7 (1,678)	0.3 (136)	19.0 (8,618)
2019	327	15.1 (6,849)	3.9 (1,769)	0.3 (136)	19.3 (8,754)
2020	332	14.6 (6,622)	4.2 (1,905)	0.3 (136)	19.0 (8,618)

SOURCE: NMFS, 2022. Reprinted with permission.

SURVEY DATA ON SEAFOOD CONSUMPTION BY AGE AND SEX GROUP

The committee was asked to review and assess evidence on nutrition and toxicology associations of seafood intake during pregnancy, lactation, and childhood with child growth and development. As a first step, the committee sought information on the amount of seafood typically consumed by children ages 2–19 years, as well as for women during pregnancy and lactation. What We Eat in America, the dietary component of the NHANES, served as a source of national continuous cross-sectional intake data. The committee also used published results from other analyses of NHANES data as referenced below.

Because of small sample sizes for pregnant and lactating women in the NHANES dataset, results are reported for all women of childbearing age in the 2011–2020 NHANES analyses. For example, Razzaghi and Tinker (2014) used the NHANES 1999–2006 surveys, which included complete interview and survey data from 1,260 pregnant women and 5,848 nonpregnant women and found no significant differences in the proportion of fish or shellfish consumption between pregnant and nonpregnant women. This finding was consistent for prevalence, amount, and type of fish and shellfish consumed, separately or combined. The findings also showed consistency between the two measures of dietary intake in the 2011–2020 NHANES analyses commissioned for this study, namely the 30-day seafood intake questionnaire and the (day 1) 24-hour recall. The committee thus interpreted the 2011–2020 data from women of childbearing age from the later cycle years examined as hypothetically representative of pregnant and lactating women in the population. However, the committee also recognizes that because of changes in dietary patterns, this interpretation has limitations.

In Canada, data were extracted from the CCHS,[7] a series of nationally representative cross-sectional surveys that includes nutrition studies in 2004 and 2015 (Béland, 2002). Each survey has two parts: a general health questionnaire and a 24-hour dietary recall. Information on respondents' sociodemographic characteristics (e.g., age, sex, marital status, income, and education), chronic health conditions, and use of vitamin and mineral supplements was collected in the general health component. The 24-hour recall portion gathers data on food and beverage consumption via a computer-assisted personal interview for the total sample (day 1) and a telephonic interview on a subsample (day 2). The study population for both surveys was Canadians living within the 10 provinces. However, the CCHS does not include Indigenous populations living on reservations.

U.S. Women of Childbearing Age

Table 3-4 reports the percentage of seafood species commonly consumed by women of childbearing age, and Table 3-5 presents this information by race and ethnicity. The sample size reported in the table represents the number of seafood meals of each type reported. The weighted frequencies represent the percentage that each type contributes to the total seafood meals consumed. For example, shrimp represents 28.2 percent of all reported seafood meals, and tuna represents 15.9 percent (Table 3-4). By comparison, consumption of shrimp, tuna, and salmon by women of childbearing age represents 59 percent of the amount consumed by the general population.

The results of the data analysis commissioned by the committee show that the most consumed seafood types by U.S. women of childbearing age are (in descending order) shrimp, tuna, salmon, other fish, and crab. The type of seafood consumed varies with racial and ethnic identity. Non-Hispanic Asian and non-Hispanic Black races most frequently consume shrimp, salmon, other fish, and other unknown fish or catfish; Hispanic, non-Hispanic White, and other races most frequently consume shrimp, tuna, salmon, and crab (Table 3-5).

Table 3-6 presents the frequency of consuming seafood meals by women of childbearing age overall, and by race and ethnicity. Based on reported monthly frequency, fewer than one in five women consume two or more seafood meals per week, whereas more than one-quarter reported consuming seafood never or less than once per month. Large variation exists by racial and ethnic background, with non-Hispanic Asian women (37 percent) most likely to consume at least two seafood meals per week, and Hispanic (16 percent) and non-Hispanic Black (17 percent) least likely. Frequency of seafood meals increased with increasing income.

---

[7] Available at https://www.canada.ca/en/health-canada/services/food-nutrition/food-nutrition-surveillance/health-nutrition-surveys/canadian-community-health-survey-cchs.html (accessed February 25, 2024).

TABLE 3-4 Seafood Species Commonly Consumed, U.S. Women of Childbearing Age, by Percentage of Seafood Meals

Seafood Species	Sample Size (n)	Frequency, Weighted (percent)
1. Shrimp	7,447	28.2
2. Tuna	4,347	15.9
3. Salmon	4,126	15.1
4. Other fish	2,762	7.4
5. Crab	1,479	5.3
6. Breaded fish	861	3.0
7. Catfish	1,315	2.8
8. Cod	759	2.7
9. Scallops	515	2.2
10. Lobster	535	2.1

SOURCE: NHANES cycle years 2011–2012 through 2017–March 2020. Data are derived from the 30-day food frequency questionnaire.

TABLE 3-5 Seafood Species Commonly Consumed, U.S. Women of Childbearing Age by Percentage of Seafood Meals, by Race and Ethnicity

Race and Ethnicity	Seafood Species	Sample Size (n)	Frequency, Weighted (percent)
Hispanic	1. Shrimp	1,756	28.6
	2. Tuna	1,160	17.5
	3. Salmon	725	15.6
	4. Other fish	702	9.7
	5. Crab	206	5.1
Non-Hispanic Asian	1. Shrimp	1,555	27.5
	2. Salmon	1,097	18.4
	3. Other fish	582	10.2
	4. Tuna	476	9.2
	5. Other unknown fish	256	4.8
Non-Hispanic Black	1. Shrimp	2,177	30.0
	2. Salmon	1,034	11.8
	3. Other fish	921	10.8
	4. Tuna	838	9.3
	5. Catfish	784	8.1
Non-Hispanic White	1. Shrimp	1,621	26.9
	2. Tuna	1,673	20.0
	3. Salmon	1,026	14.8
	4. Crab	375	5.1
	5. Other fish	441	4.3
Other Race, Multiracial	1. Shrimp	338	33.7
	2. Salmon	244	18.7
	3. Tuna	200	11.9
	4. Other fish	116	7.6
	5. Crab	92	6.1

NOTE: See NHANES Data Analysis Methodology in Appendix E.
SOURCE: NHANES cycle years 2011–2012 through 2017–March 2020.

TABLE 3-6 Weighted Seafood Meal Frequency Among Women of Childbearing Age, by Percentage of Seafood Meals

	n, Weighted	0 Meals per Month, Percent (n)	Less Than 2 Meals per Week, Percent (n)	2 or more Meals per Week, Percent (n)
Overall	145,136,708	27 (3,694)	54 (7,392)	19 (2,646)
Race/Ethnicity				
Hispanic	29,442,289	26 (936)	58 (2,064)	16 (516)
Non-Hispanic Asian	9,262,960	21 (359)	42 (749)	37 (639)
Non-Hispanic White	18,261,908	22 (727)	57 (1,858)	21 (661)
Non-Hispanic Black	82,355,531	29 (1,478)	54 (2,372)	17 (687)
Other	5,814,021	28 (194)	53 (349)	20 (143)
Income (IPR)				
Less than 1.3	39,028,154	33 (1,570)	54 (2,616)	14 (664)
1.3–4.99	75,250,923	27 (1,748)	55 (3,787)	18 (1,342)
5+	30,857,631	20 (376)	53 (989)	27 (640)

NOTES: IPR = income poverty ratio; n = sample size. Values in parentheses are unweighted sample sizes. Seafood frequency measured using a 30-day food frequency questionnaire based on the total number of meals per month for all seafood species. Respondents not reporting food frequency are not presented in this table. See NHANES Data Analysis Methodology in Appendix E.
SOURCE: NHANES cycle years 2011–2012 through 2017–March 2020.

Children and Adolescents in the United States

Table 3-7 reports the most frequently consumed seafood species by U.S. children according to NHANES 2011–2020. The weighted frequencies represent the percentage that each type contributes to the total seafood meals consumed. For example, shrimp represent 28.7 percent of all reported seafood meals, and tuna 14.4 percent (Table 3-7). The top 10 types of seafood that U.S. children most frequently consume are similar to the top 10 types consumed by U.S. women of childbearing age (Table 3-4) and by the total U.S. population (Table 3-1). One difference is that breaded fish of unspecified species contributes almost 7 percent of the overall consumed seafood among children, but only 3 percent for women of childbearing age.

TABLE 3-7 Seafood Species Frequently Consumed, U.S. Children by Percentage of Seafood Meals

Seafood Species	Sample Size (n)	Frequency, Weighted (percent)
1. Shrimp	7,168	28.7
2. Tuna	3,466	14.4
3. Salmon	3,172	12.1
4. Other fish	2,586	7.8
5. Breaded fish	1,732	6.7
6. Crab	1,292	5.2
7. Catfish	1,344	4.3
8. Cod	633	2.6
9. Other unknown	838	2.2
10. Clam	392	2.2

NOTE: See NHANES Data Analysis Methodology in Appendix E.
SOURCE: NHANES cycle years 2011–2012 through 2017–March 2020. Data are derived from the 30-day food frequency questionnaire.

Table 3-8 presents information by sex and age group, and Table 3-9 presents information by racial and ethnic group. Seafood consumption for children increased with increasing age, which is expected given the higher energy demands and greater food intake as children grow. Female children were reported as having higher consumption than males, and consumption was highest among children who identify as non-Hispanic Black or other race (including Asian), compared to those who identify as non-Hispanic White, Mexican American, or other Hispanic.

The committee also requested information on frequency of seafood consumption and portion sizes consumed for children ages 12–24 months (Tables 3-10 and 3-11). Overall, about 45 percent of 1-year-old U.S. children consume seafood never or less than once per month and 3.8 percent consume seafood at least twice per week.

Table 3-12 reports frequency of seafood consumption for children ages 2–19 years by age group, sex, race and ethnicity, and income. Compared with 1-year-old children (Table 3-10), rates of consumption were only marginally higher with 43 percent consuming seafood less than once per month and 6.4 percent consuming two or more seafood meals per week. Differences by age and sex were small, although adolescent males ate seafood somewhat more frequently compared with younger males or females at all ages (7 percent of males 12–19 years consumed

TABLE 3-8 Seafood Species Commonly Consumed, U.S. Children by Percentage, by Sex and Age Group

Age (years) Group and Sex	Seafood Species	Sample Size (n)	Frequency, Weighted (percent)
2–5 years			
Girls	1. Shrimp	866	24.5
	2. Tuna	470	17.5
	3. Breaded fish	287	11.8
	4. Salmon	368	11.8
	5. Other fish	398	10.2
Boys	1. Shrimp	673	26.0
	2. Tuna	439	16.7
	3. Breaded fish	355	14.7
	4. Salmon	343	12.6
	5. Other fish	335	11.0
6–11 years			
Girls	1. Shrimp	1,256	28.3
	2. Tuna	731	17.8
	3. Other fish	605	12.0
	4. Salmon	463	11.4
	5. Breaded fish	310	7.0
Boys	1. Shrimp	1,214	26.2
	2. Tuna	566	13.5
	3. Salmon	543	12.4
	4. Other fish	579	11.3
	5. Breaded fish	350	8.2
12–19 years			
Girls	1. Shrimp	1,640	35.1
	2. Tuna	578	12.6
	3. Salmon	698	11.2
	4. Crab	333	6.8
	5. Breaded fish	224	5.1
Boys	1. Shrimp	1,519	26.4
	2. Tuna	682	13.9
	3. Salmon	757	12.9
	4. Other fish	321	5.6
	5. Crab	307	5.2

NOTE: See NHANES Data Analysis Methodology in Appendix E.
SOURCE: NHANES cycle years 2011–2012 through 2017–March 2020.

TABLE 3-9 Seafood Species Commonly Consumed, U.S. Children, by Percentage of Seafood Meals, by Race and Ethnicity

Race and Ethnicity	Seafood Species	Sample Size (*n*)	Frequency, Weighted (percent)
Hispanic	1. Shrimp	2,468	31.4
	2. Tuna	1,377	18.0
	3. Salmon	720	11.1
	4. Other fish	847	10.0
	5. Breaded fish	443	5.3
Non-Hispanic Asian	1. Shrimp	1,570	28.9
	2. Salmon	1,030	17.7
	3. Tuna	394	9.3
	4. Other fish	565	8.7
	5. Other unknown	370	5.8
Non-Hispanic Black	1. Shrimp	2,791	31.3
	2. Catfish	1,011	11.0
	3. Other fish	1,132	10.6
	4. Tuna	865	10.0
	5. Salmon	800	8.7
Non-Hispanic White	1. Shrimp	1,384	26.0
	2. Tuna	1,174	16.6
	3. Salmon	801	12.6
	4. Breaded fish	617	8.1
	5. Crab	322	5.7
Other Race, Multiracial	1. Shrimp	552	34.6
	2. Salmon	397	15.0
	3. Tuna	291	12.2
	4. Breaded fish	171	6.2
	5. Cod	127	6.1

NOTE: See NHANES Data Analysis Methodology in Appendix E.
SOURCE: NHANES cycle years 2011–2012 through 2017–March 2020.

TABLE 3-10 Weighted Seafood Meal Frequency, U.S. Children, 12–24 Months

	n, Weighted	0 Meals per Month, Percent (*n*)	Less Than 2 Meals per Week, Percent (*n*)	2 or More Meals per Week, Percent (*n*)	Portion Size from 24-Hour Recall, Grams Mean (SD)	Unweighted n for Portion Size Analysis (*n*)
Overall	3,786,018	45 (438)	51 (466)	3.8 (47)	N/A	N/A
Age (months)						
12–14	836,724	53 (116)	43 (92)	3.7 (7)	45.1 (47.3)	32
15–17	1,049,177	44 (120)	52 (122)	4.0 (11)	33.3 (28.1)	28
18–20	908,120	40 (94)	57 (122)	2.6 (15)	36.0 (33.9)	39
21–24	991,997	42 (108)	53 (130)	4.7 (14)	39.4 (29.7)	36

NOTES: *n* = sample size; SD = standard deviation. Values in parentheses are unweighted sample sizes. Seafood frequency measured using a 30-day food frequency questionnaire based on the total number of meals per month for all seafood species. Respondents not reporting food frequency are not presented in this table. Infants less than 12 months are not included in NHANES data collection, and for older children, parents, or other proxies report consumption of seafood on the child's behalf. See NHANES Data Analysis Methodology in Appendix E.
SOURCE: NHANES cycle years 2011–2012 through 2017–March 2020.

TABLE 3-11 Weighted Average Number of Seafood Meals Per Month, U.S. children, 12–24 Months

	n, Weighted	n, Unweighted	Number of Seafood Meals (average per month)	SE
Overall	3,786,018	951	1.78	0.13
Age (months)				
12–14	836,724	215	1.67	0.21
15–17	1,049,177	253	1.81	0.22
18–20	908,120	231	1.79	0.20
21–24	991,997	252	1.82	0.23

NOTES: n = sample size; SE = standard error. Average number of seafood meals measured using a 30-day food frequency questionnaire based on the total number of meals per month for all seafood species. Infants less than 12 months are not included in NHANES data collection, and for older children, parents, or other proxies report consumption of seafood on the child's behalf. See NHANES Data Analysis Methodology in Appendix E.
SOURCE: NHANES cycle years 2011–2012 through 2017–March 2020.

TABLE 3-12 Weighted Seafood Meal Frequency, U.S. children, 2–19 Years

	n, Weighted	0 Meals per Month, Percent (n)	Less than 2 Meals per Week, Percent (n)	2 or more Meals per Week, Percent (n)
Overall	74,270,808	43 (5,372)	51 (6,631)	6.4 (926)
Males (years)				
2–5	7,908,059	46 (698)	49 (735)	5.9 (103)
6–11	12,925,783	43 (945)	50 (1,185)	6.9 (164)
12–19	17,022,525	42 (1,131)	51 (1,364)	7.0 (199)
Females (years)				
2–5	8,029,348	39 (602)	55 (828)	5.9 (124)
6–11	11,739,998	43 (909)	52 (1,183)	5.7 (163)
12–19	16,645,096	44 (1,087)	50 (1,336)	6.2 (173)
Race/Ethnicity				
Hispanic	17,869,766	44 (1,734)	50 (1,936)	5.4 (186)
Non-Hispanic Asian	3,428,654	31 (343)	50 (574)	19 (234)
Non-Hispanic White	10,429,463	36 (1,186)	56 (1,896)	8.1 (274)
Non-Hispanic Black	38,447,678	45 (1,708)	50 (1,762)	5.0 (159)
Other	4,095,247	43 (401)	48 (463)	9.1 (73)
Income (IPR)				
Less than 1.3	25,389,481	46 (2,488)	49 (2,788)	5.7 (325)
1.3–4.99	37,715,367	43 (2,448)	51 (3,172)	5.8 (455)
5+	11,165,960	36 (436)	54 (671)	9.8 (146)

NOTES: IPR = income-to-poverty ratio. Values in parentheses are unweighted sample sizes. Seafood frequency measured using a 30-day food frequency questionnaire based on the total number of meals per month for all seafood species. Respondents not reporting food frequency are not presented in this table; n = sample size. See NHANES Data Analysis Methodology in Appendix E.
SOURCE: NHANES cycle years 2011–2012 through 2017–March 2020.

at least two seafood meals per week compared with 5.9 percent of males aged 2–5 and 6.2 percent of females aged 12–19. Clear differences existed, however, among racial and ethnic groups as well as by income groups. As with women of childbearing age, non-Hispanic Asian children were most likely (19 percent) to consume at least two seafood meals per week, and Hispanic (5.4 percent) and non-Hispanic Black children (5.0 percent) were least likely. Frequency of seafood meals increased with increasing income.

Women of Childbearing Age and Children in Canada

In Canada, the usual fish consumption rate (UFCR) from the CCHS estimates intake (grams per day raw weight, edible portion) by age, sex, race, and ethnicity. Table 3-13 reports the usual fish consumption rate among women of childbearing age and among children and adolescents ages 2–21 years in Canada, based on UFCR data.

Women of Childbearing Age

According to the 24-hour dietary recall data collected by the 2015 CCHS, 81.8 percent of women of childbearing age did not consume fish, and fewer than 5 percent consumed at least two servings of fish per week (Table 3-13). The median intake was 10.3 g (0.4 oz)/day for the population and 79.7 g (2.8 oz)/day for fish consumers. Asian population groups consumed more fish, 13.5 g (0.5 oz)/day, compared with White Canadians, 8.5 g (0.3 oz)/day. Individuals of other racial and ethnic identities combined consumed the most fish, 25 g (0.9 oz)/day.

Table 3-14 presents the most frequently consumed species of seafood among women of childbearing age, children, and adolescents in Canada. These species include marine fish such as cod, haddock, salmon, and tuna; freshwater fish such as tilapia and trout; and shellfish such as clam, crab, lobster, and shrimp. Salmon is the most frequently consumed species among consumers of seafood, reported by 5.3 percent of women of childbearing age and 3.8 percent of children and adolescents. Overall, consumers of seafood reported eating approximately 36–100 g of seafood per day. The highest rate of population intake is for salmon at 5.0 g/day for women of childbearing age and 2.9 g/day for children and adolescents.

Children and Adolescents

UFCR data indicate that 87.2 percent of children in Canada did not consume fish, and only 5.0 percent consumed at least two servings per week, similar to the 6.4 percent reported for U.S. children (Table 3-13). The median fish consumption rate was 6.2 g (0.2 oz)/day for all children, and 72.3 g (2.6 oz)/day among consumers of fish, with differences between males and females. The percent of children who consume fish was highest (19.7 percent) among young children (2–3 years old) compared to older children and adolescents. The median fish consumption rate increased with age among consumers of fish, and more Asian Canadian children consumed fish (20 percent) compared with White (10.2 percent) and "Others" (unspecified racial/ethnic group) (13.1 percent). Table 3-13 reports consumption amounts for the overall population, as well as among seafood consumers.

The most frequently consumed species of seafood among children and adolescents are similar to those reported by the Canadian general population (Table 3-2). Five percent or fewer of women of childbearing age and children reported consuming at least two servings of fish per week (Table 3-13). Salmon is the most frequently consumed fish by women of childbearing age, children, and adolescents, followed by tuna, shrimp, cod, and crab. Women of childbearing age had higher intakes than children and adolescents for all the most frequently consumed species, except for tilapia and trout.

Summary of Evidence on Fish and Seafood Intake by Age and Sex Group

Taken together, the evidence indicates that few women of childbearing age, children, and adolescents in the United States and Canada consume the *Dietary Guidelines for Americans 2020–2025 (DGA)*-recommended two or more servings of fish per week. Both the type and amount of fish consumed vary by race and ethnicity, as well as income, among women of childbearing age, children, and adolescents; age and sex are not strong drivers of fish consumption among children.

TABLE 3-13 Usual Fish Consumption Rate (UFCR), Women of Childbearing Age and Children in Canada by Age, Sex, Race, and Ethnicity, 2015

Population	Population Size (in 1,000s)	Percent Never Consuming Fish	Percent Consuming at Least 2 Servings per Week (40 day)	Estimated Consumption (day) at Selected Percentiles of Intake (whole population)			Estimated Consumption (day) at Selected Percentiles of Intake (fish consumers only)		
				5th	50th	95th	10th	50th	90th
Women of Childbearing Age (13–49 years)									
All females of childbearing age	8,266	81.8	4.6	2.5	10.3	36.4	68.9	79.7	103.8
Race and Ethnicity[a]									
Caucasian	5,466	85.3	0.8	2.1	8.3	26.4	68.4	76.5	101.3
Asian	4,865	77.7	3.4	3.7	13.5	36.8	72.9	79.9	86.5
Others	896	69.3	21.1	7.6	25.0	58.4	83.0	91.5	120.4
Geographic Region									
Coastal provinces	1,586	83.5	2.9	2.4	9.5	31.3	68.9	76.6	101.9
Noncoastal provinces	6,640	81.5	4.0	2.5	10.5	37.6	69.4	81.0	104.1
Prairies	1,544	85.0	1.7	2.1	8.6	31.3	69.5	77.9	101.4
Ontario	3,249	82.2	3.8	2.4	10.1	37.0	75.6	82.9	113.5
Quebec	1,847	77.1	6.4	3.5	13.6	43.4	68.2	77.3	101.0
Adolescents									
All adolescents (less than 21 years)	7,296	87.2	5.0	0.7	6.2	39.9	33.3	72.3	145.6
Children									
Age (years)									
2–3	804	80.3	3.0	0.8	6.3	32.9	24.4	49.9	93.2
4–8	1,901	87.4	2.2	0.6	4.7	28.4	29.7	58.9	106.4
9–13	1,796	89.0	1.8	0.5	4.3	26.5	31.1	61.9	112.8
14–18	1,843	87.4	7.1	1.0	8.1	46.6	50.8	95.7	169.9
19–21	953	88.5	14.0	1.5	12.3	65.7	63.5	119.3	208.2
Sex									
Female	3,643	86.2	5.1	0.7	6.1	40.3	33.3	72.6	146.1
Male	3,653	88.1	4.9	0.7	6.2	39.6	33.3	71.9	145.0
Race and Ethnicity[a]									

	N							
Caucasian	4,654	89.8	3.2	0.6	5.1	32.4	34.3	74.6	148.0
Asian	1,697	80.0	11.2	1.5	11.3	58.0	35.2	75.0	150.0
Others	945	86.9	2.9	0.7	5.3	31.7	26.3	57.7	116.3
Geographic Region									
Coastal provinces	1,348	84.9	6.8	0.9	7.5	46.3	36.5	79.7	157.5
Noncoastal provinces	5,948	87.7	4.6	0.7	5.9	38.4	32.4	70.0	141.6
Prairies	1,410	91.4	2.1	0.4	7.5	27.0	29.5	63.5	129.3
Ontario	2,948	87.0	5.2	0.8	6.4	40.8	31.7	68.2	135.9
Quebec	1,590	85.7	5.7	1.0	7.4	42.2	36.4	77.8	156.7

NOTE: The age range for women of childbearing age is different in Canada compared to U.S. data collected through NHANES.
[a] Race/ethnic categories as defined in Canadian Community Health Survey.
SOURCE: Canadian Community Health Survey, 2015 (Statistics Canada, 2015).

TABLE 3-14 Most Commonly Consumed Seafood Species, Women of Childbearing Age, Children, and Adolescents in Canada

	Women of Childbearing Age			Children and Adolescents (2–21 years)		
Species	Population Intake, g/day (SE)	Seafood Consumers, Percent (SE)	Intake Among Seafood Consumers, g/day (SE)	Population Intake, g/day (SE)	Seafood Consumer, Percent (SE)	Intake Among Seafood Consumers, g/day (SE)
Clam	0.11 (0.06)	0.14 (0.05)	76.36 (22.31)	0.08 (0.05)	0.08 (0.04)	90.98 (28.31)
Cod	1.53 (0.51)	2.42 (0.59)	63.20 (17.58)	0.76 (0.15)	1.91 (0.36)	39.80 (8.06)
Crab	1.09 (0.30)	2.32 (0.50)	47.03 (15.57)	0.62 (0.19)	1.34 (0.30)	46.27 (13.15)
Haddock	0.41 (0.15)	0.68 (0.20)	60.86 (19.57)	0.35 (0.14)	0.48 (0.14)	74.07 (22.12)
Lobster	0.63 (0.28)	0.64 (0.29)	99.26 (31.80)	0.23 (0.07)	0.48 (0.22)	48.40 (34.14)
Salmon	5.00 (0.76)	5.31 (0.61)	94.23 (9.71)	2.93 (0.47)	3.81 (0.44)	76.71 (8.02)
Shrimp	1.50 (0.25)	4.14 (0.61)	36.24 (5.47)	1.36 (0.34)	3.01 (0.42)	45.11 (8.35)
Tilapia	0.33 (0.14)	0.60 (0.23)	54.48 (17.12)	0.54 (0.22)	0.63 (0.17)	84.90 (25.47)
Trout	0.16 (0.06)	0.19 (0.06)	87.09 (18.92)	0.23 (0.11)	0.27 (0.12)	86.01 (22.89)
Tuna	1.96 (0.33)	3.69 (0.54)	53.03 (5.88)	1.31 (0.21)	2.85 (0.38)	46.10 (5.13)

NOTE: g = grams; SE = standard error.
SOURCE: Canadian Community Health Survey, 2015. CCHS day 1 24-hour dietary recall analysis (Statistics Canada, 2015).

FACTORS INFLUENCING SEAFOOD CONSUMPTION

Geographic, sociocultural, and economic factors affect an individual's decision to consume seafood. An understanding of the array of factors that influence the decisions to consume seafood can inform strategies to advise consumers about benefits and risks associated with seafood consumption.

Govzman et al. (2021) aimed to identify the main drivers and barriers to fish consumption as well as consumers' perceptions about attributes of fish and seafood products in developed countries (Canada, United States, Australia, and European countries). The systematic review identified the main drivers of fish consumption as perceived health benefits, influences from family and social norms, availability of fresh seafood, and personal preferences. Although fish and seafood were commonly perceived as healthy foods, those perceptions alone were insufficient to explain variation in fish consumption because individual characteristics, such as interest in healthy eating, were also found to be important drivers.

The most frequently reported barriers included sensory dislike of fish, lack of convenience, health risk concerns, lack of self-efficacy in the choice and preparation of fish, lack of fish availability, and high prices of fish. Additional literature reviewed by the committee suggests that certain attributes such as quality, origin, and ecolabeling are factors that consumers value when selecting a type of seafood for purchase (Del Giudice et al., 2018; Dey et al., 2017; McClenachan et al., 2016; Nguyen et al., 2023). Consumption habits also emerged as an important factor in determining those who did and did not regularly consume fish (Honkanen et al., 2005).

Cultural and Lifestyle Factors

Multiple cultural and lifestyle factors influence seafood selection and consumption. For example, immigrants often use recipes and preparation methods derived from their home country's cuisine and cooking practices. For recreational fishers, species of fish consumed may not reflect the same species available in the commercial marketplace. Economic factors, including the affordability of culturally appropriate seafood, may affect where people acquire or purchase seafood (Govzman et al., 2021; Judd et al., 2004).

Ethnicity

Certain ethnic groups have been reported to consume more fish than the national average. For example, Jahns et al. (2014) used NHANES data from 2005 to 2010 to show that non-Hispanic Black adults reported the highest fish consumption, and Mexican American adults reported the highest shellfish consumption compared with other racial and ethnic groups. Differences were not statistically significant, however, across racial or ethnic groups.

He et al. (2021) surveyed 103 Burmese refugees resettled in Wisconsin and found that most (72.5 percent) were women of childbearing age. About 30.6 percent reported consuming one to three meals of sport-caught fish per month, while 21.2 percent reported consuming more than three meals of such fish per month. When surveying the consumption of purchased fish, 26.3 percent reported eating one to three fish meals per month. Meanwhile, 88.3 percent were unaware of Wisconsin's safe-eating sportfish guidelines, and 96.6 percent were unaware of the guidelines for Milwaukee's waterbodies.

Tsuchiya et al. (2008) investigated the fish consumption rate among 108 Korean and 106 Japanese women living in Washington State. This study found that both Korean and Japanese women of childbearing age consumed amounts of fish that exceeded the national average. U.S. consumers of fish reported mean values of less than 20 g/day, whereas the Japanese and Korean cohorts had significantly higher mean values (73 and 82 g/day, respectively). Mean consumption values for the Koreans and Japanese approached or exceeded the 95th percentile intake for NHANES and the Continuing Survey of Food Intake of Individuals (CSFII) distributions (Tsuchiya et al., 2008). Among Canadian population groups, Hu and Chan (2020) also found that Asian and other ethnic groups had a higher average fish consumption rate (24 and 22 percent, respectively) than did Whites (15 percent).

Evidence from an analysis of familial eating habits of Hispanic parents and caregivers suggests that low intake of seafood in this adult population may be influenced by limited knowledge and ability to prepare fish as well as a lack of family members and caregivers who are a role model for recommended seafood consumption (Santiago-Torres et al., 2014). In addition, seafood preferences can evolve with increasing exposure to other cuisines, changes in local culture, and fewer family meals. These factors may contribute to the low intake of fish observed among Hispanic children, despite a traditionally high fish intake in this population (Huss et al., 2013; Santiago-Torres et al., 2014).

Oken et al. (2023) analyzed data from 10,800 pregnant women who gave birth from 1999 to 2020 and were enrolled across 23 cohorts participating in the Environmental Influences on Child Health Outcomes (ECHO) consortium. About 40 percent of participants reported consuming fish less than once per week, followed by 24 percent who reported consuming fish never or less than once per month, and about 22 percent who reported consuming fish one to two times per week. Respondents with the highest reported fish consumption (about 13 percent) ate fish at least twice per week. The relative risk of ever (vs. never) consuming fish was higher among those who were older (1.14, 95% confidence interval [CI]: 1.10, 1.18 for 35–40 years vs. < 29 years) or who did not identify as non-Hispanic White (1.13, 95% CI: 1.08, 1.18 for non-Hispanic Black; 1.05, 95% CI: 1.01, 1.10 for non-Hispanic Asian; 1.06, 95% CI: 1.02, 1.10 for Hispanic).

Native Tribes and Indigenous Peoples

For many Native tribes and Indigenous peoples, traditional preparation (e.g., smoking) and sourcing (e.g., using nets in rivers at specific locations) methods are dictated by intergenerational practices. Judd et al. (2004) reviewed rates and patterns of fish and shellfish consumption among the Native tribes in the Pacific Northwest that reported much higher average consumption rates than did the total U.S. population. For example, the average Squamish tribal member reported consuming 25 times the amount of shellfish compared with the national average. Native tribes also reported eating different species and parts of seafood (e.g., hepatopancreas of crab and skin and eggs of fish) compared with the total U.S. population.

Marushka et al. (2021) analyzed data from 6,258 participants in 92 First Nations across Canada, collected for the First Nations, Nutrition and Environment Study (2008–2018). They found that 95 percent of participating First Nations adults reported consuming at least one locally harvested traditional food in the previous year, and about 71 percent reported consuming fish or seafood. First Nations participants also reported eating 15.4 grams

(0.54 oz) of fish or seafood per day whereas participants in remote fly-in only communities reported consuming 23.6 g (0.83 oz)/day of fish or seafood. Earlier studies also found variety in species of fish consumed among different First Nations groups. For example, the most frequently consumed seafood types in British Columbia were sockeye salmon, chinook salmon, and halibut, compared with walleye, lake whitefish, and lake trout in Ontario (Marushka et al., 2017, 2018).

Recreational Fishers

Patterns of fish consumption differ between recreational fishers (also known as anglers) and the general population. For example, a review of recreational fishing and its contribution to nutrition at regional, national, and international levels reported that recreational fishing in the United States in 2004 accounted for 10 percent of the total commercial, industrial, recreational, and subsistence harvest of 4,995,418 tons (Cooke et al., 2017). Additionally, recreational harvest included 396,242 tons from inland waters and 103,779 tons from marine waters. As a result, recreational anglers (who represent about 9.3 percent of the population) had access to 7.3 kg of edible fish per angler per year (Cooke et al., 2017).

Comparable values reported for Canada in 2010 indicated that recreational fishers (9 percent of the population) harvested a total of 35,941 tons of fish including 22,758 tons from inland waters. Recreational harvest represented 3.7 percent of total harvest (commercial, industrial, recreational, and subsistence), contributing 4.7 kg of edible fish per angler per year (Cooke et al., 2017). Thus, this type of fishing is not only pursued for recreational purposes but also can provide accessible and affordable seafood.

Cost

Love et al. (2022) analyzed NHANES data and found that low-income groups consume less seafood than high-income groups. Low-income groups consumed substantially less n-3 LCPUFA-rich seafood compared with high-income groups. The committee's analysis of NHANES 2011–2020 data reinforced the finding that the types of fish consumed by women of childbearing age varies with income (Table 3-15). For example, tuna is the second most consumed seafood species by those whose income is less than 1.3 times the income-to-poverty ratio (IPR), but it is the third most consumed by those whose income was more.

Another analysis of NHANES data from 2005–2010 found that a lower odds of seafood consumption was associated with participants who were younger, had lower incomes, and had lower education levels (Jahns et al., 2014).

TABLE 3-15 Seafood Species Commonly Consumed, U.S. Women of Childbearing Age, by Income-to-Poverty Ratio

Income-to-Poverty Ratio	Seafood Species	Sample Size (n)	Frequency, Weighted (percent)
Less than 1.30	1. Shrimp	1. 2,741	1. 30.7
	2. Tuna	2. 1,550	2. 14.3
	3. Salmon	3. 1,074	3. 10.8
	4. Other fish	4. 1,072	4. 8.4
	5. Crab	5. 512	5. 6.3
1.30–4.99	1. Shrimp	1. 3,997	1. 29.4
	2. Salmon	2. 2,147	2. 16.6
	3. Tuna	3. 2,237	3. 16.2
	4. Other fish	4. 1,393	4. 7.2
	5. Crab	5. 766	5. 5.2
5.0	1. Shrimp	1. 1,648	1. 26.2
	2. Salmon	2. 1,309	2. 17.0
	3. Tuna	3. 941	3. 15.2
	4. Other fish	4. 546	4. 4.6
	5. Crab	5. 364	5. 4.1

SOURCE: NHANES 2011–2012 through 2017–March 2020.

Little evidence is available on access to seafood among low-income women, but potential contributing factors to lower access include lack of physical access to acquire seafood from local vendors, low quality of available seafood, and the higher cost of some fatty fish compared with, for example, processed meats (Jones et al., 2014).

Nguyen et al. (2023) examined perceptions of U.S. consumers in terms of specific safety, health, and environment-related attributes of a seafood entrée served at restaurants, as well as how those perceptions are associated with socioeconomic and demographic characteristics. Most participants expressed a positive perception about farm-raised and sustainability-certified fish. However, the difference in perceptions were found to be ambiguous for domestic and imported fish, while perceptions of nutritional value were neutral. The primary determinants of consumer perceptions included frequency of seafood consumption and demographic characteristics, including sex, ethnicity, age, and the number of children in a household.

Brockington et al. (2023) conducted a scoping review of the literature to identify barriers and pathways linking fish as a seafood to food security among Inuit Nunangat populations in the Northwest Territories. They identified direct pathways, such as intra- and intercommunity food and knowledge networks, which increased access to fish; and indirect pathways, such as fisheries' efforts to increase household purchasing power, including employment opportunities in the fishing industry. Barriers linking seafood to food security included climate change, socioeconomic change, and the sustainability and stability of fisheries and fish-related community programs. To support the role of seafood in promoting food security in this population, the investigators suggested the improvement of metrics, shared management of fisheries resources, and an integrated policy framework.

Knowledge

The *Dietary Guidelines for Americans* (*DGA*)[8] are published every 5 years and provide advice on what to eat and drink to meet nutrient needs, promote health, and prevent disease, as well as form the basis of federal food and nutrition guidance, policies, and programs. They are also a resource for state and local governments, schools, the food industry, other businesses, community groups, and media to develop programs, policies, and communication for the general public. Similarly, Canada's *Dietary Guidelines* are written for professional audiences and serve as a resource for nutrition policies, programs, and educational resources for the Canadian population 2 years of age and older.[9] Both the U.S. and Canadian dietary guidelines recommend eating fish as part of a healthy eating pattern.

The committee did not identify any research evaluating the role of knowledge of dietary guidelines in relation to fish consumption by women or children. The specific guidance for fish consumption during pregnancy and childhood included in the *DGA* derives from guidance put out by the U.S. Environmental Protection Agency (EPA) and the U.S. Food and Drug Administration (FDA) titled *Advice* "About Eating Fish for Those Who Might Become Pregnant, Are Pregnant, or Breastfeeding, and Children."[10] The committee did not identify any recent studies evaluating knowledge of the most recent FDA/EPA Fish Advice. However, a 2004 survey conducted in New Jersey found no sex differences in awareness of the then-current FDA advisories, although differences by ethnicity were found. Specifically, a lower percentage of Asian people were aware of the advisories, and fewer Black people knew that there were benefits from consuming fish, compared with people from other ethnic groups. Awareness of both the benefits and risks of consuming fish was lower for people aged 21–45 years compared with older people (Burger, 2005).

In a follow-up cross-sectional study in a similar population, the greatest decrease in fish consumption was reported between 2004 and 2007, from an average of nearly eight meals per month in 2004 to approximately six meals per month in 2007 (Burger, 2008). This suggests that some of the warnings and advisories may have had the unintended effect of decreasing overall fish consumption rather than reducing consumption of fish species known to have high contamination levels and switching to fish species with low contamination levels.

A 2008 study among people in three coastal regions of the New York Bight[11] found that a far greater percentage of participants reported hearing nonspecific information about risks and benefits of eating fish than the percentage

---

[8] Available at https://www.dietaryguidelines.gov/ (accessed February 25, 2024).
[9] Available at https://food-guide.canada.ca/en/guidelines/#CDG-sections (accessed February 25, 2024).
[10] Available at https://www.fda.gov/food/consumers/advice-about-eating-fish (accessed February 25, 2024).
[11] The New York Bight runs along the east coast of the United States and encompasses an area that extends out from the New York–New Jersey shore to the eastern limit of Long Island and down to the southern tip of New Jersey.

who reported hearing any specific information about risks or benefits of eating fish (Burger and Gochfeld, 2009). The authors concluded that the lack of details in current fish advisories was a major component of ineffective communication.

Another study used nationally representative data pooled from the 2001 and 2006 U.S. Food Safety Surveys to examine changes in awareness and knowledge of mercury as a potential problem of contamination in fish. The study results indicated that consumers' awareness increased from 69 percent in 2001 to 80 percent in 2006. Significant predictors for consumers' awareness and knowledge included demographic characteristics (i.e., race, education, and income), region, fish preparation experiences, previous recent foodborne illness, and risk perceptions of food safety (Lando and Zhang, 2011).

In a qualitative study of pregnant women from Massachusetts, Bloomingdale et al. (2010) found that many women had knowledge that fish may contain mercury and had received advice to limit their fish consumption. Fewer women had prior knowledge that fish contains DHA or knew its function. None of the women had been advised to consume fish, and most had not been informed about the different types of fish containing lower levels of contaminants (e.g., mercury) and higher levels of DHA. Many of the women reported that they preferred to avoid fish rather than risk harm to themselves or their infants because they had received advice to limit fish intake and had been provided limited information about which types of fish they should consume (Bloomingdale et al., 2010).

Preparation Skills

Burns et al. (2023) examined whether parental confidence in preparing fish and seafood are associated with frequency of fish and seafood consumption in Canadian children. The investigators collected cross-sectional data from 28 parents (of 40 children) participating in the Guelph Family Health Study pilot, a longitudinal family-based cohort. The parents indicated that all children consumed fish and seafood at least once per year and 63 percent consumed fish and seafood at least monthly. Results of the analysis showed that the parent's cooking confidence was significantly and positively associated with the child's monthly fish and seafood consumption.

Sushi is gaining popularity in some North American subpopulations and can be an important source of seafood intake. Sushi is a preparation method that includes one or more of the fish types identified in Tables 3-4 and 3-7. A meal of eight sushi pieces for adults and adolescents could amount to an intake of 84 grams of fish, and three sushi pieces for children could amount to 31.5 grams of fish (González et al., 2021). Karimi et al. (2014) showed that tuna was consumed as steak, fillet, or sushi at least weekly by 34 percent of those surveyed in an adult population in New York.

Summary of Evidence on Factors Influencing Seafood Consumption

In summary, results from specific populations (e.g., Burmese refugees living in Wisconsin) have limited generalizability, but it is clear that amounts and types of seafood consumed vary widely across populations. Cultural traditions involving seafood and knowledge of seafood preparation methods are factors associated with greater seafood consumption. Recreational fishers are also likely to consume seafood more frequently than other populations. Individuals with lower household incomes may tend to eat fish less frequently and consume fish that are less rich in n-3 LCPUFAs, important nutrients whose roles in health are detailed in Chapter 4.

Insufficient information is available about awareness of fish consumption guidelines for women of childbearing age and children to determine any association with consumption of seafood; some evidence from previous decades suggested that no association existed between consumer awareness about prior editions of fish consumption guidelines and consumption of seafood.

SEAFOOD CONSUMPTION BY SETTING

To understand seafood consumption by setting among women of childbearing age, children, and adolescents, the committee evaluated results from analyses of NHANES 2011–2020 24-hour dietary recalls and examined evidence from the peer-reviewed published literature. The committee first discusses results from the NHANES analyses, then describes evidence from the peer-reviewed published literature.

NHANES Analyses

The committee commissioned the Johns Hopkins Center for a Livable Future at the Bloomberg School of Public Health to conduct analyses of data from NHANES 2011–2012 to 2017–March 2020 for women of childbearing age and children and adolescents up to age 19 years. The following sections report analyses of seafood consumption by these age and life-stage groups by setting.

Women of Childbearing Age

For U.S. women of childbearing age, dinner (62 percent of seafood meals) and lunch (32 percent of seafood meals) are the meal types most likely to include seafood. Together, these two meals account for 94 percent of meals at which seafood is consumed (Table 3-16). Hispanic women are somewhat more likely to consume seafood at breakfast (8 percent of seafood meals with 3 percent among all women) or lunch (45 percent vs. 32 percent among all women). No marked differences by income level were observed.

Table 3-17 shows that seafood consumption among U.S. women is primarily based on seafood purchased at retail outlets (60 percent) and from restaurants or food service locations (25 percent). All other food sources combined contribute 15 percent. A higher proportion of seafood was consumed at restaurants by non-Hispanic White (33 percent) and non-Hispanic Asian (28 percent) women compared with Hispanic (22 percent) women, non-Hispanic Black (15 percent) women, or women of another race or ethnicity (24 percent). Women with higher incomes also consumed a higher proportion of seafood meals in restaurant settings.

Children and Adolescents

For U.S. children, dinner (58 percent of seafood meals) and lunch (36 percent of seafood meals) are the meal types most likely to include seafood. Together, these two meals account for 94 percent of meals at which seafood is consumed (Table 3-18).

TABLE 3-16 Seafood Consumption by Meal Type, Women of Childbearing Age

	n, weighted	Dinner, Percent (n)	Lunch, Percent (n)	Breakfast, Percent (n)	Other, Percent (n)
Overall	22,549,512	62 (1,174)	32 (837)	3 (90)	3 (122)
Race/Ethnicity					
Hispanic	4,612,582	44 (216)	45 (240)	8 (27)	3 (30)
Non-Hispanic Asian	2,788,786	67 (241)	28 (175)	3 (23)	2 (18)
Non-Hispanic White	9,915,554	68 (273)	28 (177)	0 (6)	3 (21)
Non-Hispanic Black	4,347,238	59 (382)	34 (219)	2 (31)	5 (47)
Other	885,352	81 (62)	16 (26)	1 (3)	2 (6)
Income (IPR)					
Less than 1.3	5,856,109	60 (356)	34 (268)	3 (33)	3 (39)
1.3–4.99	11,870,966	61 (608)	32 (431)	3 (45)	4 (66)
5.0+	4,822,437	66 (210)	31 (138)	2 (12)	2 (17)

NOTES: IPR = income-to-poverty ratio; n = sample size. Values in parentheses are unweighted sample sizes. Some rows sum to greater than 100 percent because of rounding.
SOURCE: NHANES 2011–2012 through 2017–March 2020, days 1 and 2.

TABLE 3-17 Food Source of Seafood, Women of Childbearing Age, Overall and by Race/Ethnicity and Income

	n, Weighted	Retail, Percent (n)	Restaurant or Food Service, Percent (n)	Restaurant Fast Food/Pizza, Percent (n)	From Someone Else/Gift, Percent (n)	Caught by You or Someone You Know, Percent (n)	Other, Percent (n)
Overall	23,430,754	60 (1265)	25 (601)	9 (294)	5 (130)	1 (20)	1 (20)
Race/Ethnicity							
Hispanic	4,705,268	60 (298)	22 (119)	10 (63)	7 (36)	1 (5)	1 (6)
Non-Hispanic Asian	2,983,538	60 (279)	28 (145)	6 (33)	4 (24)	1 (4)	1 (6)
Non-Hispanic Black	4,572,743	66 (360)	15 (156)	14 (145)	4 (44)	1 (5)	1 (7)
Non-Hispanic White	10,233,695	57 (267)	33 (154)	6 (45)	3 (19)	1 (4)	0 (3)
Other	935,509	63 (61)	24 (27)	3 (8)	9 (7)	1 (2)	0 (1)
Income (IPR)							
Less than 1.3	6,001,777	66 (428)	19 (137)	10 (102)	4 (38)	1 (8)	1 (7)
1.3–4.99	12,456,955	57 (619)	26 (339)	10 (155)	5 (73)	1 (11)	1 (12)
5.0+	4,972,022	60 (218)	33 (125)	4 (37)	3 (19)	0 (1)	0 (1)

NOTE: IPR = income-to-poverty ratio; n = sample size.
SOURCE: NHANES 2011–2012 through 2017–March 2020, days 1 and 2.

TABLE 3-18 Seafood Consumption by Meal Type, United States, Children and Adolescents, Ages 2–19

Meal Type	Sample Size (n)	Frequency, Weighted (percent)
Dinner	1,448	58.1
Lunch	754	36.3
Snack	133	3.4
Breakfast	72	2.0

SOURCE: NHANES 2011–2012 through 2017–March 2020.

Compared with boys, girls are more likely to consume seafood at dinner and less likely at lunch. Hispanic (42 percent), non-Hispanic Asian (38 percent), and non-Hispanic White (41 percent) children are more likely to consume seafood at lunch compared with non-Hispanic Black children (21 percent of seafood meals). Lower-income children are more likely to consume seafood at lunch than higher-income children. Among children with the lowest income-to-poverty ratio (IPR), 43 percent of seafood was consumed at lunch compared with 26 percent among those with the highest IPR (Table 3-19).

Table 3-20 shows that children's seafood consumption is primarily based on seafood purchased at retail outlets (67 percent) and from restaurants of food service locations (21 percent). All other food sources combined contribute 12 percent. The committee notes that only 2 percent of seafood consumption by children occurs in school cafeterias. Compared with women of childbearing age, children consume a smaller proportion of seafood at restaurants. Older children consumed a higher proportion of seafood meals at restaurants, as did Hispanic (26 percent) or non-Hispanic White (23 percent) children compared with non-Hispanic Asian (17 percent) children,

TABLE 3-19 Seafood Consumption by Meal Type, U.S. Children and Adolescents, Overall and by Age Group, Race/Ethnicity, and Income

	n, Weighted	Dinner, Percent, (n)	Lunch, Percent, (n)	Breakfast, Percent, (n)	Other, Percent, (n)
Overall	11,837,188	58 (1,238)	36 (663)	2 (66)	4 (115)
Males (years)					
2–5	1,041,125	54 (127)	45 (68)	1 (4)	0 (3)
6–11	2,139,205	45 (227)	49 (130)	1 (9)	4 (20)
12–19	2,512,058	58 (240)	37 (129)	3 (18)	3 (23)
Females (years)					
2–5	1,218,328	48 (127)	46 (83)	2 (6)	4 (13)
6–11	1,897,216	62 (224)	30 (113)	3 (12)	4 (24)
12–19	3,029,256	67 (293)	27 (140)	1 (17)	4 (32)
Race/Ethnicity					
Hispanic	3,157,323	52 (300)	42 (206)	1 (16)	5 (42)
Non-Hispanic Asian	1,316,481	54 (221)	38 (129)	6 (26)	3 (16)
Non-Hispanic White	4,357,496	56 (214)	41 (134)	1 (6)	2 (15)
Non-Hispanic Black	2,344,908	70 (412)	21 (165)	3 (16)	6 (36)
Other	660,980	72 (91)	24 (29)	1 (2)	4 (6)
Income (IPR)					
Less than 1.3	3,823,044	50 (457)	43 (294)	2 (22)	5 (45)
1.3–4.99	5,848,239	58 (607)	35 (290)	3 (35)	4 (60)
5+	2,165,905	71 (174)	26 (79)	1 (9)	1 (10)

NOTES: IPR = income-to-poverty ratio; n = sample size. Values in parentheses are unweighted sample sizes. Some rows sum to greater than 100 percent because of rounding.
SOURCE: NHANES 2011–2012 through 2017–March 2020.

non-Hispanic Black (12 percent) children, or children of another race or ethnicity (18 percent). Higher-income children also consumed a higher proportion of seafood meals at a restaurant.

Evidence from Peer-Reviewed Published Literature

In addition to considering data from its commissioned analyses of NHANES data, the committee reviewed relevant evidence from peer-reviewed published literature on seafood consumption by women of childbearing age and children and adolescents, by setting.

Meals Eaten Away from Home

Engle et al. (2023) examined the results of an online consumer survey on seafood purchasing behavior pre- and post-COVID-19 pandemic. Fifty percent of respondents reported consuming a similar amount of seafood before and after the pandemic, whereas 31 percent reported consuming less after the pandemic, and 19 percent reported greater post-pandemic seafood consumption. The results suggested that the pandemic may have contributed to a shift in consumers eating a greater proportions of seafood meals at home compared with away from home. Among ethnic groups, no notable differences in at-home consumption of seafood were observed.

TABLE 3-20 Food Source of Seafood, U.S. Children and Adolescents, Overall and by Age Group, Race/Ethnicity, and Income

	n, Weighted	Retail, Percent (n)	Restaurant or Food Service, Percent (n)	Restaurant Fast Food/Pizza, Percent (n)	From Someone Else/Gift, Percent (n)	Cafeteria in K-12 School, Percent (n)	Caught by You or Someone You Know, Percent (n)	Other, Percent (n)
Overall	12,061,992	67 (1358)	21 (380)	4 (144)	4 (96)	2 (97)	1 (30)	1 (31)
Males (years)								
2–5	1,056,427	78 (147)	9 (25)	3 (13)	6 (10)	1 (7)	1 (1)	1 (5)
6–11	2,182,232	79 (260)	9 (55)	3 (23)	4 (18)	4 (34)	1 (6)	0 (1)
12–19	2,546,688	58 (244)	32 (93)	4 (41)	4 (14)	2 (17)	1 (4)	1 (7)
Females (years)								
2–5	1,223,417	81 (168)	5 (20)	4 (11)	4 (15)	1 (4)	3 (5)	2 (8)
6–11	1,945,333	73 (249)	14 (60)	5 (23)	4 (16)	3 (24)	1 (6)	1 (5)
12–19	3,107,895	61 (290)	27 (127)	6 (33)	4 (23)	1 (11)	1 (8)	0 (5)
Race/Ethnicity								
Hispanic	3,195,842	63 (356)	26 (106)	4 (35)	3 (20)	2 (37)	2 (12)	0 (6)
Non-Hispanic Asian	1,379,615	68 (269)	17 (83)	5 (15)	3 (17)	3 (12)	4 (8)	0 (2)
Non-Hispanic Black	2,418,008	74 (428)	12 (86)	7 (68)	3 (27)	2 (28)	0 (2)	1 (13)
Non-Hispanic White	4,385,414	67 (232)	23 (76)	3 (13)	5 (24)	1 (13)	1 (8)	0 (7)
Other	683,113	66 (73)	18 (29)	5 (13)	7 (8)	4 (7)	0 (0)	0 (3)
Income (IPR)								
Less than 1.3	3,904,123	71 (543)	16 (118)	5 (68)	4 (35)	2 (50)	1 (12)	1 (13)
1.3–4.99	5,964,264	64 (638)	21 (194)	5 (64)	5 (49)	2 (39)	2 (18)	0 (16)
5+	2,193,604	66 (177)	30 (68)	2 (12)	1 (12)	2 (8)	0 (0)	0 (2)

NOTES: IPR = income-to-poverty ratio; n = sample size. Values in parentheses are unweighted sample sizes. Income is defined as income-to-poverty ratio. Some rows sum to greater than 100 percent because of rounding.
SOURCE: NHANES 2011–2012 through 2017–March 2020.

Love et al. (2020) used NHANES data to assess U.S. seafood consumption patterns. Adults consumed 63 percent of their total seafood intake (by weight) at home. Twenty-five percent of seafood purchased from restaurants and other locations away from home was consumed in the home rather than at the point of purchase. Seafood-based dinners were primarily consumed at home compared with seafood lunches, which were more often consumed at restaurants and other venues.

School and Childcare Settings

Seafood is also consumed by children and adolescents participating in the National School Lunch Program (NSLP). From 2014 to 2019 the USDA seafood purchases represented between 1 and 2 percent of all animal food source proteins procured annually for the NSLP. The average quantity of USDA-purchased seafood for the NSLP during this time was about 3 oz per student per year and included three varieties of seafood: Alaska pollock, canned tuna, and catfish. USDA purchased only bulk Alaska pollock and breaded catfish strips during 2014–2015, and breaded Alaska pollock fish sticks were added in 2017 in response to requests from states (GAO, 2022). Figure 3-2 shows the average quantity (oz) of seafood available per student participating in the NSLP from 2014 to 2019.

Huss et al. (2013) conducted a pilot study to assess strategies to increase dietary intake of eicosapentaenoic acid (EPA) and docosahexaenoic acid (DHA) from fatty fish among preschool-age children in childcare settings in Indiana. Their analysis found that meats, such as chicken, were usually used in the lunch meals served in childcare settings, but that fatty fish could be a replacement if incorporated into familiar, well-accepted main dishes. Because fatty fish, such as salmon, herring, and sardines, are high in EPA and DHA, even a small increase in consumption of these fish results in significantly improved EPA and DHA intake. Adding fish to mixed dishes offers an opportunity to significantly improve children's EPA and DHA levels in childcare settings.

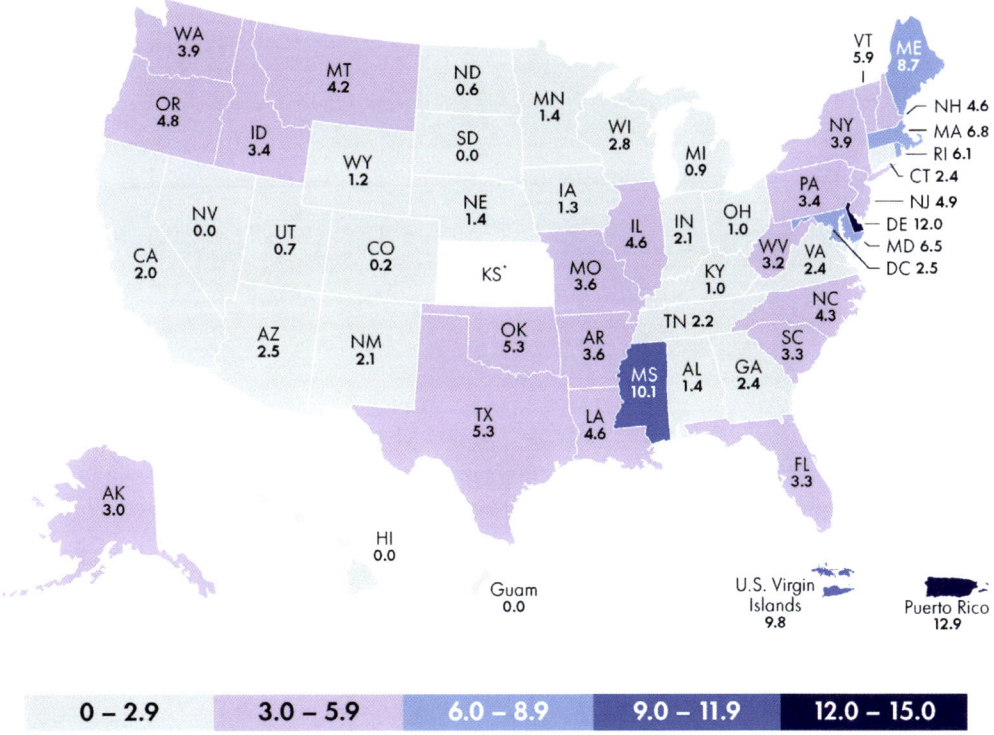

FIGURE 3-2 Average quantity of seafood that USDA purchased per student participating in the National School Lunch Program by state per fiscal year, 2014–2019.
SOURCE: U.S. Government Accountability Office analysis of USDA information; Map Resources (map). GAO-23-105179.

Geographic Consumption Patterns

Patterns of fish and shellfish consumption vary by geographic location. For example, residents who live on or near a coast differ in the types and amounts of seafood consumed compared with those who live inland, or among different regions of the United States. Fish consumption patterns also vary by specific coast. Residents near the Atlantic coast, for example, may have different consumption patterns than those residing on the Gulf of Mexico. Table 3-21 shows estimates of usual fish consumption rates, by percentile, for children and adolescents ages 1–20 years across geographic regions (EPA, 2014).

Cusack et al. (2017) analyzed data on women of childbearing age from six consecutive cycles of NHANES (1999–2010 [n = 9,597]), including frequency and type of fish and shellfish consumed across the 30-day recall period. The types consumed included tuna, predator fish (shark and swordfish), marine fish (fish sticks, haddock, salmon, sardines, mackerel, porgy, sea bass, unknown, other unknown, pollock, and flatfish), freshwater (catfish, trout, bass, perch, pike, and walleye) and marine shellfish (crab, crayfish, lobster, scallops, shrimp, mussels, oyster, other shellfish, and unknown other shellfish).

Results indicated that seafood was most frequently consumed among women of childbearing age residing in the Atlantic, Gulf of Mexico, and Pacific regions (Cusack et al., 2017). In this population, shellfish was the most frequently consumed species across all regions other than noncoastal regions of the West and Midwest. Freshwater

TABLE 3-21 Usual Fish Consumption Rate Total Fish, Children and Adolescents Less Than 21 Years, by Geographic Area

	Grams/Day Raw Weight, Edible Portion, by Percentile (95% confidence interval)	
	50th	95th
Youth (less than 21 years)	4.9 (4.0, 6.1)	34.2 (28.6, 40.8)
Geographic Region[a]		
Northeast	5.7 (4.1, 7.8)	40.4 (27.4, 59.6)
Midwest	3.3 (2.5, 4.3)	25.5 (21.9, 29.6)
South	5.7 (4.2, 7.7)	33.9 (27.4, 41.9)
West	5.9 (4.1, 8.7)	39.2 (27.3, 56.3)
Coastal Status[b]		
Noncoastal	4.5 (3.5, 5.7)	31.7 (24.3, 41.4)
Coastal	5.9 (4.7, 7.4)	38.0 (32.4, 44.6)
Coastal/Inland Region[a,b]		
Pacific	5.9 (4.3, 8.1)	40.2 (31.1, 52.0)
Atlantic	7.2 (5.4, 9.6)	40.3 (33.6, 48.3)
Gulf of Mexico	7.0 (4.3, 11.5)	41.5 (27.4, 62.9)
Great Lakes	3.9 (2.9, 5.2)	28.4 (21.7, 37.1)
Inland Northeast	5.1 (3.6, 7.2)	39.1 (21.7, 70.4)
Inland Midwest	3.1 (2.3, 4.1)	24.0 (20.4, 28.2)
Inland South	4.9 (3.7, 6.4)	30.3 (24.3, 37.6)
Inland West	6.0 (3.5, 10.1)	38.4 (22.2, 66.5)

NOTE: Sample size = 13,100.

[a] U.S. regions are the U.S. Census Bureau regions. Midwest = OH, MI, IN, WI, IL, MO, IA, MN, SD, ND, NE, KS. Northeast = PA, NY, NJ, CT, RI, MA, NH, VT, ME. South = DE, MD, DC, VA, WV, KY, TN, NC, SC, GA, AL, MS, FL, LA, AR, OK, TX. West = NM, CO, WY, MT, ID, UT, AZ, NV, CA, OR, WA, AK, HI.

[b] Coastal regions include counties bordering the three coasts (Pacific, Atlantic, and Gulf of Mexico) and the Great Lakes and estuaries and bays. Additionally, any county that did not directly border a coast, but the central point was within 25 miles of a coast, was defined as coastal. The inland regions are the remaining counties in each of the four Census regions.

SOURCE: EPA, 2014.

fish was most often consumed by women living in the coastal region of the Gulf of Mexico and the least often consumed by women in the noncoastal regions of the Northeast. Marine fish were most often consumed by women living on the Pacific Coast and least often consumed by those living in the Gulf of Mexico. Consumption of tuna was similar between women in the Great Lakes, the Midwest, and noncoastal regions of the Northeast. Shellfish was the most frequently consumed species in the Gulf of Mexico and the least frequently consumed in the Great Lakes. Fewer than 1 percent of all women in all regions consumed swordfish and shark (Cusack et al., 2017).

Residents in the Great Lakes region also reported consuming high amounts of fish. A survey of 4,452 respondents representing residents in the Great Lakes basin states of Illinois, Indiana, Michigan, Minnesota, New York, Ohio, Pennsylvania, and Wisconsin in 2017 found that the majority (92 percent) of adults living in these states had eaten at least one fish meal in the previous year (He et al., 2022). Consumption of tuna was most prevalent with 78 percent of adults reporting at least one meal in the past 12 months. Consumption of any sportfish (from Great Lakes and non–Great Lakes water bodies) was reported by 28 percent (estimated 18.6 million) of adults, while 11 percent (estimated 7.1 million) of adults reported consuming Great Lakes sportfish. The majority (64 percent, estimated 42.2 million adults) consumed exclusively commercial fish, with an average of 57.64 (54.29, 61.00) meals per year. An average of 7.89 (95% CI: 6.24, 9.54) Great Lakes sportfish meals were reported to be consumed per year (He et al., 2022).

Species of fish consumed in the past 12 months by consumers of sport-caught fish were also examined with walleye accounting for about half of all reported sportfish consumption. Other species included bluegill, sunfish, or crappie (43 percent); whitefish, perch, or smelt (39 percent); bass (39 percent); and trout (34 percent). Fewer than 25 percent of respondents reported consumption of catfish, carp, chinook and Coho salmon, northern pike, and muskellunge (He et al., 2022).

Another survey, conducted in 2014 among 1,419 women of childbearing age in the Great Lakes region, found that the average fish consumption rate was 0.93 meals per week or 20.1 g (0.71 oz)/day and did not differ by state of residence (Connelly et al., 2016). Considerable variation was present in individual daily fish consumption, with half of the women eating 15.2–17.2 g (0.5–0.6 oz)/day or less, 10 percent consuming more than 35.4–38.4 g (1.2–1.4 oz)/day; and 1 percent consuming more than 67.8–73.3 g (2.4–2.6 oz)/day. Only 5 percent reported consumption levels exceeding 340 g (12 oz)/day based on the number of meals consumed. Even though women of childbearing age in the Great Lakes reported eating more fish on average than national study estimates, their reported fish consumption was below amounts recommended for obtaining the greatest health benefits from fish consumption. A small proportion of study participants (10–12 percent) reported eating within the recommended range of 8–12 oz of fish per week, with 84–87 percent eating less than the recommended amount (Connelly et al., 2016).

In Canada, UFCR data from the 2015 CCHS (Table 3-13) indicated that more children in the coastal provinces consumed fish than the national average (15.1 compared with 12.8 percent) and the fish consumers living in the coastal provinces consumed more fish than the overall fish consumers (median intake of 79.7 g [2.8 oz]/day compared with 72.3 g [2.6 oz]/day). In contrast, women of childbearing age in the noncoastal provinces of Ontario and Quebec consumed more fish than those in the coastal provinces. Among First Nations populations, mean intake of fish or seafood varied significantly across Canadian provinces, ranging from 40.8 g (1.4 oz)/day in British Columbia to 3 g (0.1 oz)/day of fish or seafood in Alberta, Canada (Marushka et al., 2021).

Summary of Evidence on Seafood Consumption by Setting

Evidence reviewed by the committee indicates that most of the seafood consumed by women of childbearing age, children, and adolescents occurs at home, at lunch and dinner meals, followed by retail establishments and less frequently, restaurant meals. School and other institutional meals provide a negligible contribution to overall seafood intake. Residence in a geographical area closer to the Atlantic, Pacific, or Gulf of Mexico coasts or to the Great Lakes was associated with greater average seafood consumption; nevertheless, few children or women in these areas consume the recommended two servings of fish per week.

FINDINGS AND CONCLUSIONS

Seafood Consumption Patterns

Findings

1. Despite population-level increases in seafood disappearance during the past decade, seafood consumption among women of childbearing age and children and adolescents is generally low and has remained similar to that reported in *Seafood Choices: Balancing Benefits and Risks* (IOM, 2007).
2. Limited evidence is available to suggest that the public is knowledgeable about both the types and amounts of seafood that are recommended for consumption by women of childbearing age and children and adolescents.
3. Most of the seafood consumed by both women of childbearing age and children and adolescents comes from retail purchases and is consumed at home as part of lunch or dinner meals. School lunch is a negligible contributor of seafood to children's diets.

Conclusions

1. *Most women of childbearing age and children and adolescents do not consume the recommended amounts and types of seafood. Strategies to support increasing consumption toward meeting recommendations are needed.*
2. *Identification of strategies to overcome barriers to seafood consumption are needed so (1) individuals who consume some seafood will increase their intake toward recommended amounts, and (2) nonconsumers will begin consuming seafood with the goal of meeting recommended amounts.*

Factors Influencing Seafood Consumption

Findings

1. Limited evidence is available on the types and preparation methods of seafood consumed by pregnant and lactating women and children and adolescents in the general population.
2. Although few women of childbearing age and children and adolescents in the general population meet the recommended intake of two servings of seafood per week, some from certain ethnic or cultural backgrounds—such as those of Asian or Native American heritage, Indigenous peoples, and sport and subsistence fishers and their families—consume greater than average amounts of seafood.
3. Multiple factors influence patterns of seafood consumption, including residence in coastal areas or near bodies of water such as the Great Lakes, familiarity with fish preparation methods, and cultural and traditional practices.

Conclusion

1. *Insufficient evidence exists to suggest a need to revise seafood consumption guidelines, but a need does exist to identify strategies to help individuals meet current guidelines.*

RECOMMENDATIONS

Recommendation 1: The Centers for Disease Control and Prevention should identify strategies to address gaps in current *National Health and Nutrition Examination Survey* monitoring to better assess the sources, types, amounts, and preparation methods of seafood consumed by women of childbearing age, pregnant and lactating women, and children and adolescents up to 18 years of age.

Recommendation 2: The U.S. Department of Agriculture should reevaluate its federal nutrition programs, especially school meals, to support greater inclusion of seafood in meal patterns.

RESEARCH GAPS

- Research is needed to characterize the knowledge of, and responses to, current seafood consumption guidelines among women of childbearing age and children and adolescents. This should include research of seafood consumption by children, particularly in school settings and other meals consumed outside the home.
- Further research is needed to assess the types, amounts, and patterns of seafood consumed during pregnancy and lactation.
- Additional research is needed to assess the barriers to providing seafood as a component of meals served in schools and other settings frequented by children.

REFERENCES

Agriculture Canada. 2023. *Sector trend analysis—Fish and seafood trends in Canada*. https://agriculture.canada.ca/en/international-trade/market-intelligence/reports/sector-trend-analysis-fish-and-seafood-trends-canada (accessed December 7, 2023).

Asche, F., B. Yang, J. A. Gephart, M. D. Smith, J. L. Anderson, E. V. Camp, T. M. Garlock, D. C. Love, A. Oglend, and H. M. Straume. 2022. China's seafood imports—Not for domestic consumption? *Science* 375(6579):386-388.

Béland, Y. 2002. Canadian Community Health Survey—methodological overview. *Health Reports* 13(3):9-14.

Bloomingdale, A., L. B. Guthrie, S. Price, R. O. Wright, D. Platek, J. Haines, and E. Oken. 2010. A qualitative study of fish consumption during pregnancy. *American Journal of Clinical Nutrition* 92(5):1234-1240.

Brockington, M., D. Beale, J. Gaupholm, A. Naylor, T. A. Kenny, M. Lemire, M. Falardeau, P. Loring, J. Parmley, and M. Little. 2023. Identifying barriers and pathways linking fish and seafood to food security in Inuit Nunangat: A scoping review. *International Journal of Environmental Research and Public Health* 20(3).

Burger, J. 2005. Fishing, fish consumption, and knowledge about advisories in college students and others in central New Jersey. *Environmental Research* 98(2):268-275.

Burger, J. 2008. Fishing, fish consumption, and awareness about warnings in a university community in central New Jersey in 2007, and comparisons with 2004. *Environmental Research* 108(1):107-116.

Burger, J., and M. Gochfeld. 2009. Perceptions of the risks and benefits of fish consumption: Individual choices to reduce risk and increase health benefits. *Environmental Research* 109(3):343-349.

Burns, J. L. P., A. Bhattacharjee, G. P. Darlington, J. P. Haines, D. W. L. P. Ma, and The Guelph Family Health Study. 2023. Parental cooking confidence is associated with children's intake of fish and seafood. *Canadian Journal of Dietetic Practice and Research* 1-4.

Burridge, L., J. S. Weis, F. Cabello, J. Pizarro, and K. Bostick. 2010. Chemical use in salmon aquaculture: A review of current practices and possible environmental effects. *Aquaculture (Amsterdam, Netherlands)* 306(1-4):7-23.

Connelly, N. A., T. Bruce Lauber, J. Niederdeppe, and B. A. Knuth. 2016. Fish consumption among women anglers of childbearing age in the Great Lakes region. *Environmental Research* 150:213-218.

Cooke, S. J., W. M. Twardek, R. J. Lennox, A. J. Zolderdo, S. D. Bower, L. F. G. Gutowsky, A. J. Danylchuk, R. Arlinghaus, and D. Beard. 2017. The nexus of fun and nutrition: Recreational fishing is also food. *Fish and Fisheries* 19:201-224.

Cusack, L. K., E. Smit, M. L. Kile, and A. K. Harding. 2017. Regional and temporal trends in blood mercury concentrations and fish consumption in women of child bearing age in the United States using NHANES data from 1999-2010. *Environmental Health: A Global Access Science Source* 16(1):10.

Del Giudice, T., S. Stranieri, F. Caracciolo, E. C. Ricci, L. Cembalo, A. Banterle, and G. Cicia. 2018. Corporate social responsibility certifications influence consumer preferences and seafood market price. *Journal of Cleaner Production* 178:526-533.

Dey, M. M., P. Surathkal, O. L. Chen, and C. R. Engle. 2017. Market trends for seafood products in the USA: Implication for southern aquaculture products. *Aquaculture Economics & Management* 21(1):25-43.

Engle, C., J. van Senten, G. Kumar, and M. Dey. 2023. Pre- and post-pandemic seafood purchasing behavior in the U.S. *Aquaculture (Amsterdam, Netherlands)* 571:739491.

EPA (U.S. Environmental Protection Agency). 2014. *Estimated fish consumption rates for the U.S. population and selected subpopulations (NHANES 2003–2010). Final report.* https://www.epa.gov/fish-tech/reports-and-fact-sheets-about-fish-consumption-and-human-health (accessed August 22, 2023).

ERS (Economic Research Service). 2020. *Food availability (per capita) data system. Fish and shellfish.* https://www.ers.usda.gov/data-products/food-availability-per-capita-data-system/food-availability-per-capita-data-system/#Loss-Adjusted%20Food%20Availability (accessed August 16, 2023).

FAO (Food and Agriculture Organization). 2020. *The state of world fisheries and aquaculture. Sustainability in action.* https://doi.org/10.4060/ca9229en (accessed August 16, 2023).

FAO. 2022. *The state of world fisheries and aquaculture 2022. Towards blue transformation.* https://doi.org/10.4060/cc0461en (accessed August 16, 2023).

GAO (Government Accountability Office). 2022. *National School Lunch Program. USDA could enhance assistance to states and schools in providing seafood to students.* GAO-23-105179. https://www.gao.gov/products/gao-23-105179 (accessed August 16, 2023).

Gephart, J. A., H. E. Froehlich, and T. A. Branch. 2019. Opinion: To create sustainable seafood industries, the United States needs a better accounting of imports and exports. *Proceedings of the National Academy of Sciences of the United States of America* 116(19):9142-9146.

González, N., E. Correig, I. Marmelo, A. Marques, R. la Cour, J. J. Sloth, M. Nadal, M. Marquès, and J. L. Domingo. 2021. Dietary exposure to potentially toxic elements through sushi consumption in Catalonia, Spain. *Food and Chemical Toxicology* 153:112285.

Govzman, S., S. Looby, X. Wang, F. Butler, E. R. Gibney, and C. M. Timon. 2021. A systematic review of the determinants of seafood consumption. *British Journal of Nutrition* 126(1):66-80.

He, X., M. Raymond, C. Tomasallo, A. Schultz, and J. Meiman. 2021. Fish consumption and awareness of fish advisories among Burmese refugees: A respondent-driven sampling study in Milwaukee, Wisconsin. *Environmental Research* 197:110906.

He, X., M. Raymond, N. LaHue, C. Tomasallo, H. Anderson, and J. Meiman. 2022. Fish consumption and advisory awareness in the Great Lakes basin. *Science of the Total Environment* 827:153974.

Hinshaw, J. M., G. Fornshell, and R. Kinnunen. 2004. *A profile of the aquaculture of trout in the United States.* https://freshwater-aquaculture.extension.org/wp-content/uploads/2019/08/Trout_Profile.pdf (accessed February 1, 2024).

Honkanen, P., S. O. Olsen, and B. Verplanken. 2005. Intention to consume seafood—the importance of habit. *Appetite* 45(2):161-168.

Hu, X. F., and H. M. Chan. 2020. Seafood consumption and its contribution to nutrients intake among Canadians in 2004 and 2015. *Nutrients* 13(1):77.

Huss, L. R., S. McCabe, J. Dobbs-Oates, J. Burgess, C. Behnke, C. R. Santerre, and S. Kranz. 2013. Development of child-friendly fish dishes to increase young children's acceptance and consumption of fish. *Food and Nutrition Sciences* 4:78-87.

IOM (Institute of Medicine). 2007. *Seafood choices. Balancing benefits and risks.* Washington, DC: The National Academies Press.

Jahns, L., S. K. Raatz, L. K. Johnson, S. Kranz, J. T. Silverstein, and M. J. Picklo. 2014. Intake of seafood in the US varies by age, income, and education level but not by race-ethnicity. *Nutrients* 6(12):6060-6075.

Jones, N. R., A. I. Conklin, M. Suhrcke, and P. Monsivais. 2014. The growing price gap between more and less healthy foods: Analysis of a novel longitudinal UK dataset. *PLoS One* 9(10):e109343.

Judd, N. L., W. C. Griffith, and E. M. Faustman. 2004. Consideration of cultural and lifestyle factors in defining susceptible populations for environmental disease. *Toxicology* 198(1-3):121-133.

Lando, A. M., and Y. Zhang. 2011. Awareness and knowledge of methylmercury in fish in the United States. *Environmental Research* 111(3):442-450.

Karimi, R., S. Silbernagel, N. S. Fisher, and J. R. Meliker. 2014. Elevated blood Hg at recommended seafood consumption rates in adult seafood consumers. *International Journal of Hygiene and Environmental Health* 217(7):758-764.

Love, D. C., F. Asche, Z. Conrad, R. Young, J. Harding, E. M. Nussbaumer, A. L. Thorne-Lyman, and R. Neff. 2020. Food sources and expenditures for seafood in the United States. *Nutrients* 12(6).

Love, D. C., E. M. Nussbaumer, J. Harding, J. A. Gephart, J. L. Anderson, F. Asche, J. S. Stoll, A. L. Thorne-Lyman, and M. W. Bloem. 2021. Risks shift along seafood supply chains. *Global Food Security-Agriculture Policy Economics and Environment* 28:100476.

Love, D. C., A. L. Thorne-Lyman, Z. Conrad, J. A. Gephart, F. Asche, D. Godo-Solo, A. McDowell, E. M. Nussbaumer, and M. W. Bloem. 2022. Affordability influences nutritional quality of seafood consumption among income and race/ethnicity groups in the United States. *American Journal of Clinical Nutrition* 116(2):415-425.

Marushka, L., M. Batal, W. David, H. Schwartz, A. Ing, K. Fediuk, D. Sharp, A. Black, C. Tikhonov, and H. M. Chan. 2017. Association between fish consumption, dietary omega-3 fatty acids and persistent organic pollutants intake, and type 2 diabetes in 18 First Nations in Ontario, Canada. *Environmental Research* 156:725-737.

Marushka, L., M. Batal, T. Sadik, H. Schwartz, A. Ing, K. Fediuk, C. Tikhonov, and H. M. Chan. 2018. Seafood consumption patterns, their nutritional benefits and associated sociodemographic and lifestyle factors among First Nations in British Columbia, Canada. *Public Health Nutrition* 21(17):3223-3236.

Marushka, L., M. Batal, C. Tikhonov, T. Sadik, H. Schwartz, A. Ing, K. Fediuk, and H. M. Chan. 2021. Importance of fish for food and nutrition security among First Nations in Canada. *Canadian Journal of Public Health* 112(Suppl 1):64-80.

McClenachan, L., S. T. Dissanayake, and X. Chen. 2016. Fair trade fish: Consumer support for broader seafood sustainability. *Fish and Fisheries* 17(3):825-838.

NFI (National Fisheries Institute). 2023. *Top 10 list for seafood consumption.* https://www.aboutseafood.com/about/top-ten-list-for-seafood-consumption/ (accessed October 30, 2023).

Nguyen, L., Z. Gao, and J. L. Anderson. 2023. Perception shifts in seafood consumption in the United States. *Marine Policy* 148:105438.

NMFS (National Marine Fisheries Service). 2020. *Fisheries of the United States, 2018.* https://www.fisheries.noaa.gov/national/commercial-fishing/fisheries-united-states-2018 (accessed August 16, 2023).

NMFS. 2022 *Fisheries of the United States, 2020.* U.S. Department of Commerce, NOAA Current Fishery Statistics No. 2020. https://www.fisheries.noaa.gov/national/sustainable-fisheries/fisheries-united-states (accessed April 11, 2024).

NOAA (National Oceanic and Atmospheric Administration). n.d. *Aquaculture: Regulation & policy.* https://www.fisheries.noaa.gov/topic/aquaculture/regulation-&-policy (accessed February 2, 2024).

Oken, E., R. J. Musci, M. Westlake, K. Gachigi, J. L. Aschner, K. L. Barnes, T. M. Bastain, C. Buss, C. A. Camargo, J. F. Cordero, D. Dabelea, A. L. Dunlop, A. Ghassabian, A. E. Hipwell, C. W. Hockett, M. R. Karagas, C. Lugo-Candelas, A. E. Margolis, T. G. O'Connor, C. L. Shuster, J. K. Straughen, and K. Lyall. 2023. Demographic and health characteristics associated with fish and n-3 fatty acid supplement intake during pregnancy: Results from pregnancy cohorts in the ECHO program. https://doi.org/10.1101/2023.11.17.23298695.

Pulver, J. R., A. Lowther, and M. A. Yencho. 2020. Updating the NOAA fisheries per capita consumption model. NOAA Technical Memorandum NMFS-F/SPO-210. https://spo.nmfs.noaa.gov/sites/default/files/TMSPO210.pdf (accessed February 24, 2024).

Razzaghi, H., and S. C. Tinker. 2014. Seafood consumption among pregnant and non-pregnant women of childbearing age in the United States, NHANES 1999–2006. *Food & Nutrition Research* 58.

Santiago-Torres, M., A. K. Adams, A. L. Carrel, T. L. LaRowe, and D. A. Schoeller. 2014. Home food availability, parental dietary intake, and familial eating habits influence the diet quality of urban Hispanic children. *Childhood Obesity* 10(5):408-415.

Shamshak, G. L., J. L. Anderson, F. Asche, T. Garlock, and D. C. Love. 2019. U.S. seafood consumption. *Journal of the World Aquaculture Society* 50(4):715-727.

Statistics Canada. 2015. Canadian Community Health Survey 2015. https://www23.statcan.gc.ca/imdb/p2SV.pl?Function=getSurvey&Id=238854 (accessed February 26, 2024).

Tsuchiya, A., J. Hardy, T. M. Burbacher, E. M. Faustman, and K. Marien. 2008. Fish intake guidelines: Incorporating n-3 fatty acid intake and contaminant exposure in the Korean and Japanese communities. *American Journal of Clinical Nutrition* 87(6):1867-1875.

USDA/FSIS (U.S. Department of Agriculture and Food Safety Inspection Service). 2022. Catfish from farm to table. https://www.fsis.usda.gov/food-safety/safe-food-handling-and-preparation/meat-fish/catfish-farm-table (accessed December 7, 2023).

4

Dietary Intake and Nutrient Composition of Seafood

This chapter presents the committee's review of evidence on the nutrient composition of seafood and the nutrient intake from seafood, with an emphasis on nutrients of public health concern and additional nutrients for which seafood is a rich source. The chapter also describes the contribution of seafood consumption to dietary patterns and to intake of nutrients including protein, eicosapentaenoic acid (EPA) and docosahexaenoic acid (DHA), and selected micronutrients. Finally, this chapter discusses various facets of diversity, equity, and inclusion that could be associated with intake of nutrients from seafood.

NUTRIENT COMPOSITION OF SEAFOOD

Nutrients and Dietary Components of Public Health Concern

Inadequate intake of nutrient-dense foods and beverages leads to underconsumption of some nutrients and dietary components. The *Dietary Guidelines for Americans 2020–2025 (DGA)* identified vitamin D, calcium, potassium, and dietary fiber as dietary components of public health concern because low intakes are associated with health concerns (USDA and HHS, 2020). Iron was also noted as a nutrient of public health concern for infants, particularly those consuming human milk, and for women of childbearing age. Consuming sufficient amounts of these nutrients can decrease risk of heart disease, anemia, and cancer, among other diet-related diseases. The following section reviews each nutrient of public health concern in terms of its availability in seafood (Table 4-1) and its relevant relationships to intake recommendations and potential for toxicity.

Vitamin D

Vitamin D is a group of fat-soluble seco-sterols. The two major forms are vitamin D2 (ergocalciferol) and vitamin D3 (cholecalciferol). Vitamin D3 is generated from dietary cholesterol, or it is generated endogenously by ultraviolet-induced synthesis of the inactive and subcutaneously fat-stored 7-dehydrocholesterol (IOM, 2011). Because of the risks associated with sun exposure, such conversion is not sufficient to cover vitamin D needs in the bodies of many people living in the United States and Canada; therefore, consumption of vitamin D3 is recommended. Vitamin D3 occurs naturally in a few food sources, which include fatty fish, fish liver oil, and egg yolk (Benedik, 2022). Fatty fish can contain between 5 and 15 μg of vitamin D (200–600 IU) per 100 g portion.

Atlantic herring can contain as much as 41 μg (1,600 IU) per 100 g portion (USDA, 1991). Diets high in fatty fish can therefore contribute substantially toward total vitamin D intake (USDA, 1991). The highest dietary vitamin D intakes have been recorded in pesco-vegetarians who regularly consume fish. Using 24-hour recall and diet history questionnaires, Crawford et al. (2023) found 52 percent of pregnant women to be below the Estimated Average Requirement/Adequate Intake (EAR/AI) for vitamin D when diet and supplements were included. Both vitamin D2 and vitamin D3 are also synthesized commercially for use in dietary supplements and fortification of foods.

Vitamin D is stored in the liver and in adipose tissue; thus the blubber and liver of arctic marine mammals such as seal, narwhal, beluga, and walrus as well as fish (e.g., char, cisco, lake trout, loche, sculpin, whitefish) are rich sources of vitamin D. This is especially relevant for consumers of a traditional Indigenous diet. Among Indigenous Canadian populations, exchanging a traditional diet that contains vitamin D–rich foods for a westernized diet has been shown to increase risk of vitamin D deficiency (Brunborg et al., 2006; Keiver et al., 1988; Kenny et al., 2004; Kuhnlein et al., 2006). In contrast, excessive intake may lead to increased serum 25-dihydroxy vitamin D levels and consequent hypercalcemia (Jones, 2008).

Calcium

Calcium is a bivalent mineral that plays a key role in bone formation, blood clotting, muscle movement, and neural signaling. The major physiological activities of calcium include bone accretion during skeletal growth and bone mass maintenance after growth is completed. Sufficient calcium intake is usually determined by measurement of bone strength (calcium amount in bone) using dual x-ray absorptiometry. The need for calcium corresponds to life stage, skeletal growth and remodeling, and lifestyle behaviors, such as weight-bearing activity. Calcium supplementation has been shown to reduce risk of preeclampsia in pregnant women by 50 percent (Hofmeyr et al., 2019).

Calcium metabolism is largely regulated by a parathyroid hormone–vitamin D endocrine system process for which protein, vitamin D, and calcium are needed. The interchange between the dynamics of calcium and vitamin D often complicates the interpretation of data relative to calcium requirements, deficiency states, and excess intake. Excess calcium accumulation in the body is almost never attributable to calcium intake from foods, but from dysfunction of calcium excretion. In the United States, about 72 percent of dietary calcium comes from dairy products, whereas seafood contributes only about 3 percent (IOM, 2011; NIH, 2022). Calcium absorption may be reduced by insufficient dietary protein intake and low vitamin D status, both of which are provided by fatty fish. In one study of European adults, consumers of fish had the highest intake of calcium (Sobiecki et al., 2016).

Potassium

Potassium is the major intracellular cation in the human body and has a critical role through signaling pathways in neural and muscular tissue. Relatively small changes in extracellular potassium concentration significantly affect the extracellular-to-intracellular potassium ratio and thereby neural transmission, muscle contraction, and vascular tone. Potassium concentrations are regulated by the kidneys (NASEM, 2019). Evidence from observational studies, clinical trials, and meta-analyses of trials demonstrate that higher intakes of potassium are associated with lower blood pressure (Frassetto et al., 2023). Excessive potassium (hyperkalemia) can be life threatening but is rare and not usually a result of high dietary intake, but of kidney dysfunction. The *DGA* note that older infants (6 to < 12 months) and children do not consume enough potassium (USDA and HHS, 2020). Dietary sources of potassium include most fruits and vegetables; as for seafood, potassium content varies by species. For example, salmon can contain 280–535 mg/100 calories and clams offer 534 mg/100 calories (ARS, 2019).

Dietary Fiber

Dietary fiber includes soluble fiber, which supports glucose control and the lowering of blood cholesterol levels. Soluble fibers are found in oatmeal, nuts, beans, lentils, fruits, and vegetables. Dietary fiber also includes insoluble fiber, which helps promote gastrointestinal regularity. Insoluble fibers are found in whole-wheat products, brown rice, legumes, leafy greens, nuts, seeds, and fruits with edible skins. Muscle-based foods, including seafood, contain very little dietary fiber. Fiber that seafood products contain is attributed to preparation methods and the addition of breading, although breaded fish and seafood contain minimal amounts of dietary fiber (Bland et al., 2021). The USDA nutrient database[1] estimates that one 226 g serving of breaded restaurant, family style fish fillet contains approximately 2 g of fiber.

Iron

Iron functions as a key component of hemoglobin and myoglobin, which oxygenate body tissues. This active transport of oxygen from the environment to the body's tissues is critical for all aerobic bodily functions. Iron also plays a role in deoxyribonucleic acid (DNA) synthesis as well as electron transport to convert dietary energy to adenosine triphosphate (ATP). Thus, iron is critical for pregnancy, lactation, and growth. Near the end of pregnancy, absorption of 4–5 mg/day of iron is needed to maintain balance (IOM, 2001). Important subclinical and clinical consequences of iron deficiency include microcytic anemia, impaired muscle performance, adverse pregnancy outcomes, developmental delay, and cognitive impairment.

Studies of iron deficiency anemia and behavior in the developing human suggest persistent functional changes. For example, lower mental and motor test scores and behavioral alterations in infants have been associated with iron deficiency anemia (Idjradinata and Pollitt, 1993; Lozoff, 2007; Nokes et al., 1998; Walter, 2003). Additionally, increased perinatal maternal mortality is associated with anemia (Smith et al., 2019). Although high hemoglobin concentrations at the time of delivery are associated with adverse pregnancy outcomes, such as the newborn infant being small for gestational age, evidence suggests that this association is not causal or related to iron status; rather, it is attributable to hypertensive disorders of pregnancy (Yip, 2000). Iron toxicity is generally associated with excess intake from supplements and not high intake from food sources. Consequences of chronic excess iron intake include impaired zinc absorption, increased risk of vascular disease and cancer, and systemic iron overload (Kondaiah et al., 2019; Torti et al., 2018).

Dietary sources of iron are either heme iron or nonheme iron. In the United States and Canada, dietary sources of heme iron are found in meat, poultry, and fish, and dietary sources of nonheme iron are found in nuts, beans, vegetables, and fortified grain products such as breads and cereals. Muscle tissue from meat, poultry, or fish enhances absorption of bioavailable heme iron from these sources (Hurrell and Egli, 2010). Generally, absorption of dietary iron is low (approximately 1–2 mg), and daily consumption of iron-containing foods is recommended (Johnson-Wimbley and Graham, 2011). Human milk provides approximately 0.27 mg of heme iron per day (although that amount is insufficient to meet the needs of infants older than 4 to 6 months) (NIH, 2023), and levels of heme iron in milk are not significantly affected by supplementation (IOM, 2001).

Additional Nutrients in Seafood

Fish and other seafood are rich in a variety of nutrients, and many species are rich in at least some of the nutrients of public health concern, except for dietary fiber. Nutrient composition of seafood varies considerably among species obtained from marine and inland environments as well as from wild harvest and aquaculture sources. In addition to being a source of protein, fish and other seafood are a source of long-chain polyunsaturated fatty acids of the omega-3 series (n-3 LCPUFA) as well as a number of essential vitamins and minerals. The following sections review these additional nutrients that are often prominent in seafood. Health outcomes related to these nutrients in seafood and the interactions of nutrients with toxicants or other contaminants in seafood are discussed in Chapter 6.

Protein

Seafood is considered a protein source of high biological value (i.e., has all the essential amino acids, and has high absorption rates) and thus is included with other sources of dietary protein such as meat, poultry, and eggs.

---

[1] Available at https://fdc.nal.usda.gov/ (accessed October 20, 2023).

Evidence from studies on consumption patterns of seafood by U.S. and Canadian populations indicates that only about 2–4 percent of total protein intake comes from seafood (Auclair and Burgos, 2021; Gardner et al., 2019). Although protein intake from high-biological value protein foods is generally adequate across U.S. and Canadian populations (Table 4-2, Table 4-3, and Figure 4-1), replacing other animal protein sources with seafood could be expected to lead to higher nutrient intake while not reducing total protein intake. Certain Indigenous subgroups for whom seafood is a key source of complete protein, however, may be at risk of inadequate protein intake (Cisneros-Montemayor et al., 2016; Marushka et al., 2021).

Long-Chain Omega-3 Polyunsaturated Fatty Acids

Seafood can be a rich source of the n-3 LCPUFAs, EPA and DHA. Although they can be synthesized from alpha-linolenic acid (ALA), the essential short-chain n-3 fatty acid, the conversion rate is less than 10 percent in humans.[2] Thus, dietary consumption of EPA and DHA is recommended (USDA and HHS, 2020). Thus, dietary consumption of EPA and DHA is recommended (USDA and HHS, 2020). The n-3 LCPUFAs are essential for fetal development and are key components of all cell membranes. Especially in the brain and retina, both EPA and DHA serve as precursors of several metabolites that are potent lipid mediators (Swanson et al., 2012). The evidence for health effects associated with diets low in EPA and DHA is discussed in Chapter 6.

Although seafood is not the only source of EPA and DHA, it is a primary dietary source (Saini and Keum, 2018) and any dietary pattern that excludes animal foods, such as seafood, may lead to insufficient intake. The n-3 LCPUFAs are particularly abundant in fatty fish such as salmon and lake trout. Seafood varieties commonly consumed in the United States that are higher in EPA and DHA and lower in methylmercury include salmon, anchovies, sardines, Pacific oysters, trout, shrimp, crab, and flounder (USDA, 2023b).

Aquaculture is the source of about 50 percent of seafood consumed globally and Atlantic salmon is a fatty fish and a rich source of n-3 LCPUFAs. The fatty-acid content of farmed fish is influenced by the composition of the feed mixture used in farming. For farmed salmon to have a fatty-acid profile like that of wild-caught salmon, the feed must include oils containing EPA and/or DHA in finishing diets (Bell et al., 2004).

Data from the National Health and Nutrition Examination Survey (NHANES) indicate that U.S. women of childbearing age and children and adolescents do not consume sufficient levels of DHA and EPA. The Joint Food and Agriculture Organization of the United Nations (FAO) and World Health Organization (WHO) report, *Fats and Fatty Acids in Human Nutrition, Report of an Expert Consultation,* recommends a range of intake for DHA/EPA targeted at preventing chronic disease (adjusted for age to ensure sufficient DHA/EPA with increasing body mass and activity). Recommendations are 100–150 mg/day for children ages 2–4 years; 150–200 mg/day for ages 4–6 years; and 200–300 mg/day for ages 6–10 years. For pregnant and lactating women, a combined 300 mg/day of EPA and DHA is recommended, of which at least 200 mg/day should be DHA (FAO, 2010; Middleton et al., 2018).

The Dietary Reference Intakes report on macronutrients (IOM, 2002/2005) recommends 0.5 g/day as an adequate intake (AI) of total n-3 LCPUFAs for infants (up 12 month). For children and adolescents, and pregnant and lactating women, AIs are established for ALA (as well as for linoleic acid).

Selenium

As discussed in Chapter 5, selenium (Se) is an essential nutrient that functions as a component of selenoproteins, which are critical in DNA synthesis and serve as oxidative defense enzymes in the immune system. Selenoenzymes are expressed in tissue-specific distributions in all cells of vertebrates. Selenomethionine or selenocysteine are the prominent forms of selenium in human tissue. Selenomethionine, which cannot be synthesized by humans, is initially synthesized in plants and incorporated in place of methionine in a number of proteins obtained from plant and animal sources (IOM, 2000). In food sources, the amount of available Se varies depending on the selenium content of the soil for both plants and the animals that feed on them (Rayman, 2020). Meat and seafood are

---

[2] Available at https://lpi.oregonstate.edu/mic/other-nutrients/essential-fatty-acids#metabolism-bioavailability (accessed February 26, 2024).

primary sources of Se in U.S. and Canadian diets. Seafood contains Se in its functional form as selenoproteins, with levels that can range from 0.4 to 1.5 µg/g (IOM, 2000). The USDA nutrient database estimates that yellowfin tuna is high in selenium; about 92 µg per 100 g. Sardines, oysters, clams, halibut, shrimp, salmon, and crab are moderate sources of selenium with 40 and 65 µg per 100 g. By comparison, among breastfeeding women in the United States and Canada, breastmilk levels of selenium are approximately 15–20 µg/L (Guo and Hendricks, 2008). Factors that affect dietary intake of Se include geographic origin of the food and the overall meat and seafood content of the diet. The lowest Se intakes have been observed in populations that eat vegetarian diets consisting of plants grown in soils low in Se (IOM, 2000).

The Recommended Dietary Allowance (RDA) for Se for pregnant and lactating women is 60 and 70 µg/day, respectively. RDAs for Se for children range 17–45 µg/day for girls and 20–50 µg/day for boys, depending on age group (IOM, 2000). The major forms of Se in the diet are highly bioavailable. Se intake varies according to geographic location, but there is no indication that average intakes fall below the RDA in the United States or Canada.

Se deficiency symptoms include muscle weakness and impaired immune function. There is low risk of Se toxicity at the Tolerable Upper Intake Level (UL). The UL for pregnant and lactating women is 400 µg/day. The UL for infants up to age 6 months is 45 µg/day, and 60 µg/day for infants 7–12 months. For children, the UL is 90 µg/day for ages 1–3 years; 150 µg/day for 4–8 years, and 280 µg/day for 9–13 years. For adolescents the UL is 400 µg/day for 14 to 18 years (IOM, 2000). Chapter 5 includes additional discussion on the selenium interaction with MeHg.

Iodine

Iodine is an essential component of the thyroid hormones, thyroxine and tri-iodothyronine. Thyroid function is critical to regulate basal metabolism as well as brain development. Low maternal iodine status during pregnancy can lead to an underdeveloped brain in the fetus. This earliest clinical response to suboptimal iodine nutrition occurs as an adaptation to the threat of hypothyroidism. Deficiency in selenium can exacerbate the effects of iodine deficiency (Kohrle, 2015). Iodine intake may be insufficient in pregnant and lactating women, leading to adverse outcomes for the child (Griebel-Thompson et al., 2023). Observational studies have shown associations between mild maternal iodine deficiency and decreased child cognition (Cortés-Albornoz et al., 2021; de Escobar et al., 2007). Dietary trends in higher use of sea salt, which is not iodized like most table salt produced in the United States, may contribute to lower iodine intakes in at-risk groups (Hatch-McChesney and Lieberman, 2022). Current guidelines do not recommend that prenatal supplements contain iodine, as there are insufficient data to reach any meaningful conclusions about the benefits or harms of routine iodine supplementation before, during, or after pregnancy (Harding et al., 2017).

The iodine content in most food sources is low and can be affected by the iodine concentration of soil, irrigation, and fertilizers. It ranges from 3 to 75 µg per 100 g serving. Foods of marine origin, however, can have higher concentrations of iodine because marine animals concentrate the mineral from seawater. For example, cod contains about 158 µg per 100 g, scallops provide about 135 µg per 100 g, and Alaskan pollock provides around 67 µg per 100 g.

A UL for iodine for infants up to age 12 months was not determined because of inadequate data; thus the only source of iodine for this age group should be from breastmilk, formula, and complementary foods. The UL for children is 200, 300, and 600 µg/day for ages 1–3, 4–8, and 9–13 years, respectively. The UL for adolescents ages 14–18 years (including pregnant and lactating) is 900 µg/day; for pregnant and lactating women 19 years and older the UL is 1,100 µg/day. For most individuals, iodine intake from foods (and supplements) is unlikely to exceed the UL (IOM, 2001).

The nutritional status of iodine can be measured using urinary iodine concentrations. Øyen et al. (2021) used a controlled, randomized crossover study design, where participants assigned to the experimental group consumed lean seafood in accordance with the Norwegian dietary guidance and restricted intake of milk and dairy to measure urinary iodine concentrations. The objective of the study was to determine the effect of consuming lean seafood on iodine status in adult men and women. The investigators concluded that the seafood intervention increased urine iodine concentrations from suboptimal levels to adequate levels (i.e., greater than 100 µg/L).

Choline

Choline is an essential nutrient that has roles in neurotransmitter synthesis, cell-membrane signaling, methyl-group metabolism, and lipid transport. Choline functions in brain and memory development in the fetus and appears to decrease the risk of developing neural tube defects (Zeisel and da Costa, 2009). The plasma concentration of choline varies in response to diet, decreasing approximately 30 percent in humans consuming a choline-deficient diet for 3 weeks (Zeisel et al., 1991).

Owing to insufficient data to establish an RDA for choline, an AI was set based on the prevention of liver damage. The AI for choline for pregnant and lactating women is 450 mg/day and 550 mg/day, respectively (IOM, 1998). Choline crosses the placenta, and the concentration in amniotic fluid is 10-fold greater than that found in maternal blood (Zeisel, 2006). While most Americans consume below the AI, deficiencies are rare in healthy persons because choline can be synthesized (Corbin and Zeisel, 2012). The UL for choline is 1,000 mg/day for children up to age 8 years; 2,000 mg/day from 9 to 13 years; and 3,000 mg/day for 14–18 years. From 24-hour recall and diet history questionnaires, Crawford et al. (2023) found 83 percent of pregnant women were below the EAR/AI for choline when diet and supplements were included.

Choline is found in a wide variety of foods. Fish such as salmon, tuna, and cod are good sources, although eggs, milk, chicken, beef, and pork appear to be the greatest contributors of choline in the diets of women (Chiuve et al., 2007).

Vitamin B12

Vitamin B12 (cobalamin) is a water-soluble vitamin critical for central nervous system function (myelination and signaling) because it serves as a coenzyme in important steps in DNA synthesis. Adequate vitamin B12 is essential for normal erythrocyte formation and neurological function. Deficiency of B12 results in pernicious anemia. Neurological effects of deficiency include sensory and motor disturbances that include abnormal gait. Cognitive manifestations of deficiency include memory loss, disorientation, and frank dementia (IOM, 1998).

Vitamin B12 is present naturally only in animal foods and certain algae (Ford and Hunter, 1955). Fortified ready-to-eat cereals are an additional dietary source. The richest sources of vitamin B12 include shellfish—clams, oysters, mussels, crab, crayfish, scallops, and lobster. Finfish—salmon, catfish, pike, whiting, perch, swordfish, carp, porgy, and flounder—are also a rich source of B12 (IOM, 1998). To be absorbed, dietary vitamin B12 must bind to HCL-activated intrinsic factor (IF) in the stomach; the vitamin B12–IF compound is then absorbed in the small intestine. Individuals who consume high levels of antacids or who have impaired gastric function or are post-bariatric surgery are at risk for low vitamin B12 absorption. No adverse effects from high intakes of vitamin B12 have been identified in humans (IOM, 1998).

Folate

Folate is a water-soluble B-complex vitamin that is essential for brain development and function, amino acid metabolism, red blood cell production, and DNA synthesis. Sources of dietary folate are abundant and include vegetables, fruits, beans, peas, eggs, and some meats and seafood. Adequate intake of folate is particularly important for women of childbearing age because of its role in preventing neural tube defects. The RDA for folate for women of childbearing age is 400 µg/day. Folate requirements are higher during pregnancy and lactation (600 µg/day and 500 µg/day, respectively) to support the rapid growth of the fetus and newborn (IOM, 1998).

Nutrients in Seafood by Type

The following sections discuss the content of macronutrients, vitamins, and minerals in various types of seafood. Table 4-1 provides the amounts of selected nutrients in seafood, by seafood type.

Macronutrients

All seafood has approximately 20–30 percent of its total weight as protein, making it a high-quality protein source (Ariño et al., 2013). Breaded fish and seafood is also the only seafood-related source of dietary fiber, which is not naturally occurring in seafood. Because of the high consumption rate of breaded seafood by U.S. children (Table 3-7), these products become a contributor to the overall low intake of dietary fiber.

Total and saturated fat content varies greatly by species and preparation. For instance, fatty fish such as Atlantic, farmed salmon contributes 12.4 g total fat per 100 g, only 2.4 g of which are saturated fat; whereas cooked, unbreaded farmed catfish provides 7.2 g total fat per 100 g, of which 1.6 g is saturated fat. On average, the largest amount of unsaturated fat from a single seafood source is from mixed shrimp that is cooked, breaded, and fried (8.9 g/100 g). EPA and DHA intake reflect the proportion of unsaturated fatty acids from seafood with the largest amounts contained in Atlantic farmed and wild-caught salmon (1.5 and 1.4 g/100 g and 1.7 and 1.4 g/100 g, respectively) (see Table 4-1).[3]

Vitamins

Salmon is the fish with the highest concentration of vitamin D, providing more than 13.1–16.7 µg/100 g of fish, depending on the type of salmon. Catfish and shellfish, on the other hand, contain little vitamin D. Bluefish cooked tuna and clams contain the highest amount of vitamin A (757 and 171 µg/100 g, respectively). Clams have the largest concentration of vitamin B12 (98.9 µg/100 g); most other types of seafood contain very small amounts. Folate content is highest in crab (51 µg/100 g) and Atlantic farmed salmon (34 µg/100 g).

Minerals

Pink, canned salmon and shellfish are high in calcium (60–92 mg/100 g), and clams are high in iron (2.8 mg/100 g). Iron content is low in all other seafood types examined in this report, except for battered and fried or cooked fish because the grains used in the batter contain iron. Choline content is highest in cooked, unbreaded, fried shrimp (135 mg/100 g), cooked sockeye salmon (113 mg/100 g), and cooked unbreaded Alaskan pollock (92 mg/100 g). Many seafood types consumed in U.S. and Canadian diets do not contain choline. Magnesium content is highest in Alaskan pollock (81 mg/100 g), followed by bluefin tuna (64 mg/100 g) and Alaska king crab (63 mg/100 g). White canned tuna in water (65.7 µg/100 g) and clams (64 µg/100 g) are highest in selenium. Crab, clams, and catfish contain the highest concentrations of zinc.

The iodine concentration of protein sources, including various types of seafood, in the U.S. food supply is reflected in Table 4-2 in descending order. Direct comparisons between the seafood nutrient composition listed in Table 4-2 cannot be made to nutrient values reported in Table 4-1 because the USDA, the U.S. Food and Drug Administration (FDA), and the Office of Dietary Supplements (ODS)-National Institutes of Health (NIH) database (Table 4-2) has a smaller database than the USDA FoodData Central database and food codes (Table 4-1) that correspond to different preparation methods of seafood that can alter nutrient density.

The 15 most concentrated sources of iodine are seafood. Haddock has the highest concentration (227 µg/100 g), followed by dried smelt (216 µ/100 g), lobster (185 µg/100 g), and baked cod (172 µg/100 g). Contributors to iodine intake that are not seafood are pan-cooked ground beef (7.5 µg/100 g), turkey breast (4.8 µg/100 g), and beef steak (4.7 µg/100 g). Very low iodine concentrations are observed in oven-roasted chicken breast (1.2 µg/100 g). Overall, seafood has much larger iodine concentrations—by at least one order of magnitude—compared with other protein sources. However, given the RDA for iodine of 220 µg/day for pregnant women and 290 µg/day for

---

[3] Available at https://fdc.nal.usda.gov/fdc-app.html (accessed February 24, 2024).

64

TABLE 4-1 Selected Nutrients in Seafood, by Seafood Type, United States

Seafood Type	Vitamin D (μg/100g)	Calcium (mg/100g)	Iron (mg/100g)	Potassium (mg/100g)	Dietary Fiber (g/100g)	Protein (g/100g)	Total Fat (g/100g)	Saturated Fat (g/100g)	Unsaturated Fat (g/100g)	DHA (g/100g)	EPA (g/100g)	Choline (mg/100g)	Magnesium (mg/100g)	Selenium (μg/100g)	Zinc (mg/100g)	Vitamin A (μg/100g)	Vitamin B-12 (μg/100g)	Folate (μg/100g)
Finfish																		
Alaska Pollock*																		
Alaska, cooked, dry heat	1.3	72	0.56	430	0	23.5	1.18	0.16	0.72	0.423	0.086	91.6	81	44.1	0.57	17	3.66	3
Oven ready breaded fish sticks, USDA*	0	13	1.77	281	1.8	14.2	7.08	0.88	N/A	N/A	N/A	N/A	N/A	N/A	N/A	N/A	N/A	N/A
Catfish*																		
Channel, farmed, cooked, dry heat	0.3	9	0.28	366	0	18.4	7.19	1.59	4.47	0.069	0.02	N/A	23	9.9	0.58	1	2.78	12
Channel, wild, cooked, dry heat	N/A	11	0.35	419	0	18.5	2.85	0.74	1.74	0.137	0.10	N/A	23	14.3	0.61	15	2.90	10
Channel, cooked, breaded, and fried	N/A	44	1.43	340	0.7	18.1	13.3	3.29	8.93	0.222	0.119	N/A	27	13.9	0.86	8	1.9	30
Cod*																		
Atlantic, cooked, dry heat**	1.2	14	0.49	N/A	0	22.8	0.86	0.17	0.42	0.154	0.004	83.7	42	37.6	0.58	14	1.05	8
Pacific, cooked, dry heat**	0.6	10	0.2	289	0	18.7	0.50	0.11	0.29	0.118	0.042	79.7	24	28	0.39	2.0	2.31	8
Pangasius**	-	-	-	-	-	-	-	-	-	-	-	-	-	-	-	-	-	-
Salmon*																		
pink, canned, without skin and bones, drained solids	14.1	60	0.57	N/A	0	24.6	4.21	0.75	2.27	0.074	0.274	88	24	39.6	0.65	20	4.96	4
Atlantic, farmed, cooked, dry heat	13.1	15	0.34	N/A	0	22.1	12.4	2.4	8.73	1.46	0.69	90.5	30	41.4	0.43	69	2.8	34
Atlantic, wild, cooked, dry heat	N/A	15	1.03	N/A	0	25.4	8.13	1.26	5.96	1.43	0.411	N/A	37	46.8	0.82	13	3.05	29
Chum, cooked, dry heat	N/A	14	0.71	550	0	25.8	4.83	1.08	3.13	0.505	0.299	N/A	28	46.8	0.60	34	3.46	5
Sockeye, cooked, dry heat	16.7	11	0.52	436	0	26.5	5.57	0.97	3.19	0.56	0.299	113	36	35.5	0.55	58	4.47	7

Seafood Type	Vitamin D (μg/100g)	Calcium (mg/100g)	Iron (mg/100g)	Potassium (mg/100g)	Dietary Fiber (g/100g)	Protein (g/100g)	Total Fat (g/100g)	Saturated Fat (g/100g)	Unsaturated Fat (g/100g)	DHA (g/100g)	EPA (g/100g)	Choline (mg/100g)	Magnesium (mg/100g)	Selenium (μg/100g)	Zinc (mg/100g)	Vitamin A (μg/100g)	Vitamin B-12 (μg/100g)	Folate (μg/100g)
Tilapia* Cooked, dry heat	3.7	14	0.69	N/A	0	26.2	2.65	0.94	1.56	0.13	0.005	51.3	34	54.4	0.41	0	1.86	6
Tuna* White, canned in water, drained solids	2	14	0.97	N/A	0	23.6	2.97	0.79	1.89	0.629	0.233	29.3	33	65.7	0.48	6	1.17	2
White, canned in oil, drained solids	N/A	4	0.65	333	0	26.5	8.08	1.28	6.23	0.178	0.066	N/A	34	60.1	0.47	5	2.2	5
Fresh bluefin, cooked, dry heat	N/A	10	1.31	323	0	29.9	6.28	1.61	3.89	1.14	0.363	N/A	64	46.8	0.77	757	10.9	2
Shellfish																		
Clams* Mixed, cooked, moist heat	N/A	92	2.81	628	0	25.6	1.95	0.19	0.72	0.146	0.138	N/A	18	64	2.73	171	98.9	29
Crab* Alaska king, cooked, moist heat	N/A	59	0.76	N/A	0	19.4	1.54	0.13	0.72	0.118	0.295	N/A	63	40	7.62	9	11.5	51
Shrimp* Mixed, cooked, moist heat	0.1	91	0.32	N/A	0	22.8	1.7	0.52	0.95	0.141	0.135	135	37	49.5	1.63	90	1.66	24
Mixed, cooked, breaded and fried	0.1	67	1.26	225	0.4	21.4	12.3	2.09	8.89	0.124	0.109	91.2	40	41.7	1.38	56	1.87	33

* Indicates a top 10 seafood species from NFI, 2024.
** Indicates differentiation of farm-raised and wild-caught seafood species.
\# Pangasius nutrient data are not collected from the USDA (2019) database.
+ Company source: Trident Seafoods Corps [supplies pollock (fish sticks), representing an option served in the Child Nutrition Program]
SOURCE: USDA Nutrient Database Release 28, 2019.

TABLE 4-2 Iodine Content by Protein Source, United States

Portion Size[*]	Iodine mcg/100g
Seafood Sources	
Haddock[a]	227
Smelt, dried[b]	216
Lobster[c]	185
Cod, baked[d]	172
Oyster[e]	109
Fish Sticks[f]	67
Clam[g]	66
Pollock[h]	44
Tuna, fresh, bluefin[i]	23
Swordfish[j]	19
Salmon, pink, canned[k]	15
Shrimp[l]	15
Flatfish[m]	14
Salmon, steaks[n]	13
Halibut[o]	10
Scallop[p]	<10
Trout[q]	<10
Tuna, canned in water[r]	9.4
Tilapia[s]	6.9
Catfish[t]	3.2
Meat Sources	
Beef, ground, pan-cooked[u]	7.5
Turkey Breast[v]	4.8
Beef Steak[w]	4.7
Chicken breast, oven-roasted[x]	1.2

[a] Haddock, raw; [b] Smelt, dried (Alaska Native); [c] Lobster, northern, cooked, moist heat; [d] Cod, baked; [e] Oyster, eastern, wild, cooked, moist heat; [f] Fish sticks or patty, frozen, oven-cooked; [g] Clam mixed species, canned, drained solids; [h] Pollock, Alaska, raw; [i] Tuna, fresh, bluefin, cooked, dry heat; [j] Swordfish, raw; [k] Salmon, pink, canned, drained solids; [l] Shrimp. Precooked, shell removed, no tail; [m] Flatfish (flounder and sole species), raw; [n] Salmon, steaks/fillets, baked; [o] Halibut, Atlantic and Pacific, raw; [p] Scallop, mixed species, raw; [q] Trout, rainbow, wild, raw; [r] Tuna canned in water, drained; [s] Tilapia, baked; [t] Catfish, pan-cooked with oil; [u] Beef, ground, pan-cooked; [v] Turkey breast, oven-roasted; [w] Beef steak, loin/sirloin, broiled; [x] Chicken breast, oven-roasted (skin removed); [y] Pork chop, pan-cooked with oil.
SOURCE: USDA, FDA, and ODS-NIH Database for Iodine Content of Common Foods Release 3.0 (2023) (USDA, 2023a).

lactating women (IOM, 2001), even daily consumption of the most frequently consumed seafood types—shrimp at 15 μg iodine/100 g, canned salmon at 15 μg/100 g, canned tuna 9.4 μg/100 g—are not likely to achieve the RDA for iodine.

Table 4-3 shows the relative nutrient density of 4-oz portions of seafood compared with 3.5-oz portions of other protein sources (the recommended portion sizes for these different protein food sources). To approximate the energy and protein content of each serving, four different types of each protein source were selected. The four types of seafood are fatty-acid rich (salmon), canned tuna, cooked shrimp, and fried shrimp. Examples of protein sources other than seafood are ground beef (containing 25 percent fat), ground beef (containing 5 percent fat), fried chicken, and roasted chicken. Although the portion size of seafood is 0.5 oz larger than the portion of ground beef and chicken, the large difference in density of most micronutrients in these commonly consumed seafood choices is beyond the difference in nutrient density accounted for by portion size alone. These seafood types, however, contain less iron and zinc than ground beef. Total and types of fat content vary by species and by preparation method.

TABLE 4-3 Comparison of Nutrient Density Between Selected Seafood Choices and Other High-Quality Protein Sources

	Protein Source							
	Salmon Atlantic[a]	Tuna, canned[b]	Shrimp, cooked[c]	Shrimp, fried[d]	Ground beef, 25% fat[e]	Ground beef, 5% fat[f]	Chicken, fried[g]	Chicken, roasted[h]
Portion Size*	4 oz.	4 oz.	4 oz.	4 oz.	3.5 oz.	3.5 oz.	3.5 oz.	3.5 oz.
Macronutrients								
Calories, kcal	234	145	135	274	248	164	229	153
Protein, g	25.1	26.8	25.9	24.3	23.4	25.8	24.3	27.1
Total fat, g	14.1	3.4	1.9	13.9	16.4	5.9	12.7	4.1
Saturated, g	2.7	0.9	0.6	2.4	6.3	2.6	3.5	1.1
Monounsaturated, g	4.7	0.9	0.4	4.3	7.5	2.4	5.0	1.5
Polyunsaturated, g	5.2	1.3	0.7	5.8	0.5	0.3	2.9	0.9
Micronutrients								
Vitamin A, μg	78	7	1.2	64	3	3	23	8
Vitamin D, μg	15	2.3	0.1	0.1	0	0	0.1	0.1
Vitamin B12, μg	3.2	1.3	1.7	2.1	2.8	2.8	0.3	0.3
Calcium, mg	17	16	91	76	32	9	14	13
Zinc, mg	0.5	0.5	1.9	1.6	6.0	6.5	1.7	0.8
Phosphorus, mg	286	246	347	247	199	222	162	217
Iron, mg	0.4	1.1	0.4	1.4	2.5	2.9	1.2	1.1
Choline, mg	103	33	153	103	73	84	68	77

NOTES: * For seafood sources, the portion sizes represent the 2014 EPA-FDA "Advice about Eating Fish for Those Who Might Become Pregnant, Are Pregnant, or Breastfeeding, and Children" and 2020-2025 *DGA* recommendations. Seafood portion size amounts are based on a 2,000-calorie level of dietary pattern. For beef and chicken sources, portion sizes are estimates that draw on, but are not explicitly stated, in the *DGA* recommendation of 26 oz per week of lean meat and poultry for adult women and the Healthy U.S.-Style Dietary Pattern, based on a 2,000-calorie level of pattern.

[a] Salmon, Atlantic, farmed, cooked, dry heat; [b] Tuna, white, canned in water, drained solids; [c] Shrimp, mixed species, cooked, moist heat (may contain additives to retain moisture); [d] Shrimp, mixed, cooked, breaded and fried; [e] Beef, ground, 75% lean meat/25% fat, patty, cooked, pan-broiled; [f] Beef, ground, 95% lean meat/5% fat, patty, cooked, pan-broiled; [g] Chicken, broilers or fryers, meat and skin, cooked, fried, flour; [h] Chicken, roasting, light meat, meat only, cooked, roasted.
SOURCE: ARS, 2019.

DIETARY PATTERNS AND SEAFOOD CONSUMPTION

The *DGA* includes an overarching recommendation that all Americans should aim to consume at least 8 oz (about two servings of 4 oz/250 g each) of seafood per week. For children the *DGA* recommends two servings per week in amounts corresponding to total daily caloric intake.[4] For adult women of childbearing age, the *DGA* recommends at least 8 oz of seafood per week. Pregnant or lactating women are encouraged to eat at least 8 oz and up to 12 oz of seafood per week, choosing varieties that are lower in methylmercury (USDA and HHS, 2020). The *DGA* also includes dietary patterns that were developed to serve as flexible frameworks to enable policy makers, programs, and health professionals to help people at any stage of life customize and enjoy nutrient-dense food and beverage choices to reflect personal preferences, cultural foodways, and budgetary considerations as recommended in the *DGA*.

The Healthy U.S.-Style Dietary Pattern, the primary pattern, focuses on nutrient-dense foods with an emphasis on vegetables, fruits, grains, dairy, protein, and oils, while limiting saturated fat, sugar, sodium, and alcohol. A variation on this pattern, the Healthy Mediterranean-Style Dietary Pattern, includes a range of 16–20 oz of seafood per week for adults (DGAC, 2015). In the following sections, the committee discusses various facets of diversity, equity, and inclusion that could affect dietary patterns and thus be associated with the intake of nutrients from seafood.

---

[4] Available at https://www.dietaryguidelines.gov/sites/default/files/2020-12/Dietary_Guidelines_for_Americans_2020-2025.pdf (accessed October 15, 2023).

The Contribution of Seafood to Diet and Nutrient Intake by Race and Ethnicity

The committee was charged to consider diversity, equity, and inclusion in its assessment of associations between seafood intake, in consideration of the nutritional contributions to the diet from seafood. Love et al. (2022) analyzed NHANES data and reported relationships between race and ethnicity and seafood. Overall, rates of seafood intake were significantly lower among non-Hispanic White adults than non-Hispanic Black ($P = 0.001$) or non-Hispanic Asian ($P < 0.001$) adults. Non-Hispanic Asian adults routinely met *DGA* recommendations to consume 227 g (8 oz) of seafood.

A cross-sectional analysis of 2011–2014 NHANES was performed to examine associations between food insecurity and diet quality, and variations by sex and race/ethnicity compared with adults living in food-secure households, and adults living in food-insecure households with a 2.22-unit lower Healthy Eating Index-2015 score (95% confidence interval [CI] –3.35 to –1.08). Food insecurity among non-Hispanic Whites was associated with lower scores for total protein foods, including seafood. There were no such associations among non-Hispanic Black or Hispanic adults with food insecurity and no differences by sex (Leung and Tester, 2019).

Kranz et al. (2017) used a nationally representative sample from the UK National Diet and Nutrition Survey Rolling Program (2008–2012) to describe fish consumption among children ages 2–18 years. Data were collected from four consecutive 24-hour estimated diet diaries (records) from the children surveyed. Analysis of the data found that eating any amount of fish was associated with better diet quality than not eating any fish, in that consuming any amount of fish was strongly and positively associated with being in the medium or highest tertile of vegetable intake and negatively associated with eating the medium or highest tertile of meat (odds ratio [OR] = 1.55, 95% CI 1.19–2.12; OR = 1.88, 95% CI 1.39–2.58; OR = 0.72, 95% CI 0.55–0.98; OR = 0.47, 95% CI 0.34–0.66, respectively). Consuming the recommended amount of two servings of fish per week was significantly and positively predicted by consuming the highest tertile of vegetables (OR = 2.51, 95% CI 1.30–4.84) and significantly but negatively associated with consuming the highest tertile of meat (OR = 0.32, 95% CI 0.16–0.64).

Changes in food availability among population groups that traditionally depend on seafood affects seafood-based dietary patterns. Slater et al. (2013) showed that transitioning from a nutrient-dense traditional seafood-based diet to nutrient-poor market foods in a Canadian Dene Indigenous population resulted in inadequate vitamin D intake. Their study found that only 11 and 13 percent of the study population had adequate vitamin D intake in winter and summer, respectively. Milk and local fish were the major dietary sources of vitamin D for this population group.

Kenny et al. (2018) examined data derived from 24-hour recalls collected by the Inuit Health Survey from 2007 to 2008. Their analysis of dietary patterns across all regions showed that the most frequently consumed Arctic foods were caribou (18–39 percent, by region) and fish (7–22 percent by region). The most frequently reported market food items were coffee and tea, (granulated) sugar, sweetened beverages, and bread. At the regional level, Arctic foods represented a modest contribution to total dietary intake (6.4–19.6 percent of total energy) but they were a major source of both micro- and macronutrients. For example, Arctic foods contributed significantly to intakes of protein (23–52 percent), iron (28–54 percent), niacin (24–52 percent), and vitamins D (73 percent), B6 (18–55 percent), and B12 (50–82 percent) by total dietary energy intake. This study concluded that although traditional Arctic foods are a rich source of micronutrients, the decreased use of micronutrient-rich animal food sources, combined with a pattern of substituting micronutrient-poor market foods for Arctic foods, places Inuit communities at risk of poor nutrition.

Similarly, Sharma et al. (2015) analyzed dietary patterns from three 24-hour recalls from Yup'ik women aged 18 years and older, not including pregnant and lactating women. Sweetened juices, drinks, and soda were among the leading contributors for total energy intake (8.2 percent), carbohydrates (16.1 percent), and sugar (32.7 percent), while traditional foods contributed significantly to intakes of protein, iron, and vitamin A. This study also found that a dietary transition away from traditional foods has resulted in a decrease in diet quality among Alaskan Native populations.

Seafood Contribution to Protein Intake by Race and Ethnicity Among Women of Childbearing Age

To identify the contribution of seafood to protein intake across racial and ethnic groups the committee commissioned an analysis of data from NHANES 2011–2020, as detailed in Chapter 3. As shown in Table 4-4, less than 10 percent of protein among women of childbearing age was from seafood (13.5 out of a total of 144.8 g/day) and consumption of seafood high in n-3 LCPUFAs was only 4.0 g/day. Even among the top consumers (95th percentile), only 36.9 g/day of protein consumed were from seafood. Although total protein intake was similar between racial and ethnic groups (ranging 140.9–159.4 g/day), non-Hispanic Asian and non-Hispanic White individuals had the highest proportion of protein intake from seafood at 24.8 and 20.6 g/day, respectively. Non-Hispanic Black individuals had the lowest proportions at 10.0 g/day. Accordingly, non-Hispanic Asian women had the highest intakes of seafood high in n-3 LCPUFAs at 9.5 g/day, but those of non-Hispanic White women were less than half that level (4.1 g/day).

Table 4-4 shows only small differences in daily consumption of total protein or protein from seafood between women by income group, but total protein and protein intake from seafood increased slightly with increasing income. Even in the highest-income groups, the greatest amount of protein consumed (95th percentile) from seafood was only 37.4 g/day (37.3 and 36.5 g/day in the lowest- and middle-income groups, respectively). Total seafood high in n-3 LCPUFAs was highest in the high-income groups at 4.4 g/day compared with 3.0 and 3.4 g/day in the lowest- and middle-income groups, respectively.

Data from the NHANES food frequency questionnaire (FFQ), which provides the average seafood intake over the previous 30 days, shows that among 7,355 intake records, 25.5 percent ($n = 1,878$) did not consume any seafood. Because the time frame of the FFQ did not necessarily include the days of 24-hour recall and the episodic intake of seafood for most individuals, the data still show that 2.3 g/day of protein intake was from seafood in women classified as "nonconsumers" based on their intake in the 30 days prior to completing the FFQ. Among women who reportedly eating at least some seafood in the prior 30 days, seafood contributed 17.4 g/day of protein and 4.6 g/day of high n-3 LCPUFAs. Women classified as seafood consumers had higher total protein intakes than nonconsumers (153.1 vs. 120.9 g/day), and almost 10 times greater intake of n-3 LCPUFAs (4.6 g/day compared with 0.5 g/day). For the top consumers of seafood (95th percentile), seafood contributed an average of 40 g/day of protein.

Seafood Contribution to Protein Intake by Race and Ethnicity Among Children and Adolescents

Table 4-5 shows the contribution to children and adolescents' total protein intake by seafood from low– and high–n-3 LCPUFA sources compared with other animal sources as well as total protein sources by race and ethnicity. The data indicate that even in the highest consumption tertile, seafood accounts for only an estimated 27.3 g (0.96 oz) of protein per day. Increasing age was associated with increasing amounts of protein consumed; however, girls consistently consumed less protein from seafood per day compared with the age-matched boys. Total protein intake from seafood ranged from 4.3–8.3 g (0.15–0.29 oz)/day in males and 4.4–7.8 g (0.16–0.29 oz)/day in females, respectively. Only a small fraction of the seafood consumed was from fatty fish (or high–n-3 LCPUFA), and therefore protein intake from those fish was only 0.7–1.8 g (0.2–0.6 oz)/day in males and 0.8–1.8 g/day (0.3–0.6 oz)/day in females.

Although total protein intake increases with increasing income, protein intake from seafood was highest (8.5 g/day) in the highest-income group, followed by the lowest-income group (6.9 g/day) and lowest in the middle-income group (6.1 g/day). Data from the FFQ showed that of 13,177 records, 40.8 percent ($n = 5,372$) did not consume any seafood. Because the time frame of the FFQ did not necessarily include the days of 24-hour recall, the data still show that 1.4 g/day of protein intake was from seafood among children classified as "nonconsumers" based on their intake in the 30 days prior to completing the FFQ.

Data from NHANES 24-hour recalls (Table 4-5) show that only a small portion of daily protein intake among U.S. children is from seafood (6.7 g of 118.9 g/day); protein intake from seafood with high n-3 LCPUFA is extremely low with 1.3 g/day on average. Individuals at the 95th percentile consume 27.3 g/day of protein

TABLE 4-4 Estimated Usual Mean Intake and Percentiles for Protein Intake from Seafood and Other Sources, U.S. Women of Childbearing Age

		Source of Protein						Total Protein from Seafood (g/day)		
	N	Total Protein Foods (g/day)	Total Protein from Meat, Poultry, and Seafood (g/day)	Total Protein from Seafood (g/day)	Total Protein from Seafood Low n-3 (g/day)	Total Protein from Seafood High n-3 (g/day)[a]		5th Percentile	50th Percentile	95th Percentile
Overall	7,355	144.8	110.1	13.5	9.9	4.0		0.9	10.8	36.9
Race/Ethnicity										
Hispanic	1,927	146.9	114.2	14.6	11.1	3.7		1.2	12.5	36.8
Non-Hispanic Asian	911	147.2	110.2	24.8	15.9	9.5		2.7	23.2	54.5
Non-Hispanic Black	2,354	140.9	104.0	10.1	7.2	2.6		0.8	8.3	26.9
Non-Hispanic White	1,812	159.4	132.4	20.6	16.3	4.1		2.0	18.5	47.6
Other	351	134.5	98.9	14.2	10.4	3.8		1.2	12.3	35.3
Income (IPR)[b]										
Less than 1.3	2,736	138.8	110.8	13.1	10.1	3.0		0.9	10.0	37.3
1.3–4.99	3,604	146.8	111.1	13.4	9.9	3.4		0.9	10.8	36.5
≥5	1,015	148.1	106.5	14.3	9.6	4.4		1.1	11.7	37.4
Seafood Consumption in the Previous 30 Days from FFQ[c]										
None	1,878	120.9	92.1	2.3	1.9	0.5		0.5	2.9	6.1
Some	5,473	153.1	116.3	17.4	12.7	4.6		4.6	14.5	40.0

NOTES: Usual seafood consumption modeled using 24-hour recall data. FFQ = food frequency questionnaire; IPR = income-to-poverty ratio.
[a] Refers to grams per day. Cooked seafood containing 500 mg or more n-3 fatty acids (EPA and DHA) per 3 oz was assigned as seafood high in n-3 fatty acids.
[b] Income-to-poverty ratio.
[c] Seafood consumers and nonconsumers defined as any/no intake of seafood in the previous 30 days in the food frequency questionnaire.
SOURCE: NHANES 2011–2012 through 2017–March 2020.

from seafood, approximately 25 percent of the daily total protein intake. Children consumed more seafood with increasing age, and boys had higher protein intake from seafood compared with girls; nonetheless, the proportion of protein intake from seafood was less than 25 percent in all age groups. Non-Hispanic Asian children consumed more protein (4.3 g/day) from seafood high in n-3 LCPUFAs than all other children, followed by Hispanic (1.5 g/day) and "other" (1.5 g/day).

Using these data from NHANES 2011–2012 through 2017–March 2020, the committee was able to estimate for children ages 2–19 years a percentage of protein intake that came from seafood compared with other animal sources and total protein sources.

A technical report from the American Academy of Pediatrics (Bernstein et al., 2019) reviewed the benefits and potential risks associated with the consumption of fish and shellfish by children and concluded that, despite the nutritional benefits, children in the United States eat relatively small amounts of fish and shellfish compared with other protein sources. The authors noted that evidence-based expert guidance, such as the *DGA*, advises that seafood should have a larger place in the American diet.

Seafood Contribution to Nutrient Intake by Age and Sex Group

Figure 4-1 shows that among children ages 2–5 years old, boys consume a higher proportion of protein from seafood than girls, and the proportion of intake from seafood is higher in this age group (2.82 percent of total protein intake) than in children ages 6–11 and 12–19 (2.3 percent of total intake). In those two older age groups, girls consume a higher proportion of protein from seafood than boys.

Seafood Contribution to EPA and DHA Intake Among Women of Childbearing Age and Children and Adolescents

To understand the contribution of seafood to daily intake of EPA and DHA, the committee compared intake of these n-3 LCPUFAs for seafood consumers and seafood nonconsumers.

Tables 4-6, 4-7, 4-8, and 4-9 show the total daily intake of EPA and DHA from all sources among U.S. individuals by age and sex group. For women of childbearing age, total intake of n-3 LCPUFAs was low, at 57 mg/day, and seafood consumers had double the intake (64 mg/day) compared with nonconsumers of seafood (36 mg/day). Children and adolescents had even lower intakes of total n-3 LCPUFAs (33 mg/day), and seafood consumers had higher intakes (39 mg/day) than nonconsumers of seafood (26 mg/day).

Kranz (2015) studied EPA and DHA consumption from seafood using 24-hour recall data from NHANES 2003–2010 (primary analysis) and 30-day FFQ data from the same NHANES cycles (secondary analysis). These analyses found that fewer than 50 percent of U.S. children and adolescents ages 2–18 years reported any consumption of fish or shellfish; only 0.3 percent of the study population reported consumption of fish high in EPA and DHA. Furthermore, among fish consumers, an average of fewer than 25 percent achieved the recommended intake of EPA and DHA. Among the full surveyed population, the fish that contributed the highest amounts of dietary EPA and DHA (on average) were canned sardines, cooked salmon, and fried carp.

Kranz et al., (2017) also used National Diet and Nutrition Survey Rolling Program data from 2008 to 2012 to examine national fish consumption trends for UK children ages 2–5, 6–11, and 12–18 years. Among all participants, 55 percent reported consumption of fish during a 4-day period, but only 4.5 percent met the recommended intake levels for fatty fish. Logistic regression models found no associations of income or ethnic group with either total fish or fatty fish consumption in the UK population. Similarly, an analysis of dietary fish consumption among U.S. children ages 1–5 years found very low intake of fish and n-3 LCPUFAs (Maguire and Monsivais, 2015).

Table 4-6 presents average mean amounts of fat consumed by women of childbearing age stratified by percentile of the seafood intake amounts and by age group, race and ethnicity, income-to-poverty ratio, and seafood consumers versus nonconsumers. Overall fat intake was 68 g/day, 25 g/day saturated and 44 g/day unsaturated. Intake of n-3 LCPUFAs was 57 mg/day with 16 mg/day from EPA and 43 mg/day from DHA. Younger women tended to consume less total fat and subtypes of fat, including n-3 LCPUFAs, compared to women 25 years and older. Non-Hispanic Asian women consumed the lowest amount of saturated fat (21 g/day) but the highest amount

TABLE 4-5 Estimated Usual Mean Intake and Percentiles for Protein Intake from Seafood and Other Sources, U.S. Children, Ages 2–19 Years

		Source of Protein					Total Protein from Seafood (g/day)		
	N	Total Protein Foods (g/day)	Total Protein from Meat, Poultry, and Seafood (g/day)	Total Protein from Seafood (g/day)	Total Protein from Seafood Low in n-3 LCPUFA (g/day)	Total Protein from Seafood High in n-3 LCPUFA (g/day)[a]	5th Percentile	50th Percentile	95th Percentile
Overall	13,177	118.9	95.2	6.7	5.4	1.3	0.3	3.4	27.3
Males (years)									
2–5	1,567	101.4	76.0	4.3	3.6	0.7	0.2	2.1	15.7
6–11	2,344	127.0	101.1	6.6	5.6	1.1	0.3	3.4	23.4
12–19	2,739	148.6	123.1	8.3	6.5	1.8	0.4	4.3	29.3
Females (years)									
2–5	1,584	81.3	59.8	4.4	3.5	0.8	0.2	2.3	15.3
6–11	2,299	102.7	80.6	6.2	5.2	1.1	0.3	3.3	21.9
12–19	2,644	120.4	98.6	7.8	6.1	1.8	0.3	4.1	27.7
Race/Ethnicity									
Hispanic	3,912	117.2	94.7	7.9	6.4	1.5	0.4	4.2	27.7
Non-Hispanic Asian	1,196	115.7	93.0	13.4	9.3	4.3	0.8	9.5	39.8
Non-Hispanic Black	3,688	118.3	92.2	5.0	4.0	1.1	0.2	2.4	18.2
Non-Hispanic White	3,430	127.4	110.1	9.1	8.1	0.9	0.4	5.6	29.6
Other	951	114.0	89.7	6.1	4.4	1.5	0.3	3.3	21.2
Income (IPR)[b]									
Less than 1.3	5,690	117.3	97.1	6.9	5.7	1.2	0.3	3.3	25.1
1.3–4.99	6,195	119.6	94.9	6.1	4.9	1.2	0.2	3.0	22.1
5 or greater	1,292	120.6	91.9	8.5	6.5	2.1	0.4	5.0	28.8

Seafood Consumption in the Previous 30 Days from FFQ[c]

None	5,372	106.0	84.4	1.4	1.2	0.2	0.2	0.9	4.3
Some	7,799	128.4	103.0	10.6	8.4	2.2	1.5	7.5	30.0

NOTE: Usual seafood consumption modeled using 24-hour recall data.

[a] Refers to grams per day. Cooked seafood containing 500 mg or more n-3 fatty acids (EPA and DHA) per 3 oz was assigned as seafood high in n-3 fatty acids.
[b] Income-to-poverty ratio.
[c] Seafood consumers and nonconsumers defined as any/no intake of seafood in the previous 30 days in the food frequency questionnaire (FFQ).

SOURCE: NHANES 2011–2012 through March 2017–2020.

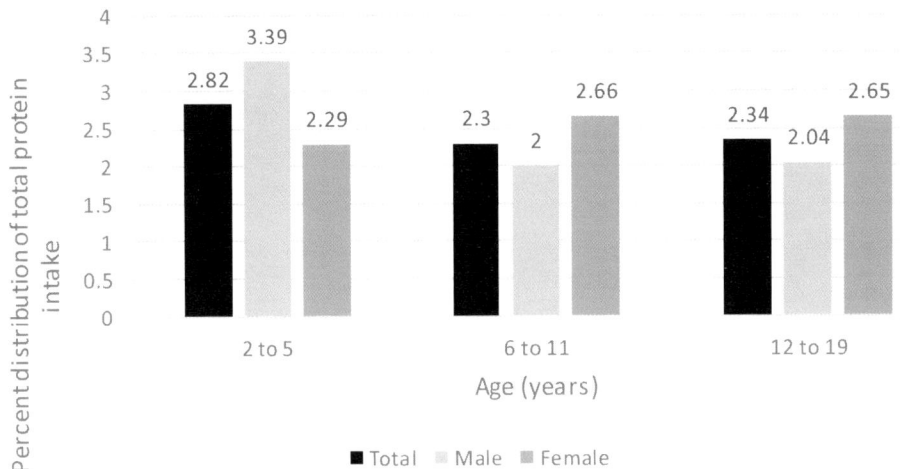

FIGURE 4-1 Total seafood as a distribution of total protein intake (percentage): children by age and sex, United States.
SOURCE: DGAC, 2020.

of n-3 LCPUFA (80 mg/day), EPA (22 mg/day), and DHA (72 mg/day). Increasing income was associated with increased amount of total fat, saturated fat, and unsaturated fat but intake of n-3 LCPUFAs and of DHA was slightly higher in the middle-income group than the lowest- and highest-income groups. Intakes of total fat, saturated fat, and unsaturated fat were similar between seafood consumers and nonconsumers, but intakes of n-3 LCPUFA, EPA, and DHA among seafood nonconsumers were 33 percent, 7 percent, and almost 50 percent lower, respectively, compared to intake among seafood consumers.

Table 4-7 shows mean daily consumption of fatty acids by children and adolescents (ages 2–19 years). On average, they consumed 67 g/day total fat, 26 g/day saturated fat, and 41.g/day unsaturated fat, and boys had higher intakes of total fat than girls in every age group. Only 33 mg/day were n-3 LCPUFAs, of which 11 mg/day were EPA and 22 mg/day were DHA. Seafood consumers at the highest percentile of intake consumed 71 mg/day. Thus, no subgroup of the population age 2–19 years met recommendations for combined intake of EPA/DHA (100–150 mg/day for 2- to 4-year-olds; 150–200 mg/day for 4- to 6-year-olds; 200–300 mg/day for ages 6–10 years; and 300 mg/day for all older children) (NHANES 2011–2020). Even individuals with the highest intakes of n-3 LCPUFAs achieved intakes around 50 percent of recommended levels. For males, increasing age was associated with higher EPA and DHA intake levels. For females intakes were higher in ages 6–19 years (11 mg/day EPA and 22 mg/day DHA) than ages 2–5 years (7 mg/day EPA and 17 mg/day DHA).

Total and saturated fat intake was highest in non-Hispanic Black and Other (unspecified race/ethnicity) children, but intakes of n-3 LCPUFAs were highest among non-Hispanic Asians. Non-Hispanic Asians consumed 45 mg/day, followed by non-Hispanic Whites (37 mg/day), Hispanics (36 mg/day), and non-Hispanic Blacks (30 mg/day). At the lowest percentiles of fat intake, little differences existed by racial/ethnic group in n-3 LCPUFA intake levels, whereas at the highest percentiles of fat intake, non-Hispanic Asian children had the highest n-3 LCPUFA intake (94 mg/day), followed by non-Hispanic White (77 mg/day) and Hispanic children (75 mg/day). Intakes of total fat, saturated fat, and unsaturated fat increased with increasing income, but n-3 LCPUFA intakes did not differ among income groups.

Table 4-8 presents population representative data from the Canadian Community Health Survey for seafood-consuming women of childbearing age and children ages 1–19 years in terms of intake of EPA, DHA, and EPA+DHA. Women of childbearing age (20–54 years old) had mean intakes of 298.7 mg/day of EPA, 515.7 mg/day of DHA, and 814.4 mg/day of EPA+DHA. Compared with pregnant women, lactating women had more than three-fold higher EPA, DHA, and EPA+DHA intake (358.1 vs. 95.7 mg/day EPA; 651.1 vs. 160.0 mg/day DHA; and 1,009.2 vs. 255.8 mg/day EPA+DHA.

TABLE 4-6 Estimated Usual Mean Intake and Percentiles of Fatty Acids by Women of Childbearing Age, by Age Group, Race/Ethnicity, Income, and Seafood Consumption Status

	N	Total Fat (g)	Total Saturated Fat (g)	Total Unsaturated Fat (g)	Total Long Chain n-3 Fatty Acid (mg)	EPA (mg)	DHA (mg)	5th Percentile	50th Percentile	95th Percentile
Overall	7,355	68.2	24.5	43.8	57	16	43	0.014	0.047	0.134
Age Group (years)										
16–25	2,465	66.4	24.3	42.1	50	16	36	0.013	0.041	0.118
25–40	2,918	70.2	25.1	45.3	61	17	46	0.016	0.050	0.143
41–50	1,972	67.1	23.8	43.3	59	16	46	0.015	0.049	0.136
Race/Ethnicity										
Hispanic	1,927	66.9	23.9	43.1	60	16	45	0.016	0.050	0.138
Non-Hispanic Asian	911	60.9	20.9	39.9	80	22	72	0.019	0.066	0.186
Non-Hispanic White	1,812	71.3	24.7	46.6	69	20	52	0.019	0.058	0.158
Non-Hispanic Black	2,354	68.8	25.1	43.8	51	15	37	0.013	0.042	0.117
Other	351	67.7	24.4	43.2	55	16	40	0.014	0.046	0.127
Income-to-Poverty Ratio										
Less than 1.3	2,724	65.6	23.7	41.8	54	16	41	0.013	0.044	0.129
1.3–4.99	3,613	68.8	24.7	44.1	59	16	45	0.015	0.049	0.139
≥5.0	1,018	70.6	25.1	45.7	56	17	41	0.015	0.046	0.128
Seafood Consumption Status										
Nonconsumer of seafood	1,878	67.8	24.5	43.3	36	11	24	0.010	0.030	0.082
Seafood consumer	5,473	68.4	24.5	43.9	64	18	49	0.019	0.054	0.145

NOTES: Seafood consumers and nonconsumers defined as any/no intake of seafood in the previous 30 days in the food frequency questionnaire (FFQ). Excludes intake of dietary supplements. Variables used to predict n-3, EPA, and DHA consumption included sex, age, race, income category; and seafood consumption in the FFQ; for other fatty acids FFQ consumption was not included in the model.
SOURCE: NHANES 2011–2012 through 2017–March 2020.

TABLE 4-7 Estimated Usual Mean Intake and Percentiles of Fatty Acids by Children and Adolescents, by Age Group, Race/Ethnicity, Income Status, and Seafood Consumption Status

	N	Total Fat (g)	Total Saturated Fat (g)	Total Unsaturated Fat (g)	Total Long-Chain n-3 Fatty Acid (mg)	EPA (mg)	DHA (mg)	5th Percentile	50th Percentile	95th Percentile
Overall	13,177	66.6	25.6	41.0	33	11	22	0.011	0.029	0.071
Males (years)										
2–5	1,567	58.2	23.0	35.3	28	9	19	0.010	0.024	0.058
6–11	2,344	74.0	28.9	45.2	37	13	24	0.013	0.032	0.077
12–19	2,739	75.9	28.7	47.0	39	14	25	0.013	0.034	0.081
Females (years)										
2–5	1,584	49.6	19.4	30.3	24	7	17	0.008	0.021	0.049
6–11	2,299	63.8	26.7	39.2	31	11	21	0.011	0.027	0.065
12–19	2,644	65.6	24.5	40.9	33	11	22	0.011	0.028	0.068
Race/Ethnicity										
Hispanic	3,912	63.8	24.4	39.3	36	11	24	0.012	0.031	0.075
Non-Hispanic Asian	1,196	61.2	23.5	37.6	45	14	35	0.015	0.039	0.094
Non-Hispanic White	3,430	66.2	24.1	42.0	37	13	24	0.012	0.032	0.077
Non-Hispanic Black	3,688	68.5	26.6	41.9	30	11	19	0.010	0.026	0.063
Other	951	67.5	26.3	41.1	32	12	21	0.011	0.027	0.068
Income-to-Poverty Ratio										
Less than 1.3	5,690	64.5	24.7	39.7	33	11	22	0.011	0.029	0.071
1.3–4.99	6,195	67.3	25.8	41.5	33	(11)	22	0.011	0.029	0.071
≥5	1,292	69.2	26.6	42.5	33	(12)	23	0.011	0.029	0.071
Seafood Intake Status										
Nonconsumer of seafood	5,372	66.6	25.6	41.0	26	(10)	15	0.009	0.023	0.053
Seafood consumer	7,799	66.6	25.4	41.1	39	(13)	27	0.014	0.034	0.079

NOTES: Seafood consumers and nonconsumers defined as any/no intake of seafood in the previous 30 days in the food frequency questionnaire (FFQ). Excludes intake of dietary supplements. Variables used to predict n-3, EPA, and DHA consumption included sex, age, race, income category, and seafood consumption in the FFQ; for other fatty acids, FFQ consumption was not included in the model.
SOURCE: NHANES 2011–2012 through 2017–March 2020.

TABLE 4-8 Daily EPA and DHA Intake by Age, Sex, and Pregnancy/Lactating Status for Seafood Consumers in Canada, 2015

	EPA			DHA		EPA+DHA	
	Weighted (%)	Mean (mg/day)	SE[c] (mg)	Mean (mg/day)	SE (mg/day)	Mean (mg/day)	SE (mg/day)
Male (years)[a]							
1–5	4.77	124.9	25.8	235.5	41.9	360.4	66.3
6–11	4.82	302.0	88.5	583.4	182.1	885.4	270.0
12–19	5.02	298.7	39.1	581.7	72.2	880.4	105.3
Female (years)[b]							
1–5	4.90	95.3	27.0	179.7	40.7	275.0	67.5
6–11	3.47	131.8	30.3	273.0	73.9	404.9	103.1
12–19	7.06	322.6	64.2	518.5	93.1	841.1	154.5
20–54	50.05	298.7	61.6	515.7	89.7	814.4	151.1
Pregnant	1.03	95.7	25.1	160.0	53.2	255.8	75.2
Lactating	1.62	358.1	108.2	651.1	195.6	1009.2	300.8

[a] 17.1% of the total surveyed male population are seafood consumers.
[b] 17.9% of the total surveyed male population are seafood consumers.
[c] SE = standard error.
SOURCE: Canadian Community Health Survey, 2015 (Statistics Canada, 2015).

Among children consuming seafood, boys ages 6–11 years consumed more EPA, DHA, and EPA+DHA than boys ages 1–5 or 12–19 years. Girls consumed less EPA, DHA, and EPA+DHA than boys at every age group; they consumed more fatty acids with increasing age.

Table 4-9 presents the same data as Table 4-8, but for nonconsumers of seafood. Women of childbearing age consumed an average 5.9 mg/day of EPA, 28.4 mg/day of DHA, and 34.3 mg/day of EPA+DHA. Pregnant women consumed approximately twice as much EPA, DHA, and EPA+DHA compared with lactating women. For both boys and girls, increasing age was associated with increasing EPA, DHA, and EPA+DHA intake. Overall, boys consumed more than girls, except girls ages 1–5 years consumed slightly more DHA than boys in that age group.

A comparison of seafood consumers and nonconsumers indicates that individuals of all ages and sex groups who were seafood consumers had much higher intakes of EPA, DHA, and EPA+DHA. For instance, 12–19-year-old boys who consumed seafood had 880.4 mg/day of EPA+DHA, whereas nonconsumer boys of the same age had only 48.1 mg/day, a 20-fold difference.

Seafood Contribution to Micronutrient Intake Among Women of Childbearing Age and Children and Adolescents

According to Table 4-10, women age 16–25 years consumed lower amounts of micronutrients compared to older women of childbearing age, except for vitamin B12, which was consumed in lowest amounts by women age 41–50 years. No large differences in average intakes of any of the micronutrients were observed by race or ethnicity. Increasing income was associated with increased intake for all micronutrients, except for vitamin D, which was the same in women from middle- and high-income households (3.9 µg/day compared to 3.7 µg/day in the low-income group). The RDA for vitamin D for adult and pregnant and lactating women is 15 µg/day. Only small differences were observed in intake of any micronutrient between seafood consumers and nonconsumers.

Table 4-11 shows average consumption of micronutrients among children age 2–19 years. Among boys, increasing age is associated with increased consumption of selenium, zinc, and magnesium. Boys age 6–11 years had the highest intake of iron (15.8 mg/day), folate (405.0 µg/day), vitamin B12 (5.4 µg/day), choline (5.4 µg/day),

TABLE 4-9 Daily EPA and DHA Intake by Age, Sex, and Pregnancy/Lactating Status for Nonconsumers of Fish in Canada, 2015

	Weighted (%)	EPA		DHA		EPA and DHA	
		Mean (mg/day)	SE[c] (mg/day)	Mean (mg/day)	SE (mg/day)	Mean (mg/day)	SE (mg/day)
Male (years)[a]							
1–5	5.69	4.7	0.3	18.7	1.3	23.5	1.5
6–11	7.31	5.9	0.4	23.1	1.7	29.1	2.0
12–19	10.18	10.2	1.1	37.9	5.5	48.1	6.6
Female (years)[b]							
1–5	6.00	4.0	0.4	18.8	1.5	22.8	1.7
6–11	6.85	5.6	0.4	19.8	1.5	25.4	1.8
12–19	8.57	7.6	0.6	25.1	1.5	32.7	1.8
20–54	46.46	5.9	0.2	28.4	1.3	34.3	1.5
Pregnant	1.18	11.8	3.5	51.5	15.7	63.3	19.0
Lactating	1.58	5.9	0.8	26.6	3.8	32.5	4.4

[a] 82.9% of the total surveyed male population are seafood consumers.
[b] 82.1% of the total surveyed male population are seafood consumers.
[c] SE = standard error.
SOURCE: Canadian Community Health Survey, 2015 (Statistics Canada, 2015).

potassium (2,367.5 mg/day), and calcium (1,157.3 mg/day). Older boys (12–19 years) consumed lower levels of these nutrients, and younger boys (2–5 years) had the lowest intake levels.

Similarly, among girls, intakes were also highest among ages 6–11 years for iron (13.3 mg/day), folate (350.8 µg/day), vitamin B12 (4.3 µg/day), choline (4.3 µg/day), potassium (2,037.3 mg/day), and calcium (981.6 mg/day). Older girls consumed lower levels of these nutrients, and younger girls had the lowest intakes.

Vitamin D intake decreased among both boys and in girls as age increased. No large differences existed in consumption of any of the nutrients by racial or ethnic group except calcium, which was the highest in non-Hispanic Black children (1,055.4 mg/day) and lowest in non-Hispanic White children (842.9 mg/day). Intakes of selenium and zinc increased with increasing household income level, and the highest intakes of magnesium, iron, folate, potassium, calcium, and vitamin D were found in the highest-income group. Only small differences were observed in nutrient intake of any micronutrient between seafood consumers and nonconsumers.

Summary of Evidence on Dietary Patterns and Seafood Consumption

Children and women of childbearing age consume very small amounts of seafood, which contributes less than 25 percent of their total protein intake. Different types of seafood vary greatly in nutrient density. For example, fatty fish such as salmon have much higher n-3 LCPUFA content, vitamin D, and calcium, while shrimp, salmon, and Alaskan pollock are high in choline. Compared with other types of seafood, Alaskan pollock has the highest content of magnesium. Overall, both women of childbearing age and children and adolescents have low intake of n-3 LCPUFAs from seafood, particularly EPA and DHA in all age groups. Non-Hispanic Asian women and children and adolescents have higher consumption compared to the other racial and ethnic groups. Household income was not associated with intake levels of EPA and DHA.

Both women of childbearing age and children and adolescents classified as seafood consumers were 40.8 and 25.6 percent, respectively, of the NHANES sample population. Seafood nonconsumers had much lower intakes of EPA and DHA. Total fat, saturated fat, and nutrient intakes either did not differ at all or only slightly differed between individuals classified as consumers, and nonconsumers.

TABLE 4-10 Estimated Usual Mean Intake of Micronutrients by Women of Childbearing Age by Age Group, Race/Ethnicity, Income Status, and Seafood Consumption Status

	N	Selenium (µg)	Zinc (mg)	Magnesium (mg)	Iron (mg)	Folate (µg)	B12 (µg)	Choline (mg)	Potassium (mg)	Calcium (mg)	Vitamin D (µg)
Overall	7,355	98.7	9.4	268.5	12.6	351.9	4.0	280.0	2,272.5	879.3	3.9
Age Group (years)											
16–25	2,465	94.7	8.9	240.6	12.1	338.2	4.0	252.7	2,056.0	855.0	3.7
25–40	2,918	102.4	9.8	282.0	13.0	362.4	4.1	294.7	2,371.3	904.9	4.0
41–50	1,972	97.4	9.4	278.5	12.4	350.9	3.9	287.0	2,355.0	867.1	3.9
Race/Ethnicity											
Hispanic	1,927	102.0	9.7	275.8	13.1	359.2	4.1	292.9	2,319.6	903.6	4.1
Non-Hispanic Asian	911	105.7	9.3	290.8	12.9	402.4	3.8	297.3	2,443.2	788.5	4.2
Non-Hispanic White	1,812	99.9	8.7	237.9	12.0	313.0	3.8	271.3	2,080.4	767.9	3.4
Non-Hispanic Black	2,354	96.5	9.5	271.6	12.5	354.1	4.1	276.6	2,291.3	910.2	3.9
Other	351	95.7	8.9	258.5	12.0	333.9	4.2	263.2	2,151.5	849.2	3.5
Income-to-Poverty Ratio											
Less than 1.3	2,724	96.5	9.0	246.2	12.3	335.7	3.9	267.0	2,136.8	847.1	3.7
1.3–4.99	3,613	99.2	9.4	268.6	12.5	351.3	4.0	284.4	2,274.1	880.6	3.9
≥ 5.0	1,018	100.3	10.0	301.2	13.2	376.9	4.2	286.9	2,464.0	936.9	3.9
Seafood Consumption Status											
Nonconsumer of seafood	1,878	97.9	9.4	264.1	12.5	350.2	4.0	275.8	2,240.8	881.4	3.8
Seafood consumer	5,473	98.9	9.4	270.0	12.6	352.5	4.0	281.4	2,283.5	878.6	3.9

NOTES: Seafood consumers and nonconsumers defined as any/no intake of seafood in the previous 30 days in the food frequency questionnaire. Excludes intake of dietary supplements.
SOURCE: NHANES 2011–2012 through 2017–March 2020.

TABLE 4-11 Estimated Usual Mean Intake of Micronutrients by U.S. Children and Adolescents, by Age Group, Race/Ethnicity, Income Status, and Seafood Consumption Status

	N	Selenium (μg)	Zinc (mg)	Magnesium (mg)	Iron (mg)	Folate (μg)	B12 (μg)	Choline (mg)	Potassium (mg)	Calcium (mg)	Vitamin D (μg)
Overall	13,177	95.8	9.8	236.0	13.7	356.0	4.6	4.6	2,144.6	1,009.6	5.3
Males (years)											
2–5	1,567	83.9	9.1	224.8	12.5	325.9	4.7	4.7	2,166.3	1,054.0	6.8
6–11	2,344	106.1	11.1	258.6	15.8	405.0	5.4	5.4	2,367.5	1,157.3	6.4
12–19	2,739	113.3	11.1	260.0	15.3	390.1	5.2	5.2	2,321.7	1,061.6	4.9
Females (years)											
2–5	1,584	68.7	7.4	195.5	10.4	280.5	3.7	3.7	1,855.9	893.0	5.6
6–11	2,299	87.9	9.1	225.2	13.3	350.8	4.3	4.3	2,037.3	981.6	5.2
12–19	2,644	94.2	9.2	225.6	12.9	337.4	4.1	4.1	1,994.9	896.7	4.0
Race/Ethnicity											
Hispanic	3,912	95.3	9.8	237.8	14.0	365.6	4.7	4.7	2,201.0	1,024.7	5.6
Non-Hispanic Asian	1,196	102.3	9.8	249.6	13.6	385.9	4.4	4.4	2,243.4	951.0	5.7
Non-Hispanic White	3,430	92.9	8.9	213.1	13.1	329.7	4.1	4.1	1,995.2	842.9	4.3
Non-Hispanic Black	3,688	96.4	10.0	240.9	13.8	357.5	4.8	4.7	2,157.5	1,055.4	5.4
Other	951	94.0	9.6	229.4	13.4	342.4	4.6	4.6	2,074.6	987.9	5.2
Income-to-Poverty Ratio											
Less than 1.3	5,690	94.7	9.6	224.8	13.7	351.7	4.7	4.7	2,098.5	977.2	5.3
1.3–4.99	6,195	95.4	9.7	236.5	13.6	353.4	4.6	4.6	2,135.9	1,004.4	5.1
≥ 5.0	1,292	99.8	10.1	257.8	14.1	374.5	4.7	4.7	2,278.7	1,101.2	5.6
Seafood Intake Status											
Nonconsumer of seafood	5,372	95.7	9.8	235.7	13.7	355.8	4.7	4.7	2,142.6	1,012.9	5.3
Seafood consumer	7,799	95.9	9.7	236.3	13.7	356.2	4.6	4.6	2,146.0	1,007.2	5.3

NOTES: Seafood consumers and nonconsumers defined as any/no intake of seafood in the previous 30 days in the food frequency questionnaire (FFQ). Excludes intake of dietary supplements.
SOURCE: NHANES 2011–2012 through 2017–March 2020.

FINDINGS AND CONCLUSION

Findings

Nutrient Composition of Seafood

1. Current evidence on the nutrient content of seafood indicates that seafood is a rich source of multiple nutrients, including vitamin D, calcium, potassium, and iron, which are identified as nutrients of public health concern by the *Dietary Guidelines for Americans* and play roles in supporting pregnancy and lactation as well as growth and development.
2. Seafood is an important source of n-3 LCPUFAs, which are key nutrients for the prenatal period, during lactation, and throughout childhood. Choline, iodine, and magnesium are additional nutrients that are provided by seafood and have important functions throughout childhood and adolescence.
3. Individuals who do not consume seafood likely have intakes of n-3 LCPUFAs below recommended amounts.

Dietary Patterns

1. Seafood is one component of healthful dietary patterns described in the *Dietary Guidelines for Americans*. The majority of the U.S. and Canadian population has lower-than-recommended intakes of n-3 LCPUFAs from seafood. Intakes are highest among high-income women and children, but income status, however, is not consistently associated with intake levels of other nutrients.
2. Among Native and Indigenous populations who are transitioning away from traditional diets, limiting seafood consumption increases the risk of not achieving optimal intake of a range of nutrients, including n-3 LCPUFAs. Low seafood consumption may also contribute to inadequate nutrient intakes among other at-risk populations who are low consumers, such as non-Hispanic Black and Hispanic Americans, and especially among those with lower incomes or experiencing food insecurity.

Conclusion

1. *Taken together, the committee concludes that nutrient intakes from seafood by women of childbearing age and children are low.*

RESEARCH GAPS

- Data are needed on levels of nutrient intake by seafood consumers who meet current seafood intake recommendations compared to nonconsumers and low consumers of seafood.
- Additional data are needed on the nutrient composition of types of seafood frequently consumed in different geographic regions in the United States and Canada.

REFERENCES

Ariño, A., J. Beltrán, A. Herrera, and P. Roncalés. 2013. Fish and seafood: Nutritional value. In *Encyclopedia of human nutrition,* 3rd ed. Pp. 254-261.

ARS (Agricultural Research Service). 2019. *FoodData Central.* http://fdc.nal.usda.gov (accessed February 27, 2024).

Auclair, O., and S. A. Burgos. 2021. Protein consumption in Canadian habitual diets: Usual intake, inadequacy, and the contribution of animal- and plant-based foods to nutrient intakes. *Applied Physiology, Nutrition, and Metabolism* 46(5):501-510.

Bell, J. G., R. J. Henderson, D. R. Tocher, and J. R. Sargent. 2004. Replacement of dietary fish oil with increasing levels of linseed oil: Modification of flesh fatty acid compositions in Atlantic salmon (*Salmo salar*) using a fish oil finishing diet. *Lipids* 39(3):223-232.

Benedik, E. 2022. Sources of vitamin D for humans. *International Journal for Vitamin and Nutrition Research* 92(2):118-125.

Bernstein, A. S., E. Oken, S. de Ferranti, Council on Environmental Health, and Committee on Nutrition. 2019. Fish, shellfish, and children's health: An assessment of benefits, risks, and sustainability. *Pediatrics* 143(6):e20190999.

Bland, J. M., C. C. Grimm, P. J. Bechtel, U. Deb, and M. M. Dey. 2021. Proximate composition and nutritional attributes of ready-to-cook catfish products. *Foods* 10(11):2716. https://doi.org/10.3390/foods10112716.

Brunborg, L. A., K. Julshamn, R. Nortvedt, and L. Frøyland. 2006. Nutritional composition of blubber and meat of hooded seal (*Cystophora cristata*) and harp seal (*Phagophilus groenlandicus*) from Greenland. *Food Chemistry* 96(4):524-531.

Chiuve, S., E. Giovannucci, S. Hankinson, S. H. Zeisel, L. W. Dougherty, W. C. Willett, and E. B. Rimm. 2007. The association between betaine and choline intakes and the plasma concentrations of homocysteine in women. *American Journal of Clinical Nutrition* 86:1073-1081.

Cisneros-Montemayor, A. M., D. Pauly, L. V. Weatherdon, and Y. Ota. 2016. A global estimate of seafood consumption by coastal Indigenous peoples. *PLoS One* 11(12):e0166681.

Corbin, K. D., and S. H. Zeisel. 2012. Choline metabolism provides novel insights into non-alcoholic fatty liver disease and its progression. *Current Opinion in Gastroenterology* 28(2):159.

Cortes-Albornoz, M. C., D. P. Garcia-Guaqueta, A. Velez-van-Meerbeke, and C. Talero-Gutierrez. 2021. Maternal nutrition and neurodevelopment: A scoping review. *Nutrients* 13(10).

Crawford, S. A., A. R. Brown, J. Teruel Camargo, E. H. Kerling, S. E. Carlson, B. J. Gajewski, D. K. Sullivan, and C. J. Valentine. 2023. Micronutrient gaps and supplement use in a diverse cohort of pregnant women. *Nutrients* 15(14).

de Escobar, G. M., M. J. Obregon, and F. E. del Rey. 2007. Iodine deficiency and brain development in the first half of pregnancy. *Public Health Nutrition* 10(12A):1554-1570.

DGAC (Dietary Guidelines Advisory Committee). 2015. Scientific Report of the 2015 Dietary Guidelines Advisory Committee: Advisory Report to the Secretary of Health and Human Services and the Secretary of Agriculture. U.S. Department of Agriculture, Agricultural Research Service, Washington, DC.

DGAC. 2020. Data Supplement for Food Category Sources: All Life Stages. 2020 Dietary Guidelines Advisory Committee Project. Washington, DC: U.S. Department of Agriculture and U.S. Department of Health and Human Services.

FAO (Food and Agriculture Organization of the United Nations). 2010. *Fats and fatty acids in human nutrition. Report of an expert consultation*. https://www.fao.org/documents/card/en?details=8c1967eb-69a8-5e62-9371-9c18214e6fce (accessed February 27, 2024).

Ford, J. E., and S. H. Hutner. 1955. Role of vitamin B12 in the metabolism of microorganisms. *Vitamins and Hormones* (13):101-136.

Frassetto, L. A., A. Goas, R. Gannon, S. A. Lanham-New, and H. Lambert. 2023. Potassium. *Advances in Nutrition* 14(5):1237-1240.

Gardner, C. D., J. C. Hartle, R. D. Garrett, L. C. Offringa, and A. S. Wasserman. 2019. Maximizing the intersection of human health and the health of the environment with regard to the amount and type of protein produced and consumed in the United States. *Nutrition Reviews* 77(4):197-215.

Griebel-Thompson, A. K., S. Sands, L. Chollet-Hinton, D. Christifano, D. K. Sullivan, H. Hull, J. T. Camargo, and S. E. Carlson. 2023. Iodine intake from diet and supplements and urinary iodine concentration in a cohort of pregnant women in the United States. *American Journal of Clinical Nutrition* 118(1):283-289.

Guo, M., and G. M. Hendricks. 2008. Chemistry and biological properties of human milk. *Current Nutrition and Food Science* 4(4):305-320.

Harding, K. B., J. P. Peña-Rosas, A. C. Webster, C. M. Yap, B. A. Payne, E. Ota, and L. M. De-Regil. 2017. Iodine supplementation for women during the preconception, pregnancy and postpartum period. *Cochrane Database of Systematic Reviews*(3). 3(3):CD011761.

Hatch-McChesney, A., and H. R. Lieberman. 2022. Iodine and iodine deficiency: A comprehensive review of a re-emerging issue. *Nutrients* 14(17).

Hofmeyr, G. J., A. P. Betrán, M. Singata-Madliki, G. Cormick, S. P. Munjanja, S. Fawcus, S. Mose, D. Hall, A. Ciganda, and A. H. Seuc. 2019. Prepregnancy and early pregnancy calcium supplementation among women at high risk of pre-eclampsia: A multicentre, double-blind, randomised, placebo-controlled trial. *Lancet* 393(10169):330-339.

Hurrell, R., and I. Egli. 2010. Iron bioavailability and dietary reference values. *American Journal of Clinical Nutrition* 91(5):1461S-1467S.

Idjradinata, P., and E. Pollitt. 1993. Reversal of developmental delays in iron-deficient anaemic infants treated with iron. *Lancet* 341(8836):1-4.

IOM. 1998. *Dietary Reference Intakes for thiamin, riboflavin, niacin, vitamin B6, folate, vitamin B12, pantothenic acid, biotin, and choline*. Washington, DC: National Academy Press.

IOM. 2000. *Dietary Reference Intakes for vitamin C, vitamin E, selenium, and carotenoids.* Washington, DC: National Academy Press.

IOM. 2001. *Dietary Reference Intakes for vitamin A, vitamin K, arsenic, boron, chromium, copper, iodine, iron, manganese, molybdenum, nickel, silicon, vanadium, and zinc.* Washington, DC: National Academy Press.

IOM. 2002/2005. *Dietary Reference Intakes for water, potassium, sodium, chloride, and sulfate.* Washington, DC: The National Academies Press.

IOM. 2011. *Dietary Reference Intakes for calcium and vitamin D.* Washington, DC: The National Academies Press.

Johnson-Wimbley, T. D., and D. Y. Graham. 2011. Diagnosis and management of iron deficiency anemia in the 21st century. *Therapeutic Advances in Gastroenterology* 4(3):177-184.

Jones, G. 2008. Pharmacokinetics of vitamin D toxicity. *American Journal of Clinical Nutrition* 88(2):582S-586S.

Keiver, K., K. Ronald, and H. Draper. 1988. Plasma levels of vitamin D and some metabolites in marine mammals. *Canadian Journal of Zoology* 66(6):1297-1300.

Kenny, D. E., T. O'Hara, T. C. Chen, Z. Lu, X. Tian, and M. F. Holick. 2004. Vitamin D content in Alaskan arctic zooplankton, fishes, and marine mammals. *Zoo Biology* 23(1):33-43.

Kenny, T. A., X. F. Hu, H. V. Kuhnlein, S. D. Wesche, and H. M. Chan. 2018. Dietary sources of energy and nutrients in the contemporary diet of Inuit adults: Results from the 2007-08 Inuit health survey. *Public Health Nutrition* 21(7):1319-1331.

Kohrle, J. 2015. Selenium and the thyroid. *Current Opinion in Endocrinology, Diabetes, and Obesity* 22(5):392-401.

Kondaiah, P., P. S. Yaduvanshi, P. A. Sharp, and R. Pullakhandam. 2019. Iron and zinc homeostasis and interactions: Does enteric zinc excretion cross-talk with intestinal iron absorption? *Nutrients* 11(8).

Kranz, S. 2015. Food sources of EPA and DHA in the diets of American children, NHANES 2003–2010. *BAOJ Nutrition* 1(1):1-12.

Kranz, S., N. R. V. Jones, and P. Monsivais. 2017. Intake levels of fish in the UK paediatric population. *Nutrients* 9(4).

Kuhnlein, H. V., V. Barthet, A. Farren, E. Falahi, D. Leggee, O. Receveur, and P. Berti. 2006. Vitamins A, D, and E in Canadian arctic traditional food and adult diets. *Journal of Food Composition and Analysis* 19(6-7):495-506.

Leung, C. W., and J. M. Tester. 2019. The association between food insecurity and diet quality varies by race/ethnicity: An analysis of National Health and Nutrition Examination Survey 2011–2014 results. *Journal of the Academy of Nutrition and Dietetics* 19(10):1676-1686.

Love, D. C., A. L. Thorne-Lyman, Z. Conrad, J. A. Gephart, F. Asche, D. Godo-Solo, A. McDowell, E. M. Nussbaumer, and M. W. Bloem. 2022. Affordability influences nutritional quality of seafood consumption among income and race/ethnicity groups in the United States. *American Journal of Clinical Nutrition* 116(2):415-425.

Lozoff, B. 2007. Iron deficiency and child development. *Food and Nutrition Bulletin* 28(4):0S560-S571.

Maguire, E. R., and P. Monsivais. 2015. Socio-economic dietary inequalities in UK adults: An updated picture of key food groups and nutrients from national surveillance data. *British Journal of Nutrition* 113(1):181-189.

Marushka, L., M. Batal, C. Tikhonov, T. Sadik, H. Schwartz, A. Ing, K. Fediuk, and H. M. Chan. 2021. Importance of fish for food and nutrition security among First Nations in Canada. *Canadian Journal of Public Health* 112(Suppl 1):64-80.

Middleton, P., J. C. Gomersall, J. F. Gould, E. Shepherd, S. F. Olsen, and M. Makrides. 2018. Omega-3 fatty acid addition during pregnancy. *Cochrane Database of Systematic Reviews* 11(11):CD003402.

NASEM (National Academies of Science, Engineering, and Medicine). 2019. *Dietary Reference Intakes for sodium and potassium.* Washington, DC: The National Academies Press. https://doi.org/10.17226/25353.

NFI (National Fisheries Institute). 2024. *Top 10 list for seafood consumption.* https://aboutseafood.com/about/top-ten-list-for-seafood-consumption/ (accessed April 16, 2024).

NIH (National Institutes of Health). 2022. *Calcium: Fact sheet for professionals.* https://ods.od.nih.gov/factsheets/Calcium-HealthProfessional/ (accessed October 31, 2023).

NIH. 2023. *Iron: Fact sheet for professionals.* https://ods.od.nih.gov/factsheets/Iron-HealthProfessional/ (accessed February 23, 2024).

Nokes, C., C. van den Bosch, and D. A. Bundy. 1998. *The effects of iron deficiency and anemia on mental and motor performance, educational achievement, and behavior in children: An annotated bibliography.* Washington, DC: International Nutritional Anemia Consultative Group.

Øyen J., E. Aadland, B. Liaset, E. Fjære, L. Dahl, and L. Madsen. 2021. Lean-seafood intake increases urinary iodine concentrations and plasma selenium levels: A randomized controlled trial with crossover design. *European Journal of Nutrition* 60:1679–1689. https://doi.org/10.1007/s00394-020-02366-2.

Rayman, M. P. 2020. Selenium intake, status, and health: A complex relationship. *Hormones (Athens)* 19(1):9-14.

Saini, R. K., and Y. S. Keum. 2018. Omega-3 and omega-6 polyunsaturated fatty acids: Dietary sources, metabolism, and significance - A review. *Life Sciences* 203:255-267.

Sharma, S., E. Mead, D. Simeon, G. Ferguson, and F. Kolahdooz. 2015. Dietary adequacy among rural Yup'ik women in western Alaska. *Journal of the American College of Nutrition* 34(1):65-72.

Slater, J., L. Larcombe, C. Green, C. Slivinski, M. Singer, L. Denechezhe, C. Whaley, P. Nickerson, and P. Orr. 2013. Dietary intake of vitamin D in a northern Canadian Dene First Nation community. *International Journal of Circumpolar Health* 72.

Smith, C., F. Teng, E. Branch, S. Chu, and K. S. Joseph. 2019. Maternal and perinatal morbidity and mortality associated with anemia in pregnancy. *Obstetrics and Gynecology* 134(6):1234-1244.

Sobiecki, J. G., P. N. Appleby, K. E. Bradbury, and T. J. Key. 2016. High compliance with dietary recommendations in a cohort of meat eaters, fish eaters, vegetarians, and vegans: Results from the European Prospective Investigation into Cancer and Nutrition-Oxford study. *Nutrition Research* 36(5):464-477.

Statistics Canada. 2015. Canadian Community Health Survey 2015. https://www23.statcan.gc.ca/imdb/p2SV.pl?Function=getSurvey&Id=238854 (accessed February 26, 2024).

Swanson, D., R. Block, and S. A. Mousa. 2012. Omega-3 fatty acids EPA and DHA: Health benefits throughout life. *Advances in Nutrition* 3(1):1-7.

Torti, S. V., D. H. Manz, B. T. Paul, N. Blanchette-Farra, and F. M. Torti. 2018. Iron and cancer. *Annual Review of Nutrition* 38:97-125.

USDA (U.S. Department of Agriculture). 1991. *Provisional table on the vitamin D content of foods.* Washington, DC: USDA.

U.S. Department of Agriculture, Agricultural Research Service. 2019. FoodData Central. fdc.nal.usda.gov (accessed October 20, 2023).

USDA. 2023a. USDA, FDA and ODS-NIH Database for the Iodine Content of Common Foods. https://www.ars.usda.gov/northeast-area/beltsville-md-bhnrc/beltsville-human-nutrition-research-center/methods-and-application-of-food-composition-laboratory/mafcl-site-pages/iodine/ (accessed March 1, 2024).

USDA. 2023b. *Why is it important to eat seafood and how often should I eat it?* https://ask.usda.gov/s/article/How-often-should-I-eat-seafood (accessed February 1, 2024).

USDA and HHS (U.S. Department of Health and Human Services). 2020. *Dietary Guidelines for Americans, 2020–2025,* 9th ed. http://www.dietaryguidelines.gov/ (accessed August 17, 2023).

Walter, T. 2003. Effect of iron-deficiency anemia on cognitive skills and neuromaturation in infancy and childhood. *Food and Nutrition Bulletin* 24(4 Suppl):S104-S110.

Yip, R. 2000. Significance of an abnormally low or high hemoglobin concentration during pregnancy: Special consideration of iron nutrition. *American Journal of Clinical Nutrition* 72(1 Suppl):272s-279s.

Zeisel, S. H. 2006. Choline: Critical role during fetal development and dietary requirements in adults. *Annual Review of Nutrition* 26:229-250.

Zeisel, S. H., and K. A. da Costa. 2009. Choline: An essential nutrient for public health. *Nutrition Review* 67(11):615-623.

Zeisel, S. H., K.-A. Da Costa, P. D. Franklin, E. A. Alexander, J. T. Lamont, N. F. Sheard, and A. Beiser. 1991. Choline, an essential nutrient for humans. *FASEB Journal* 5(7):2093-2098.

5

Exposure to Contaminants Associated with Consumption of Seafood

This chapter discusses the committee's review and assessment of evidence on exposure to toxins and toxicants of concern in seafood, sources of contaminants in seafood, and biomarkers of exposure, including evidence published after the report *Seafood Choices: Balancing Benefits and Risks* (IOM, 2007). The chapter reviews all contaminants for which seafood consumption may be an important route of either chronic exposures or acute (episodic) exposures, although the latter were not reviewed in detail owing to being acute in nature. This chapter also provides further information about the extent to which seafood is likely to be a primary route of exposure, compared with other foods or nondietary exposure routes.

It was not within the scope of the committee's work to review contaminants associated with consumption of other animal sources of protein or other foods beyond seafood. The committee recognizes, however, that multiple dietary and nondietary exposures exist for many of the contaminants reviewed.

TOXINS AND TOXICANTS OF CONCERN IN SEAFOOD

As noted in Chapter 4, the *Dietary Guidelines for Americans 2020–2025* includes recommendations for including seafood in a healthful dietary pattern. Some seafood may contain contaminants or microorganisms that could pose a health risk, particularly to pregnant and lactating women and children. The following sections discuss evidence on contaminants of concern, including variant isoforms identified by the committee as potentially relevant to its task.

Estimates of exposure to contaminants of concern through consumption of seafood depend principally on two factors: the amount of the seafood consumed (discussed in Chapter 3), and the amount of the contaminant in seafood. Using the reported consumption rate from national surveys such as the National Health and Nutrition Examination Survey (NHANES) and the Canadian Community Health Survey (CCHS), along with data on evaluation of exposure or risk assessment reported in the literature, it is possible to estimate quantitatively the exposure to different contaminants from seafood consumption among women of childbearing age and children and adolescents. The concentrations of contaminants in seafood depend on many factors, including species, age, region of origin, preparation method, and parts of the species consumed. These factors are discussed in this chapter as they relate to different classes of contaminants, but it is beyond the committee's task to perform quantitative exposure estimates of how concentrations of contaminants could change based on variations in such factors.

CONTAMINANTS RESULTING IN CHRONIC EXPOSURES

Metals, Metalloids, and Other Elements

Both essential and non-essential elements "are found naturally in the Earth's crust, and their compositions vary among different localities, resulting in spatial variations of surrounding concentrations. Metals are substances with high electrical conductivity, malleability, and luster, which voluntarily lose their electrons to form cations" (Jaishankar et al., 2014, p. 60). A metalloid is a chemical element with a predominance of properties that are a mixture of those found in metals and nonmetals. Typical metalloids are metallic in appearance but are brittle and are only fair conductors of electricity that behave chemically mostly as nonmetals (Vernon, 2013). The metals, metalloids, and other trace elements of human health concern that are discussed in this chapter are mercury, cadmium, lead, arsenic, and selenium.

Mercury

Mercury (Hg) is generated as a gaseous element that is released into the atmosphere from natural (volcanic) and anthropogenic (fossil fuel combustion) sources and deposited onto land or water (Driscoll et al., 2013).

Ocean fish and marine mammals are major sources of dietary intakes of mercury. The potential for human exposure from seafood is related to the magnitude of regional and global emissions and deposition but also the ability of watersheds and oceans to convert Hg to methylmercury (MeHg) and biomagnify up the food chain. In general, fish that are higher on their respective food chains (e.g., marlin, sea bass, shark, orange roughy, swordfish, some tuna), tend to have higher total Hg levels.

Hg accumulates in the muscle of fish and is assumed to exist primarily as MeHg as an earlier study reported that, on average, 95 percent of the Hg detected in muscle tissue from 12 fish species was MeHg (Hight and Cheng, 2006). In contrast, only an estimated 45 percent of shellfish Hg is in the form of MeHg (FDA, 2014).The percentage of MeHg in seafood can vary by species and size of the organism (Lescord et al., 2018); for instance, the percentage can be lower in smaller and younger fish, as well as freshwater fish, accounting for approximately 60–80 percent of total Hg (Lescord et al., 2018). Therefore, using total Hg concentrations to estimate MeHg concentrations would likely result in an overestimation of exposure. In addition, the analytical methods for detecting total Hg are simpler and less expensive than for MeHg. Therefore, it is common to use total Hg concentrations as a proxy for MeHg concentrations in fish muscle tissues. Most Hg databases for fish and shellfish report only total Hg; therefore, total Hg is often used as a proxy for MeHg. Because industrial processing of fish and domestic cooking generally do not alter Hg concentrations (Goyer and Clarkson, 2001), the total concentration in raw fish serves as a reasonable approximation of that in prepared fish (Health Canada, 2007).

Although not covered in this report, consumption of marine mammals is also a source of exposure to MeHg, particularly in regions with high consumers such as populations living in western and eastern Canadian Arctic regions (Dietz et al., 2021). Hg concentrations have been detected in numerous marine mammals from these areas, including beluga whales, narwhal, white-toothed dolphins, pilot whales, walruses, harp seals, and ringed seals (Wagemann et al., 1995).

Karimi et al. (2012) created a seafood database of Hg data from federal and state governmental reports as well as the peer-reviewed scientific literature. The database focused on fish and shellfish from sources marketed in the United States, but it is not an exact model of the composition of the seafood market. Furthermore, although Hg is primarily associated with muscle tissue, the data compiled include fillets as well as whole fish. In the analysis, MeHg was used where available instead of total Hg. Overall, the levels of Hg detected varied widely across individual seafood samples, and the amount of variability differed by species. Hg concentrations were generally higher in wild-caught than farmed fish owing to differences among species and other factors.

Hg levels were understudied in farmed seafood and in some major imported fisheries as well as Asia and South America. The mean Hg values in the database tended to be greater than the values reflected in the U.S. Food and Drug Administration (FDA) Hg Monitoring Program data (FDA, 2011; Karimi et al., 2012).

Data on Hg concentrations in popular fish sold in Canada are reported by the Canadian Food Inspection Agency. It found most fish species (e.g., oyster, clams, scallops, mussels, shrimp, salmon, cod, flounder, trout, herring, lobster, crab, lake whitefish) to contain total average Hg levels less than 0.2 parts per million (ppm) (Health Canada, 2007).

FDA reported results from its Total Diet Study (TDS) from 2018 to 2020 for a range of contaminants including Hg (FDA, 2022a). Total Hg concentrations in the collected samples were below 1 ppm, the FDA action level for MeHg in fish, shellfish, crustaceans, and other aquatic animals. The five fish with the highest Hg concentrations were canned tuna (0.230 ppm),[1] baked cod (0.084 ppm), baked salmon (0.021 ppm), pan-cooked catfish, and precooked shrimp.

As discussed in Chapter 3, the most frequently consumed seafood species among women of childbearing age and children and adolescents in the United States are shrimp, tuna, salmon, other fish, crab, breaded fish, catfish, cod, scallops, lobster, and clam (Table 3-4 and Table 3-7). All of those have relatively low Hg concentrations and are classified by FDA in the good choice category (less than 0.23 μg/g [ppm]) or the best choice category (0.15 μg/g [ppm]). Thus, consumers can eat up to two servings of fish per week from the good choice category, or three servings per week from the best choice category without exceeding the reference dose.

Tuna is the only exception in that average Hg concentrations range from 0.13 μg/g [ppm] for canned light tuna to 0.35 μg/g [ppm] for yellowfin tuna and canned white tuna, to 0.36 μg/g [ppm] for fresh or frozen albacore tuna, and to 0.69 μg/g [ppm] for bigeye tuna. Bigeye tuna is in the avoid category (higher than 0.46 μg/g [ppm]) or not recommended to be consumed by women of childbearing age and children. Other fish are in the good choice category (less than 0.46 μg/g [ppm]) and can be consumed once per week (FDA, 2022b). As discussed in Chapter 3, only 19 percent of women of childbearing age (Table 3-6) and 6.4 percent of children (Table 3-12) consume more than two meals of fish per week. Therefore, these groups are estimated to have a low risk from Hg exposure through consumption of fish. Groups that frequently consume tuna make up the primary at-risk group.

In Canada, the most frequently consumed species among women of childbearing age and children are clam, cod, crab, haddock, lobster, salmon, shrimp, tilapia, trout, and tuna (Table 3-14). All of these species except tuna had relatively low Hg concentrations of less than 0.2 μg/g [ppm] according to the Canadian Food Inspection Agency and reported by Health Canada (2007). The concentrations of Hg in tuna ranged from 0.14 μg/g [ppm] in canned light tuna and 0.26 μg/g [ppm] in canned albacore (white) tuna to 0.65 μg/g [ppm] in bigeye tuna, and 1.27 μg/g [ppm] in fresh/frozen tuna.

As discussed in Chapter 3, the average fish consumption rates for women of childbearing age and children and adolescents in Canada are low. The daily consumption rate ranged from 0.08 g of clam per day for children to 5 g of salmon per day for women of childbearing age (Table 3-14). Therefore, like in the United States, most consumers will not be at risk from Hg exposure through the consumption of fish although frequent tuna consumers are at increased risk.

Health Canada advises women who are or may become pregnant and breastfeeding mothers to consume up to 150 g of frozen tuna per month (Health Canada, 2019a). Young children between age 5 and 11 years can consume up to 125 g per month. Younger children (between age 1 and 4 years) are advised to consume no more than 75 g per month. Health Canada issued separate advice for canned albacore (white) tuna and light (e.g., skipjack or yellowfin) tuna. Breastfeeding women and those who are or may become pregnant may consume up to 300 g per week of albacore tuna, the equivalent to about two 170-g cans of albacore tuna per week. Children between age 5 and 11 years may consume up to 150 g (about one 170-g can per week), and younger children age 1–4 years may consume up to 75 g (about half of a 170-g can per week). This advice does not extend to non-albacore, canned tuna, as those species contain significantly less mercury (Health Canada, 2019b).

It is important to note that the above-mentioned hazard identification for Hg exposure applies only to the general population. Sex, age, and proximity to coastal regions influences seafood consumption. Ethnicity is also an important factor in consumption rates, with Asians, Native Americans, Pacific and Caribbean Islanders, and mixed races having the highest consumption rates of fish and shellfish (Mahaffey et al., 2004).

As discussed in Chapters 3 and 4, certain populations such as Native American tribes and Indigenous peoples, as well as subsistence and sport fishers and their families, can consume different fish species or fish parts, or

---

[1] The FDA Total Diet Study Food/Analyte Matrix identifies tuna as canned in water or canned in oil.

consume species from locations with potentially higher Hg. In a national study, Chan et al. (2021) found that 1.9 percent of First Nations women of childbearing age, mostly living in northern Ontario and northern Quebec, who consumed large predatory fish had Hg intake levels exceeding the reference dose.

Hg concentrations in fish are not static and can vary over time. For example, trend data for North American freshwater species collected and analyzed by Grieb et al. (2020) identified an overall trend for decreasing Hg concentrations in fish tissue sampled from North American lakes between 1972 and 2016. This trend is consistent with reported Hg emission declines and soil and water deposition trends across the United States and Canada. More recently, a plateau in the rate of change in Hg concentrations in fish tissue has been reported, possibly caused by increased emissions from global sources between 1990 and 1995.

Schartup et al. (2019) collected data for more than 30 years in ecosystem modeling of MeHg concentrations in Atlantic cod. The model estimated a 23 percent increase in MeHg concentrations detected in Atlantic cod, and a 56 percent increase in Atlantic bluefin tuna, in part attributable to increases in seawater temperatures since 1969. This increase in MeHg concentrations in fish tissue is a trend in the opposite direction of the 22 percent reduction that was modeled in the 1990s. Taken together with the plateau that was reported in 2020 for global Hg emissions, these data suggest that ocean warming may become a driver of MeHg concentrations in fish species at the high end of the food chain.

The pattern of Hg exposure can change over time because of changes in the pattern of fish consumption. For example, Sunderland et al. (2018) found that shifts in the edible seafood supply between 2000–2002 and 2010–2012 affected MeHg exposure. These shifts resulted in changes in consumer preference (e.g., away from canned light tuna), global ecosystem shifts (e.g., northern migration of cod stocks), and an increase in the supply of fish from aquaculture (e.g., shrimp and salmon). The data showed that 37 percent of the U.S. population-wide exposure to MeHg in this time frame was primarily from domestic coastal systems: 45 percent was from open ocean ecosystems and 38 percent was from fresh and canned tuna. The Pacific Ocean is estimated to supply more than half the total MeHg exposure. In the United States, aquaculture and freshwater fisheries account for an estimated 18 percent of the total MeHg intake (Sunderland et al., 2018).

Cadmium

Cadmium (Cd) is naturally found in soil, water, and air; activities such as mining, smelting, and fuel combustion can increase human exposure through food chain biomagnifications processes.

While generally low in finfish muscle, shellfish such as oysters and scallops have higher Cd concentrations, ranging from 1 to 4 µg/g in the Pacific Northwest (Bendell, 2010; Pacific Shellfish Institute, 2008). Additionally, Cd can bioaccumulate in the hepatopancreas of crustaceans, including crab and lobster, owing to this organ's detoxifying function (Chavez-Crooker et al., 2003; Lordan and Zabetakis, 2022). Therefore, heavy consumers of oysters, scallops, and the hepatopancreas may have higher risk of Cd exposure.

Using the data from FDA's Total Diet Study (TDS, 2014–2016) and food consumption data from What We Eat In America (WWEIA)—the food survey portion of the NHANES—Spungen (2019) estimated that mean Cd exposures for children (age 1–6 years) ranged from 0.38 to 0.44 µg/kg body weight per day, with primary contributions from grains, mixtures (e.g., hamburgers, pizza, soups), and vegetables. The combined daily intake of meat, poultry, and seafood (66 g/day) contributed to 0.25 µg/day of Cd exposure or 3.8 percent of the total cadmium intake of 6.6 µg/day. These estimates are limited because Cd concentrations were only measured in 268 TDS foods compared to the approximately 8,000 foods reported to be consumed by WWEIA/NHANES respondents.

Lead

Pb is ubiquitous in aquatic environments, and it is one of the most accumulative toxic metals owing to its ability to easily bind oxygen and sulfur atoms in proteins to form a stable complex, leading to accumulation in fish tissues (Lee et al., 2019). The Pb concentrations in fish in the United States vary depending on the species, region of origin, and environmental factors (Frank et al., 2019). Fish usually have higher Pb levels than shellfish.

Using data from FDA's TDS (2014–2016) and food consumption data from WWEIA, Spungen (2019) estimated the mean Pb exposures for children (age 1–6 years) ranged from 1.0 to 3.4 µg/day, with major contributions from fruit, grains, dairy, and mixtures (e.g., hamburgers, pizza, soups). The combined daily intake of meat, poultry, and seafood (66 g/day) was estimated to contribute 0.03 µg/day of lead exposure or 3 percent of the total Pb intake of 1.2 µg/day.

Gavelek et al. (2020) used the same approach and estimated the mean Pb exposure to range from 1.4 to 4.0 µg/day for older children (age 7–17 years), from 1.6 to 4.6 µg/day for women of childbearing age (16–49 years), and from 1.7 to 5.3 µg/day for adults (age 18 years and older). The estimated 90th percentile for lead exposures ranged from 2.3 to 5.8 µg/day for older children, 2.8 to 6.7 µg/day for women of childbearing age, and 3.2 to 7.8 µg/day for adults. Meat, poultry, and fish together contributed to only about 3 percent of the Pb intake. These results suggest that Pb exposure from fish consumption is lower than the interim reference level of 3 µg/day.

Arsenic

Arsenic (As) is a metalloid element globally present in both natural and anthropogenic sources, including commercial uses. Seafood and seaweed are primary dietary sources of total As and are present in marine-derived foods. Seafood consumption is estimated to account for 90 percent of total As exposure in the United States (Borak and Hosgood, 2007).

As is present in seafood primarily in the form of organic compounds. Two exceptions are freshwater fish from Thailand (Jankong et al., 2007), and blue mussel from Norway (Sloth et al., 2016), which are not known to contain As although the element may be found in other types. Arsenobetaine is the major As compound in most fish. It is generally nontoxic and not metabolized. Other organic As compounds include arsenosugars and arsenolipids, which are also present at significant quantities in some types of seafood and are metabolized in humans. Whereas taxonomic group affects the proportion of inorganic As in seafood, elevated levels have been found in bivalves and gastropods (Taylor et al., 2017). These group effects have also been the source of consumption guidelines in the Pacific United States (OHA, 2015).

Luvonga et al. (2020) analyzed total As and As compounds that are commonly consumed in aquatic species to better understand As speciation. The fish and shellfish samples collected were geoduck clam (*Panopea generosa*) from Alaska, wild-caught brown shrimp (*Farfantepenaeus aztecus*) from South Carolina, aquacultured white leg shrimp (*Litopenaeus vannamei*) from Alabama, and wild-caught and aquacultured coho salmon from Alaska and Washington state, respectively. The overall study results identified kelp, wild-caught shrimp, and geoduck clam as the species with the highest total As content.

In a review by Taylor et al. (2017) the presence and distribution of organic As compounds was evaluated in seafood and in combination with human consumption data. They reported that arsenosugars are associated largely with marine algae. The algae accumulate As from seawater and store it as arsenosugars, usually at high concentrations. Mollusks and crustaceans that are predominantly filter feeders are the marine species that contain arsenosugars, although at lower concentrations than algae. Arsenobetaine was reported as the major source in finfish and shellfish.

A paucity of information exists on the distribution of arsenolipids in seafood; however, levels of 50–62 percent have been found in fatty fish, with the higher concentrations in pelagic fish (Lischka et al., 2013). Methylated As compounds in seafood occur from the enzymatic methylation of inorganic As, such as arsenosugars. These compounds generally occur at low levels in seafood, with dimethylarsinate (DMA) the most prominent. Mollusks can contain from 3 to 46 percent of DMA, which is more than usually measured in finfish or algae (Taylor et al., 2017).

Selenium

As discussed in Chapter 4, selenium (Se) is an essential nutrient that functions through selenoproteins, several of which are oxidant defense enzymes. Se can be taken up through various dietary sources, but in quantities greater than the Tolerable Upper Intake Level (UL), potential for toxicity exists (see Chapter 4). Typical total Se concentrations in marine fish species from various origins range from about 0.1 mg Se per kg wet mass to almost

1 mg Se per kg wet mass (Cabañero et al., 2005; Murphy and Cashman, 2001; Navarro-Alarcon et al., 2008; Olmedo et al., 2013). Naturally occurring selenoneine (SeN) occurs in abundance in several marine fish species.

Species of fish that are sources of selenoamino acids and SeN include tuna, swordfish, and deep-sea greeneye (Cabañero et al., 2005; Yamashita et al., 2011). Kroepfl et al. (2015) reported that a methylated form of Se, Se-methylselenoneine, has been reported in human blood and urine where it was thought to result from methylation of SeN ingested from fish and was also found in muscle tissue of mackerel, sardine, and tuna. Kroepfl et al. (2015) also identified a selenosugar (selenosugar 1, methyl-2-acetamido-2-deoxy-1-seleno-β-D-galactopyranoside) in marine fish.

The characterization of Se compounds in fish and how they are stored and metabolized is important for understanding the dose–response from fish consumption. For example, SeN, found in tuna and marine mammals, is a powerful antioxidant (Achouba et al., 2016). SeN may protect against MeHg toxicity by increasing its demethylation in red blood cells and in turn decreasing its distribution to target organs. Moreover, Drobyshev et al. (2021) demonstrated that SeN can cross the blood–brain barrier and may reach brain tissue in humans, potentially making it more significant in protecting against MeHg toxicity.

Persistent Organic Pollutants

Persistent organic pollutants (POPs) are a class of synthetic carbon-based chemicals that are characterized by their persistence in the environment owing to their resistance to degradation. They are semi-volatile and accordingly, move long distances and are ubiquitous throughout the environment. POPs are lipophilic substances that sequester in fatty tissue, allowing them to bioaccumulate and biomagnify through the food chain (WHO, 2010). Therefore, organisms at the top of the food chain, including some pelagic fish and humans, have the highest concentrations of these chemicals (EPA, 2023a). POPs traditionally included polychlorinated biphenyls (PCBs), polybrominated diphenyl ethers (PBDEs), and some pesticides (e.g., dichlorodiphenyltrichloroethane [DDT]). However, in 2023, per- and poly(fluoroalkyl) substances (PFAS, e.g., perfluorooctane sulfonic acid [PFOS] and perfluorooctanoic acid [PFOA]) were included as POPs by the Stockholm Convention,[2] the global treaty targeting POPs. Additionally, perfluorinated compounds share many of the same chemical properties, including their persistence and propensity to bioaccumulate.

Polychlorinated Biphenyls

PCBs consist of 209 congeners, which are composed of two linked benzene rings with between 1 and 10 chlorine substitutions, which dictates their chemical structure and properties (von Stackelberg, 2011). Because of their stability and insulating properties, PCBs were used in a variety of industrial applications until the late 1970s when they were regulated and restricted by the Toxic Substances Control Act (updated in 2016) and the U.S. Environment Protection Agency (EPA) rulemaking.[3] However, because of their environmental persistence, PCB contamination is still widespread. Whether released in water from industrial waste or leaching into water from landfills, PCBs sequester in sediment owing to their lipophilicity. PCBs bioaccumulate in aquatic food chains and biomagnify (i.e., the increase in concentration of a substance) in predators that consume contaminated prey (Petersen and Kristensen, 1998).

In humans, the rate of individual[4] congener metabolism depends on the number and position of chlorine atoms. For example, a study of initial body burden, low serum levels, ongoing environmental exposure, and congeners with very long half-lives found that for congeners Aroclor 1242 and Aroclor 1254, the estimated half-lives during a period of high internal dose were 1.74 years and 6.01 years, respectively. During a period of low internal dose,

---

[2] Available at https://www.pops.int/TheConvention/ThePOPs/TheNewPOPs/tabid/2511/Default.aspx (accessed February 27, 2024).

[3] Public Law 114-182, June 22, 2016. Available at https://www.congress.gov/114/plaws/publ182/PLAW-114publ182.pdf (accessed February 27, 2024).

[4] Bioaccumulation occurs when chemicals become concentrated at levels that are higher in an organism than in open water. Biomagnification occurs when the chemicals become concentrated at higher levels in an organism than in the food chain. See https://www.epa.gov/sites/default/files/documents/bioaccumulationbiomagnificationeffects.pdf (accessed February 27, 2024).

the half-lives for Aroclor 1242 and Aroclor 1254 were estimated to be 21.83 years and 133.33 years, respectively (Hopf et al., 2013).

While occupational exposure routes include inhalation and dermal exposure, the majority of nonoccupational exposure to PCBs comes from dietary sources. A targeted literature review of PCB concentrations in environmental media examined the relative contribution of PCB exposure from different exposure pathways based on studies published since 2007 (Weitekamp et al., 2021). Analysis of data from the studies reviewed indicated that for adults, dietary intake accounted for 88 percent of exposure across the population (ranging from 1.8 to 3.6 ng/kg/day).

Among populations who consume large amounts of fish, particularly from the North American Great Lakes region, PCB exposure from fish may be more substantial (EPA, 2023b). This region supports one of the world's largest freshwater fisheries, which supplies fish to more than 4 million adults (and their children) in the United States and approximately 1 million adults in Canada, including Native American populations who rely on fish as a primary food source (Gandhi et al., 2017). Currently, concern about PCB exposure accounts for the majority of fish consumption advisories for the Great Lakes (Gandhi et al., 2017). Governmental agencies typically monitor contaminants in fatty fish (e.g., lake trout, lake whitefish, rainbow trout, and chinook salmon) and bottom feeders (e.g., brown bullhead, white sucker, and common carp), as these are the fish that are most likely to accumulate these hydrophobic chemicals (Gandhi et al., 2017). While concentrations of PCBs have been declining over time (Gandhi et al., 2017), for those who consume substantial quantities of fish from the Great Lakes, PCB exposure may still be an important concern (EPA, 2023b).

The National Study of Chemical Residues in Lake Fish Tissue (EPA, 2009), a national freshwater fish contamination survey, estimated the national distribution of selected persistent, bioaccumulative, and toxic chemical residues in fish tissue from 500 lakes and reservoirs in the contiguous 48 states. This 4-year study provided the first national estimates of median concentrations for 268 chemicals in lake fish, defined a baseline for national fish contamination to track progress of pollution control activities, and identified areas where further investigation of contaminants is warranted.

Specifically, 486 predator (fillet) and 395 bottom-dweller (whole-body) samples were collected and analyzed for chemicals including Hg, 17 dioxins and furans, five forms of As, 159 PCB congeners, 46 pesticides, and 40 semi-volatile organic compounds. Overall, the analysis showed that mercury, PCBs, and dioxins and furans are widely distributed in lakes and reservoirs in the contiguous 48 states. However, 43 of the 268 selected chemicals were not detected in any samples, including all nine organophosphate pesticides, 1 PCB congener, and 16 of the 17 polycyclic aromatic hydrocarbons analyzed as semi-volatile chemicals. Forty-eight percent of the sampled lakes had predator Hg tissue concentrations above the 0.3 ppm human health screening value (SV), and 16.8 percent had total PCB concentrations above the 12 parts per billion (ppb) SV. More than 7 percent of the sampled lakes had dioxin and furan concentrations greater than the 0.15 parts per trillion (ppt) SV, 1.7 percent had DDT concentrations over 69 ppb SV, and 0.3 percent had chlordane concentrations greater than 67 ppb SV.

Polybrominated Diphenyl Ethers

Polybrominated diphenyl ethers (PBDEs) are also a family of 209 congeners, which were primarily used as flame retardants in a variety of consumer products, including furniture, electronics, and clothing. PBDEs were phased out of use from 2004 through 2013, largely owing to their persistence and neurotoxicity (Washington State Department of Health, 2024a). Many consumer products that contain PBDE are still in use, however, and when these products are discarded, PBDE may leach from landfills into the watershed and bioaccumulate in the food chain (similar to PCBs). Therefore, it is plausible that as more of these PBDE-containing products are discarded, food, including fish, will become an increasingly important source of exposure (Schecter et al., 2010a). For example, in a recent report of seafood obtained from Puget Sound (Washington State) including both locally captured and nonlocal sources, a variety of finfish as well as bivalves contained the highest levels of PBDE and their metabolites. Finfish including English sole, sablefish, and trout, and shellfish including calamari and shrimp had the highest levels of parent PBDE while bivalves had higher levels of metabolites than parent compounds (Cade et al., 2018).

Human PBDE exposure, like PCB, can be measured in fat-containing tissue and fluids (e.g., blood and breast milk) (ATSDR, 2017; CDC, 2017). Current literature suggests that most important routes of PBDE exposure vary by amount of exposure and age, such that among young children, inhalation and inadvertent ingestion of house dust is likely the most important source of exposure owing to high hand-to-mouth activity. Among children and adolescents with relatively low exposure, ingestion of PBDE-containing food is estimated to be the most important. Among children and adolescents with high exposure, ingestion of dust is the dominant exposure route (ATSDR, 2017). Although consumption of PBDE-containing seafood is an important source of dietary exposure among high fish consumers, one study estimated dietary intake of PBDE using the 2007 U.S. Department of Agriculture loss-adjusted food availability report and a market basket survey estimating PBDE exposure in 31 food types (in 310 samples) (Schecter et al., 2010b). The study found that fish contain relatively high amounts of PBDE, with canned sardines containing the highest concentration of all foods measured (on a pg/g wet weight basis) excepting butter, which contained roughly four times more PBDE. In addition to sardines, salmon also had high concentrations of PBDE, followed by catfish fillets. Despite these figures, the study estimated that on average, fish consumption accounts for a small fraction of total dietary PBDE exposure, which is primarily contributed by dairy and meat.

Per- and Poly(fluoroalkyl) Substances

Per- and poly(fluoroalkyl) substances (PFAS) are a class of synthetic chemicals widely used in various industrial and consumer products. They are more persistent than PCBs in the aquatic and terrestrial environment where they can contaminate drinking water and seafood, among other pathways, resulting in dietary exposure. In the 2020 scientific opinion released by the European Food Safety Authority (EFSA), seafood was identified as the most important contributor to dietary exposure for perfluorooctane sulfonic acid (PFOS), which biomagnifies in aqueous and marine food chains, and for perfluorooctanoic acid (PFOA) (EFSA, 2020).

Young et al. (2022) examined PFAS levels in eight seafood types, including both wild-caught (canned tuna, pollock, cod, crab, and clam) and aquacultured (shrimp, salmon, and tilapia) species. Packaging materials were also analyzed but were not found to contribute to PFAS concentrations observed in seafood. Clams had the highest total PFAS values across all seafood analyzed with PFOA ranging from 4 to 23 μg/kg. All samples were labeled as products of China. Crabs were found to have the second highest total PFAS levels. Total PFAS levels in cod ranged from below the method detection limit (MDL) to 0.96 μg/kg, while in salmon perfluorododecanoic acid was the only analyte detected above the MDL with all values fewer than 0.045 μg/kg. In pollock the sum of total PFAS ranged from not detected to 0.73 μg/kg. The sum of PFAS in tuna (primarily canned and one soft package or pouch) ranged from 0.083 to 1.75 μg/kg, while in tilapia the lowest values with sum of PFAS ranged from not detected to 0.09 μg/kg. Shrimp was found to have the lowest PFAS levels among all types of seafoods tested with only one sample detected at 0.027 μg/kg. This study showed similar trends as a Netherlands study that detected the highest PFAS levels among clams and crab (Zafeiraki et al., 2019).

While levels of PFAS in freshwater fish typically exceed those of fish from commerce, these levels have declined 30 percent (using PFOS as an indicator) between 2008–2009 and 2013–2014 (Barbo et al., 2023). Data from the EPA 2018–2019 National Rivers and Streams Assessment further indicate that PFOS in fish fillet composite samples declined an additional 6.7 percent from 2013–2014 (EPA, 2023c). Given these data were just posted at the time of this report preparation (December 2023), future work examining the data in detail will permit a deeper understanding of current PFAS exposure in fish from freshwater sources.

Microplastics

Microplastics are complex materials with chemical and physical characteristics that can be classified as either contaminants or toxicants. Emerging evidence indicates that microplastic particles may be toxic because of their physical and toxicologic effects as well as acting as vectors that transport toxic chemicals, such as PBDEs and bacterial pathogens, into tissues and cells (MacLeod et al., 2021). At present, no epidemiological evidence exists to indicate that microplastics are toxic to human populations. A summary of current evidence on microplastics from seafood sources is shown in Box 5-1.

> **BOX 5-1**
> **Microplastics**
>
> Plastic waste is present in practically all ecosystems. Recent estimates suggest there are between 82 and 358 trillion plastic particles in global ocean systems, weighing approximately 1.1 to 4.9 million tonnes (Eriksen et al., 2023). Larger plastics degrade into microplastics and nanoplastics (MNPLs) that range in size from < 1 μm to 5 mm and < 1 nm to 1,000 nm, respectively. They can undergo ingestion, bioaccumulation, and gastrointestinal tract obstruction, and they can transfer associated chemicals to host organisms (MacLeod et al., 2021).
>
> Human exposure to microplastic particles occurs through ingestion, inhalation, and dermal contact. Domenech and Marcos (2021) reported that seafood consumption is a major source of exposure. They conducted a systematic review of studies published between 2018 and 2020 and estimated that the mean concentration of these particles in seafood was 0.98 particles per gram and an annual intake of 22.04 x 10^3 particles per year assuming a consumption level of 22.41 kg per capita.
>
> Zuri et al. (2023) conducted a scoping review and identified that oysters, mussels, and fish were major seafood sources with microplastic concentrations. High concentrations of microplastics were identified specifically in mussels of the species *Mytilus edulis* from the Pearl River Estuary in China.

Summary of Evidence on Contaminants Resulting in Chronic Exposures

Seafood contains a broad range of toxicants and toxins. Concentrations of metals, metalloids, and other trace elements along with organic compounds such as PCBs, PBDEs, and PFAS can result in chronic exposure through seafood consumption. Concentrations vary widely between species, geographic region, size, and age of the organism, and whether they are wild caught or cultivated, among other factors. Hg is the most studied contaminant in seafood. Because levels of seafood consumption are generally lower than recommended levels, and concentrations of Hg for commonly consumed seafood tend to be relatively low, except for tuna, human exposure is not expected to exceed guideline values. Certain subgroups of the population, owing to their pattern of seafood intake or source of seafood, could be at greater risk of exposure to seafood toxicants.

CONTAMINANTS RESULTING IN ACUTE OR EPISODIC EXPOSURE

Infectious Organisms

Many different toxins of biological origin that can have potentially deleterious effects on consumers have been detected in various types of seafood. Contamination with such infectious organisms tends to be specific to geographic location and time of year, and risk areas or periods are captured as state and local advisories.

Algal Blooms

A number of different toxins are associated with harmful algal blooms that naturally occur when environmental conditions are conducive for the organisms to proliferate at high densities and produce toxic metabolites that may enter various marine organisms destined for human consumption. Although the specific combinations of water and other environmental conditions that promote excessive algal blooms are not well known, bivalve molluscan shellfish such as clams, geoduck, mussels, oysters, and scallops are most likely to incorporate toxic compounds produced by microorganisms due to their filter feeding behavior (Washington State Department of Health, 2024b).

Amnesic Shellfish Poisoning from Domoic Acid

Human exposure to domoic acid (DA), an excitatory neurotoxin produced by marine algae, can lead to amnesic shellfish poisoning. This condition is caused by diatoms of the genus *Pseudonitzchia* that produce DA. DA becomes concentrated in filter feeding bivalves, especially razor clams, but they also can occur in crustaceans and fish such as sardines and anchovies (OEHHA, 2017). DA is not destroyed by cooking or freezing and inhibits neurochemical processes, resulting in short-term memory loss, and potentially brain damage in humans consuming contaminated seafood (Ansdell, 2019; Grant et al., 2010). Recent studies have reported that year-round consumption of large quantities of razor clams has been associated with persistent memory problems. FDA and EPA established an action level for notifying consumers of 20 mg/kg [ppm] or greater in shellfish tissue (FDA, 2021).

The committee's evidence review identified one study in humans and one in nonhuman primates relevant to exposure to DA from seafood consumption. Ferriss et al. (2017) examined consumption rates of razor clams by recreational razor clam harvesters. They used food frequency surveys to determine if the harvesters were exposed to DA levels above the regulatory reference levels and/or chronically exposed to low levels of DA. The survey collected data on the daily consumption of clams and the frequency over the past 2 years. Each survey included up to six members of a household and recorded age, sex, and race of household members. The survey results showed that children and young adults (ages 10–20 years) had the highest predicted DA exposure as a result of their lower body weights, and despite lower consumption rates than other age groups. Collectively, about 7 percent of total acute exposures calculated exceeded the regulatory reference dose (0.075 mg DA/kg body weight/day. These exposures were attributed to higher than previously reported consumption rates, lower body weights, and/or consumption of clams at the upper range of the regulatory reference levels for DA.

Petroff et al. (2019) explored how tremors in female *Macaca fascicularis* monkeys with chronic, low-level oral exposure to DA were related to changes in brain structure and neurochemistry. The exposure period included a pre-pregnancy, pregnancy, and postpartum period. Although the study found considerable variability in DA-related tremors among individual animals, overall results suggested that chronic, low-level DA oral exposure at levels below those previously shown to be asymptomatic were related to significantly greater behavioral tremors compared to nonexposed control animals.

Ciguatera Poisoning

Ciguatera fish poisoning (CFP) is a foodborne disease that results from consuming predatory ocean fish contaminated with ciguatoxins. Similar to ciguatera, neurotoxic or paralytic shellfish poisoning is a neurological disturbance that arises from consumption of tropical reef fish and shellfish. The condition is produced by naturally occurring marine biotoxins such as saxitoxin and other potent neurotoxins associated with certain species of microalgae, which are consumed by fish, as well as single-cell dinoflagellates.

In the United States, up to 5 to 70 cases per 10,000 are estimated to occur annually in endemic states and territories. Symptoms of CFP include nausea, vomiting, abdominal cramps, or diarrhea and occur within a few hours after fish consumption (CDC, 2009). Exposure to these toxins by consuming contaminated seafood affects the nervous system and results in temporary paralysis. Neurologic symptoms can include fatigue, muscle pain, tingling, itching, and reversal of hot and cold sensation (Dickey and Plakas, 2009). In the United States, ciguatera-contaminated fish have been found in coastal waters as far north as North Carolina. Research from previous decades demonstrated CFP is considered one of the most common illnesses related to fish consumption in the United States (Anderson et al., 2021; Pennotti et al., 2013).

Detection of ciguatera is based on clinical presentation as diagnostic tests do not exist. Lopez et al. (2016) conducted a study to identify relevant biomarkers and investigate factors that may contribute to clinical presentation and gene expression in peripheral blood leukocytes. This study found significant differences in plasmablastic lymphoma gene expression patterns among participants with ciguatera poisoning compared with controls, but significant differences in gene expression were not seen when participants with recurrent symptoms were compared with those with acute symptoms.

Based on the proximity of Florida to the geographic distribution of ciguatera, Radke et al. (2015) administered a survey to recreational fishermen and carried out an analysis of reported ciguatera to identify high-risk demographic groups, high-risk fish types, and catch locations that are linked to CFP in Florida. The survey results identified barracuda, grouper, and amberjack as the most frequently consumed species linked to CFP in Florida. The study further found that Hispanics had higher rates of CFP than non-Hispanics, which was likely attributable to more frequent consumption of barracuda. The majority of CFP cases identified were caused by fish caught in the Bahamas and the Florida Keys.

Vibriosis

Twelve different species of bacteria of the genus *Vibrio* cause human illness known as vibriosis, which is characterized by gastrointestinal problems marked by symptoms such as watery diarrhea, fever, nausea, and vomiting that may either precede or follow septicemia. This condition is most encountered when raw oysters or undercooked seafood having high concentrations of *Vibrio* are consumed (Baker-Austin et al., 2018; Leng et al., 2019).

Norovirus

This single-stranded RNA virus is commonly associated with the stomach flu. Shellfish are one of the most common types of food that have been associated with norovirus outbreaks.

Micro-organisms

The committee's commissioned evidence review of primary studies identified evidence about various microorganisms in seafood, but most of the studies were conducted outside of the United States and Canada. The following sections discuss current evidence from exemplar studies that examined salmonella, *Escherichia coli* (*E. coli*), and hepatitis A in seafood and aquatic food sources. Foodborne pathogens of special concern for pregnant women include *Listeria monocytogenes* and *Salmonella enterica* because of the increased risk of adverse pregnancy outcomes (Smith, 1999).

Salmonella

The majority of studies in the committee's evidence review, many of them case study reports, identified salmonella as a microorganism of concern in seafood. From 2011 to 2015, up to three cases per month of *Salmonella javiana* were reported in restaurants sporadically across Arizona. Venkat et al. (2018) investigated these outbreaks and conducted a case–control study to assess risk factors for the infection. The analysis included 21 laboratory-confirmed cases. Whole genome sequencing demonstrated that all *Salmonella* isolates were genetically related, signifying that the illnesses were linked to a common source. The analysis further showed that outbreaks could be propagated in a restaurant even when no health violations are noted. The study concluded that the outbreak of *Salmonella javiana* could have been caused by *Salmonella* contamination of prepared, uncooked shrimp and that the *Salmonella* survived the minimum cooking temperatures that are required for seafood in the Arizona Food Code and the FDA Food Code.

Huang et al. (2012) carried out a study to evaluate the prevalence of *Salmonella* and *Vibrio* species in seafoods obtained in Singapore. Seafood samples were purchased from three major supermarkets and nine wet markets in Singapore. Results of bacterial counts showed that the highest mean counts were found in thawed-frozen shellfish, although this was not significantly different from fresh shellfish, and fresh prawn. Overall, the study found that seafood sold in Singapore had the potential to be contaminated with *Vibrio parahaemolyticus* and *Salmonella lexington*, implicating unsanitary conditions in the markets as a causal factor. However, the final product may also have been contaminated through cross-contamination from raw materials due to mishandling by both vendors and customers.

A study by Hamilton et al. (2018) carried out a quantitative microbial risk assessment for wastewater-fed aquaculture to examine the relative importance of aquaculture practices for microbiological health risks. The premise of the study was that aquaculture-produced seafood products are more likely to contain *Salmonella* species than wild-caught seafood. A variety of industrial and consumer processing scenarios were identified to assess the relative risks caused by *Salmonella* species exposure from consumption of shrimp raised in aquaculture ponds in the United States. The United States has a zero-tolerance policy for the presence of *Salmonella* species on raw, ready-to-eat, and cooked shrimp.

The results of this analysis found that improper cooking times in non-gamma-irradiated shrimp were associated with the highest risk of infection. Importantly, in each risk scenario, *Salmonella* species levels in aquaculture ponds had only a moderate effect, indicating that other management points for reducing risks may be more effective. The largest difference between microbiological risks for the scenarios tested was seen for proper versus improper cooking and gamma irradiation of shrimp. The scenarios identified less than one order of magnitude of risk for peeling and deveining versus peeling only.

Escherichia coli

Viganò et al. (2007) evaluated the microbiological quality of ready-to-eat foods in Pemba Island, Tanzania. This study identified thermotolerant coliforms in 34 percent of seafoods and 58 percent of household meals that were tested. Among these, *E. coli* was the most frequently isolated species found in seafood (15 percent), except for boiled or fried seafood.

Hepatitis A

Filter feeding bivalve shellfish are common vehicles for the transmission of enteric viruses, including hepatitis A virus (HAV), primarily via the fecal–oral route. In 2005, an outbreak of HAV occurred across a four-state region of the United States among individuals who had consumed oysters. Shieh et al. (2007) described an approach using reverse transcription polymerase chain reaction (RT-PCR) to identify a single HAV strain among infected consumers who consumed oysters identified as the outbreak source. This was the first direct evidence to link infected consumers from the outbreak to HAV.

To understand the relationship between two subsequent HAV outbreak incidences from imported coquina clams and the likelihood of the infection coming from the contaminated clams, Pintó et al. (2009) used RT-PCR analysis to estimate the genome copy number of virus particles per gram of tissue in clams associated with the outbreaks. This analytical approach showed a dose–response relationship between the number of infectious particles detected and the probability of infection.

Summary of Evidence on Contaminants Resulting in Acute or Episodic Exposure

Exposure to pathogens and microbial toxins tends to occur episodically as "outbreaks" at a specific time and location or as food poisoning cases among individuals who consume contaminated seafoods. Such risks are often mitigated by closure of harvest at specific time or locations, withdrawing the sales of contaminated seafood from the market, or public health advice to avoid the contaminated seafood.

HUMAN BIOMARKERS OF TOXICANT EXPOSURE ASSOCIATED WITH SEAFOOD CONSUMPTION

Metals and Metalloids

Davis et al. (2014) analyzed NHANES data from 2007 to 2008 to examine dietary intake of mercury, cadmium, lead, and arsenic. The study populations included children younger than 18 years of age and adults. The analysis included whole blood for mercury, cadmium, and lead; urinary lead; and total arsenic and arsenic speciation. Dietary intake was assessed from the NHANES 24-hour recall questionnaire. The study results found significant associations between seafood consumption and mercury, total As, arsenobetaine, and dimethylarsinate (DMA) among both adults and children. Placental tissue and human milk both contain metals and metalloids, but these biomarkers are not used extensively in studies relating exposures to seafood consumption.

Mercury

Blood Hg is a mixture of both methylmercury and inorganic mercury but is primarily composed of MeHg among seafood-eating populations. Umbilical cord blood Hg concentrations are almost exclusively MeHg. Likewise, hair is largely MeHg and can be subject to external contamination. Nails, like hair, also accumulate MeHg. Inorganic Hg is the dominant type of urinary Hg reflecting exposure to primarily elemental Hg from inhalation and ingestion (i.e., silver-mercury dental amalgams). The transport of MeHg from the maternal bloodstream to human milk is lower than what is transferred via the placenta.

Karagas et al. (2012) reviewed the published literature to assess current evidence on the human health effects of low-level exposure to MeHg, including biomarkers of exposure. As noted by other investigators, total hair or blood Hg levels are regarded as more accurate measures of exposure than dietary assessment. While cord blood Hg may be a better marker of fetal exposure than maternal hair, variability remains a concern.

The Agency for Toxic Substances and Disease Registry and EPA, in their most recent draft "Toxicological Profile for Mercury" (ATSDR, 2022), reviewed Hg levels in blood and urine reported in NHANES, which draws from survey data collected in 2015–2016. Overall, the mean total blood Hg level in the adult U.S. population was estimated to be $0.810\,\mu g/L$ (95% confidence interval [CI] 0.740, 0.886), whereas the 50th percentiles for total blood Hg in children age 1–5 years was less than $0.28\,\mu g/L$. For the 2015–2016 collection period, the 50th percentiles of total urinary mercury were below the detection limit ($0.13\,\mu g/L$) in children ages 3–5 years.

In Canada, the geometric mean of blood Hg concentrations for women of childbearing age (18–49 years) in the general population (2009–2011) was $0.67\,\mu g/L$ (Health Canada, 2021), and the geometric mean for children (3–19 years) ranged from 0.27 to $0.3\,\mu g/L$ from 2007–2017, depending on age and sex (Health Canada, 2019c).

The EPA reference level of $5.8\,\mu g/L$ Hg in blood is the equilibrium blood Hg level that is associated with a dietary intake of Hg at the current reference dose of $0.1\,\mu g/kg$ body weight/day. Health Canada uses a blood guideline of $8.0\,\mu g/L$, based on the existing provisional tolerable daily intakes for children, pregnant women, and women of childbearing age.

Seafood consumption has been specifically related to biomarkers of total Hg (THg) in pregnancy. Schaefer et al. (2019) examined concentrations of THg from pregnant women in coastal Florida along with a validated dietary questionnaire with a 3-month recall period. Among the 299 women examined, 19 (8.3 percent) had hair Hg concentrations exceeding the EPA reference dose of $1.0\,\mu g/g$. Seafood was consumed once per week or more by 35.5 percent of respondents, while 17.1 percent did not consume seafood in the previous 3 months. The highest concentration of THg in hair was observed in women who reported eating seafood three times per week. In a pregnancy cohort study reported by Emeny et al. (2019), prenatal toenail Hg concentrations correlated with the amount of fish/seafood consumption reported on a validated food frequency questionnaire.

Cusack et al. (2017) used data from six consecutive cycles of NHANES (1999–2010) to determine trends in blood Hg levels among women aged 16–49 years and residing in different U.S. regions. Population characteristics examined included age, race/ethnicity, income level, and fish consumption using geographic variables. This study found that women of childbearing age living in coastal regions consumed more fish per month and had higher whole blood Hg concentrations compared with women living in the Midwest after controlling for other confounders. Compared with the results of a previous study by Mahaffey et al. (2009), who examined women of childbearing age using NHANES data from 1999–2004, a modest decrease in the geometric mean blood mercury concentrations was found for women residing in the Atlantic coast (1.55 to $1.35\,\mu g/L$) and the Gulf of Mexico (0.96 to $0.88\,\mu g/L$). However, after including data from the 2005–2010 NHANES survey cycles, a modest increase in blood Hg concentration was found for women residing in the Inland Northeast (0.77 to $0.85\,\mu g/L$) and no change was identified in other regions.

In addition to the NHANES study that included children (Davis et al., 2014), studies of preschool to adolescent children have been conducted in Spain where seafood consumption is higher than the United States. Among 4-year-old children, fish intake was associated with hair Hg concentrations, especially swordfish, lean fish, and canned tuna (Llop et al., 2014). Similar findings were observed among 9-year-old children in Spain (Soler-Blasco et al., 2019). Likewise, fish intake was associated with hair mercury concentrations among 11-year-old children, with the highest hair Hg concentrations among those who reported eating swordfish (López-González et al., 2023).

Cadmium

Cadmium accumulates in the kidneys; therefore, urinary Cd reflects long-term or cumulative exposure. In contrast, blood Cd represents recent exposure. Cd also binds to nail tissue, and as with urine, it correlates with smoking exposure during pregnancy, the primary source of Cd exposure. Epidemiologic studies of Cd biomarkers and seafood consumption are scant. In a randomized clinical trial testing the Mediterranean diet versus a conventional diet, fish intake was associated with urinary Cd concentrations (Rempelos et al., 2022). However, no association was found between urinary Cd and seafood intake in NHANES (Davis et al., 2014) in adults or children, nor in a Spanish cohort of children (Notario-Barandian et al., 2023).

Lead

Measurements of Pb in blood, urine, and tissues are used to assess exposures among individuals, although blood is most widely used. However, blood makes up less than 2 percent of the total Pb body burden (Levin-Schwartz et al., 2020). Because Pb is eliminated from blood faster than from bone, blood Pb reflects the previous few months of exposure (ATSDR, 2020). Additionally, slow release of Pb from bone can add to blood Pb levels after exposure ends. The use of time-integrated blood Pb measures, however, can mitigate concerns about the magnitude of exposure for both acute and chronic exposure, and can measure long-term exposure.

Urine reflects recent Pb exposure, but interpretation requires measuring the glomerular filtration rate and estimating volume. Urine Pb measures can also exhibit high intraindividual variability. Other tissues that can be used include tooth, saliva and sweat, hair, nails, and semen, although these tissues are not widely used (ATSDR, 2020).

While Pb exposure was unrelated to seafood consumption in the NHANES study by Davis et al. (2014), Pb concentration in urine was associated with shellfish but not with other seafood consumed in a study of 4-year-old children from Spain (Junqué et al., 2022). Thus, Pb exposure is a potential concern in populations with higher intakes of fish.

Arsenic

Urine is the primary biomarker of As. Identification of specific As metabolites in urine is required to measure exposure to inorganic As in fish and seafood from the metabolites of As, monomethylarsonic acid (MMA) and DMA which may be present in seafood and other foods as mentioned previously. Arsenobetaine had not been considered toxic because it is generally excreted unchanged. Evidence suggests, however, that metabolism to inorganic As (iAs) may occur based on mouse studies and *in vitro* studies which suggests metabolism to other arsenocompounds by the microbiome. Furthermore, both arsenolipids and arsenosugars present in seafood break down to form DMA as the major metabolite in urine (Raml et al., 2009; Schmeisser et al., 2006).

Studies frequently sum As, MMA, and DMA as the measure of total urinary iAs. While urine reflects short-term As exposure, urinary As can be consistent over time among those individuals with consistent exposures (i.e., through drinking water or diet). Blood is a potential exposure marker, but because As is rapidly cleared from the blood and is more complicated to analyze it is rarely used in epidemiologic studies.

In addition to the work mentioned previously from NHANES (Davis et al., 2014), studies in the draft *Scientific Opinion on the Update of the EFSA Scientific Opinion on Inorganic Arsenic in Food* (EFSA Panel on Contaminants in the Food Chain, 2024) reported elevated urinary total As, arsenobetaine, and DMA concentrations among those who consumed cod, salmon, and mussels, and elevated MMA among those who consumed mussels.

Hair and nails are used as a measure of longer-term As exposure in epidemiologic studies, although hair is susceptible to external contamination, whereas carefully washed nails are typically not. Hair provides an estimate of As exposure over time whereas toenails represent exposure over the previous 6 to 12 months (in adults) and thus are considered a reliable long-term biomarker of exposure (Signes-Pastor et al., 2021). Cottingham et al. (2013) examined associations between the As body burden, as indicated by toenail As concentration, and potential dietary exposure from seafood with exposure through drinking water. The investigators found elevated toenail As, which is primarily inorganic, in those who consumed greater amounts of dark meat fish (tuna steak, sardines, mackerel, salmon, bluefish, or swordfish), but not more fish overall.

Currently, the dominant compounds of As in human milk are not fully understood, and the concentrations of As are typically considered relatively low (Carignan et al., 2016; Tillett, 2008). A study of repeated measures of human milk following salmon consumption found that As levels peaked in about 8 hours following consumption and comprised arsenolipids (mainly As hydrocarbons for lipid fraction) and arsenobetaine (Xiong et al., 2020).

Persistent Organic Pollutants

As described above, POPs including PCBs, dioxins and dioxin-like compounds (DLCs), and PBDEs can be measured in lipophilic biomatrices (e.g., blood serum or plasma and breast milk) to assess human exposure. PFAS can also be measured in blood and breast milk. Many studies describe human exposure, but fewer studies in North America elucidate exposure attributable to fish and seafood consumption. A notable exception includes some Indigenous populations who, owing to a combination of environmental injustice and cultural practices that include dietary reliance on and importance of local fish, are generally more highly exposed (Cordier et al., 2020).

Polychlorinated Biphenyls

While prior research indicated that fish consumers generally have higher serum PCBs than fish nonconsumers (ATSDR, 1996; Humphrey et al., 2000; Tee et al., 2003), updated analyses indicate that this association is strongest in ethnic groups that consume higher amounts of fish (e.g., Asian, Pacific Islander, Native American, other multiracial ethnicities) (Xue et al., 2014).

In an analysis applying EPA's Stochastic Human Exposure and Dose Simulation (SHEDS) dietary exposure model to NHANES 2001–2002 and 2003–2004 cycle data, predictors of higher concentrations of PCB include age (older participants have higher concentrations than younger participants ages 12–30 years), ethnicity (individuals from Asian, Pacific Islander, Native American, or other multiracial ethnicities have higher concentrations than other ethnicities), and fish consumption (Xue et al., 2014).

An important limitation of this SHEDS-NHANES analysis is it was unable to estimate PCB from other dietary sources, including meat, skin, fat, and milk. Despite the observation that fish and seafood contain the highest levels of PCBs relative to other food sources, in a recent study of mothers and children from the Midwest, researchers found that among dietary sources of PCB, meat accounts for the majority of exposure and fish and seafood accounts for fewer than a quarter of dietary PCB exposure among both mothers and children (Saktrakulkla et al., 2020).

Dioxins

As described above, limited data are available to estimate dioxin body burden attributable to fish and seafood in the United States and in Canada, with the notable exception of populations relying on fish from the Great Lakes or from contaminated sites. For example, Wattigney et al. (2019) found that urban anglers who consume fish from the Detroit River, which flows between the Great Lakes, did not have higher body burdens of dioxins. However, they did have elevated levels of some PCBs and total blood Hg.

Polybrominated Diphenyl Ethers

Fraser et al. (2009) conducted an analysis evaluating dietary sources of PBDEs using both food frequency questionnaire data, which is meant to approximate a broad picture of average intake, as well as 24-hour recall data prior to blood concentrations in the NHANES 2003–2004 cycle, in which PBDE concentrations were measured.

The study found that poultry and red meat consumption are significant sources of PBDE body burdens, whereas other dietary sources including seafood were not associated with PBDE exposure.

A systematic review (Bramwell et al., 2016) identified two studies, both in European populations, that used duplicate diets to relate dietary exposure to body burden. Neither study found an association between diet and exposure but noted that stronger associations may have been observed only in cases where contaminated food is a regular or major dietary component (e.g., consumption of fish from a contaminated lake).

Per- and Poly(fluoroalkyl) Substances

Christensen et al. (2017) evaluated the association between fish consumption in the past 30 days (assessed via dietary interview) and blood concentration of PFAS in the NHANES 2007–2008, 2009–2010, 2011–2012, and 2013–2014 cycles. The study found that while fish consumption was generally low, consumption of both fish and shellfish was associated with higher levels of almost all PFAS compounds measured, though associations varied by each PFAS and by specific types of fish and shellfish, and those relationships were stronger in higher-income households. While this investigation focuses on recent fish consumption and blood concentrations, PFAS bioaccumulate in human blood and tissue and likely reflect past as well as recent exposure.

A review by McAdam and Bell (2023) focused on the determinants of PFAS exposure among pregnant mothers and neonates. Out of 35 studies reviewed, 14 evaluated dietary determinants for fish or shellfish. Findings from the review were inconsistent for individual PFAS compounds. Approximately half of the studies reported positive findings and half reported null findings, although most of the studies in the review were not from North America.

Among the U.S. and Canadian studies identified in the review that examined fish as a predictor of exposure, the two Canadian studies (Caron-Beaudoin et al., 2020; Fisher et al., 2016) and one U.S. study (Kingsley et al., 2018) reported no associations. Another U.S. study used a principal components analysis and reported a positive association between fish consumption and the principal component characterized by the high concentrations of PFOS and perfluorononanoic acid (Kalloo et al., 2018). Since the time that the review was completed, an additional study of children living in the Boston area used a food frequency questionnaire to evaluate dietary intake and patterns (Seshasayee et al., 2021). This study reported that individual food items were not associated with PFAS exposure. However, a dietary pattern that included high consumption of packaged foods and fish (excluding canned tuna and fried fish) was associated with higher concentrations of all PFAS measured.

Summary of Evidence on Biomarkers of Exposure

Epidemiological studies relating seafood intake during pregnancy to biomarkers of contaminant exposure have largely focused on Hg, with findings of higher blood, hair, and toenail Hg concentrations. Using NHANES data, higher seafood food intake was positively correlated with blood levels of Hg and urinary concentrations of total As, DMA, and arsenobetaine both among adults and children. Studies of the biomarker concentrations of other contaminants associated with seafood consumption are relatively scarce, and for all contaminants very little data exist on biomarker associations with seafood intake during lactation, infancy, and childhood.

FINDINGS AND CONCLUSIONS

Findings

Contaminants of Concern

1. Toxins, toxicants, and microbes, including persistent bioaccumulative chemicals, metals and metalloids, infectious organisms, microplastics, and microorganisms, may be present in seafood at levels hazardous to consumers. The concentration of these various contaminants in seafood depends on many factors, including species, trophic position, size, age, geographic location, and origin—wild caught or farm raised.

2. With the exception of some types of tuna, the most commonly consumed seafood species in the United States and Canada contain relatively low concentrations of methylmercury, and concentrations of other metals and metalloids tend to be limited to certain species and geographic areas.[5]

Acute and Episodic Exposure to Contaminants in Seafood

3. Among adults and children, seafood consumption is associated with higher blood, hair, and toenail levels of Hg, and urinary concentrations of certain forms of As, particularly those common to seafood such as arsenobetaine.
4. Average intake levels of MeHg from seafood are below the FDA Closer to Zero recommended limits among women of childbearing age, infants, and children, except for those who frequently consume tuna.[6]
5. Polychlorinated biphenyls (PCBs) and Hg are the key drivers for fish consumption advisories and PCBs are particularly relevant in the Great Lakes region.
6. Certain population groups, in particular Native Americans and Indigenous peoples, as well as subsistence and sport fishers and their families, may consume more seafood species or seafood components from geographic locations that could have high concentrations of Hg and PCBs than individuals in the general population, thereby exceeding recommended limits.[7]

Conclusions

1. *The committee found insufficient evidence to assess exposure to most consumers associated with emerging contaminants in seafood, including PFAS, microplastics, and domoic acids.*
2. *PBDE exposure is not due primarily to seafood consumption; however, as PBDEs migrate into aquatic environments, risk of increased exposure through seafood may emerge.*
3. *Although seafood consumption is generally low across population groups, it continues to be an important predictor of MeHg, As, and PCB exposure and may be important for assessing PFAS exposure, where evidence is beginning to emerge. Therefore, if fish intake were to increase to DGA recommended levels, then exposures would likely increase.*

RESEARCH GAPS

- Additional research is needed to assess geographic and temporal trend data for levels of MeHg, Hg, and other contaminants in seafood, and to monitor intake levels of these contaminants among women of childbearing age, infants, and children. Special attention should be given to at-risk population groups such as Native Americans and Indigenous peoples, and to other at-risk groups, such as subsistence and sport fishers and their families.
- Research is needed for specific studies that examine As and Se in fish. Additional research is needed to assess the potential protective role of nutrients and other factors, such as selenoneine effects on Hg toxicity.
- More quantitative characterization is needed to assess the risk of chronic exposure to less studied contaminants such as PFAS, arsenic species, microplastics, and DA to assess bioaccumulation in food chains at the levels of exposure and toxicity.
- Research is needed to characterize biomarkers of exposure to contaminants in seafood among women of childbearing age, infants, children, and adolescents. This research is needed to identify and characterize dose–response relationships between contaminants and contaminant mixtures in seafood and adverse outcomes among the children of women exposed during pregnancy and lactation.

---

[5] The sentence was revised after release of the report to the study sponsor to clarify that concentrations of methylmercury vary in different types of tuna.

[6] This sentence was modified after release of the report to the study sponsor to clarify that recommended limits of contaminant exposure are based on the Closer to Zero Action Plan.

[7] This phrase was modified after release of the report to the study sponsor to reference recommended limits rather than acceptable risk levels.

REFERENCES

Achouba, A., P. Dumas, N. Ouellet, M. Lemire, and P. Ayotte. 2016. Plasma levels of selenium-containing proteins in Inuit adults from Nunavik. *Environment International* 96:8-15.

Anderson, D. M., E. Fensin, C. J. Gobler, A. E. Hoeglund, K. A. Hubbard, D. M. Kulis, J. H. Landsberg, K. A. Lefebvre, P. Provoost, and M. L. Richlen. 2021. Marine harmful algal blooms (HABS) in the United States: History, current status and future trends. *Harmful Algae* 102:101975.

Ansdell, V. 2019. Seafood poisoning. In *Travel medicine*, 4th ed. Edited by J. S. Keystone, B. A. Connor, H. D. Nothdurft, M. Mendelson, and K. Leder. New York: Elsevier. Pp. 449-456.

ATSDR (Agency for Toxic Substances and Disease Registry). 1996. *Public health implications of PCB exposures*. https://semspub.epa.gov/work/02/68681.pdf (accessed February 6, 2024).

ATSDR. 2017. *Public health statement for PBDEs*. https://wwwn.cdc.gov/TSP/PHS/PHS.aspx?phsid=1449&toxid=183 (accessed February 4, 2024).

ATSDR. 2020. *Toxicological profile for lead*. Atlanta, GA: HHS, Public Health Service. https://www.atsdr.cdc.gov/toxprofiles/tp13.pdf (accessed February 4, 2024).

ATSDR. 2022. *Toxicological profile for mercury (draft for public comment)*. Atlanta, GA: HHS, Public Health Service. https://www.atsdr.cdc.gov/ToxProfiles/tp46.pdf (accessed February 4, 2023).

Baker-Austin, C., J. D. Oliver, M. Alam, A. Ali, M. K. Waldor, F. Qadri, and J. Martinez-Urtaza. 2018. Vibrio spp. infections. *Nature Reviews Disease Primers* 4(1):1-19.

Barbo, N., T. Stoiber, O. V. Naidenko, and D. Q. Andrews. 2023. Locally caught freshwater fish across the United States are likely a significant source of exposure to PFOS and other perfluorinated compounds. *Environmental Research* 220:115165.

Bendell, L. 2010. Cadmium in shellfish: The British Columbia, Canada experience—A mini-review. *Toxicology Letters* 198(1):7-12.

Borak, J., and H. D. Hosgood. 2007. Seafood arsenic: Implications for human risk assessment. *Regulatory Toxicology and Pharmacology* 47(2):204-212.

Bramwell, L., S. V. Glinianaia, J. Rankin, M. Rose, A. Fernandes, S. Harrad, and T. Pless-Mulolli. 2016. Associations between human exposure to polybrominated diphenyl ether flame retardants via diet and indoor dust, and internal dose: A systematic review. *Environment International* 92:680-694.

Cabañero, A. I., C. Carvalho, Y. Madrid, C. Batoréu, and C. Cámara. 2005. Quantification and speciation of mercury and selenium in fish samples of high consumption in Spain and Portugal. *Biological Trace Element Research* 103:17-35.

Cade, S. E., L. J. Kuo, and I. R. Schultz. 2018. Polybrominated diphenyl ethers and their hydroxylated and methoxylated derivatives in seafood obtained from Puget Sound, WA. *Science of the Total Environment* 630:1149-1154.

Carignan, C. C., M. R. Karagas, T. Punshon, D. Gilbert-Diamond, and K. L. Cottingham. 2016. Contribution of breast milk and formula to arsenic exposure during the first year of life in a US prospective cohort. *Journal of Exposure Science & Environmental Epidemiology* 26(5):452-457.

Caron-Beaudoin, É., P. Ayotte, C. Blanchette, G. Muckle, E. Avard, S. Ricard, and M. Lemire. 2020. Perfluoroalkyl acids in pregnant women from Nunavik (Quebec, Canada): Trends in exposure and associations with country foods consumption. *Environment International* 145:106169.

CDC (Centers for Disease Control and Prevention). 2009. *Cluster of ciguatera fish poisoning—North Carolina*. https://www.cdc.gov/mmwr/preview/mmwrhtml/mm5811a3.htm (accessed February 6, 2024).

CDC. 2017. *Polybrominated diphenyl ethers (PBDEs) and polybrominated biphenyls (PBBs) factsheet*. https://www.cdc.gov/biomonitoring/PBDEs_FactSheet.html (accessed February 4, 2024).

Chan, H. M., K. Singh, M. Batal, L. Marushka, C. Tikhonov, T. Sadik, H. Schwartz, A. Ing, and K. Fediuk. 2021. Levels of metals and persistent organic pollutants in traditional foods consumed by First Nations living on-reserve in Canada. *Canadian Journal of Public Health* 112(Suppl 1):81-96.

Chavez-Crooker, P., P. Pozo, H. Castro, M. S. Dice, I. Boutet, A. Tanguy, D. Moraga, and G. A. Ahearn. 2003. Cellular localization of calcium, heavy metals, and metallothionein in lobster (*Homarus americanus*) hepatopancreas. *Comparative Biochemistry and Physiology: Toxicology & Pharmacology* 136(3):213-224.

Christensen, K. Y., M. Raymond, M. Blackowicz, Y. Liu, B. A. Thompson, H. A. Anderson, and M. Turyk. 2017. Perfluoroalkyl substances and fish consumption. *Environmental Research* 154:145-151.

Cordier, S., E. Anassour-Laouan-Sidi, M. Lemire, N. Costet, M. Lucas, and P. Ayotte. 2020. Association between exposure to persistent organic pollutants and mercury, and glucose metabolism in two Canadian Indigenous populations. *Environmental Research* 184:109345.

Cottingham, K. L., R. Karimi, J. F. Gruber, M. S. Zens, V. Sayarath, C. L. Folt, T. Punshon, J. S. Morris, and M. R. Karagas. 2013. Diet and toenail arsenic concentrations in a New Hampshire population with arsenic-containing water. *Nutrition Journal* 12:1-10.

Cusack, L. K., E. Smit, M. L. Kile, and A. K. Harding. 2017. Regional and temporal trends in blood mercury concentrations and fish consumption in women of childbearing age in the United States using NHANES data from 1999–2010. *Environmental Health* 16(1):10.

Davis, M. A., D. Gilbert-Diamond, M. R. Karagas, Z, Li, J. H. Moore, S. M. Williams, and H. R. Frost. 2014. A dietary-wide association study (DWAS) of environmental metal exposure in US children and adults. *PLoS One* 9(9):e104768.

Dickey, R. W., and S. M. Plakas. 2009. Ciguatera: A public health perspective. *Toxicon* 56(2):123-136.

Dietz, R., J. Fort, C. Sonne, C. Albert, J. O. Bustnes, T. K. Christensen, T. M. Ciesielski, J. Danielsen, S. Dastnai, and M. Eens. 2021. A risk assessment of the effects of mercury on Baltic Sea, greater North Sea and North Atlantic wildlife, fish and bivalves. *Environment International* 146:106178.

Domenech, J., and R. Marcos. 2021. Pathways of human exposure to microplastics, and estimation of the total burden. *Current Opinion in Food Science* 39:144-151.

Driscoll, C. T., R. P. Mason, H. M. Chan, D. J. Jacob, and N. Pirrone. 2013. Mercury as a global pollutant: Sources, pathways, and effects. *Environmental Science & Technology* 47(10):4967-4983.

Drobyshev, E., S. Raschke, R. A. Glabonjat, J. Bornhorst, F. Ebert, D. Kuehnelt, and T. Schwerdtle. 2021. Capabilities of selenoneine to cross the in vitro blood-brain barrier model. *Metallomics* 13(1):Mfaa007.

EFSA (European Food Safety Authority) Panel on Contaminants in the Food Chain, D. Schrenk, M. Bignami, L. Bodin, J. K. Chipman, J. del Mazo, B. Grasl-Kraupp, C. Hogstrand, L. Hoogenboom, and J. C. Leblanc. 2020. Risk to human health related to the presence of perfluoroalkyl substances in food. *EFSA Journal* 18(9):e06223.

EFSA Panel on Contaminants in the Food Chain, D. Schrenk, M. Bignami, L. Bodin, J. K. Chipman, J. del Mazo, B. Grasl-Kraupp, C. Hogstrand, L. Hoogenboom, J.-C. Leblanc, C. S. Nebbia, E. Nielsen, E. Ntzani, A. Petersen, S. Sand, C. Vleminckx, H. Wallace, L. Barregård, L. Benford, K. Broberg, E. Dogliotti, T. Fletcher, L. Rylander, J. C. Abrahantes, J. Á. Gómez Ruiz, H. Steinkellner, T. Tauriainen, and T. Schwerdtle. 2024. Update of the risk assessment of inorganic arsenic in food. *EFSA Journal* 22(1):e8488.

Emeny, R. T., S. A. Korrick, Z. Li, K. Nadeau, J. Madan, B. Jackson, E. Baker, and M. R. Karagas. 2019. Prenatal exposure to mercury in relation to infant infections and respiratory symptoms in the New Hampshire birth cohort study. *Environmental Research* 171:523-529.

EPA (U.S. Environmental Protection Agency). 2009. *The national study of chemical residues in lake fish tissue*. https://www.epa.gov/sites/default/files/2018-11/documents/national-study-chemical-residues-lake-fish-tissue.pdf (accessed February 4, 2024).

EPA. 2023a. *Persistent organic pollutants: A global issue, a global response*. https://www.epa.gov/international-cooperation/persistent-organic-pollutants-global-issue-global-response (accessed December 8, 2023).

EPA. 2023b. *Great Lakes open lakes trend monitoring program: Polychlorinated biphenyls (PCBs)*. https://www.epa.gov/great-lakes-monitoring/great-lakes-open-lakes-trend-monitoring-program-polychlorinated-biphenyls (accessed February 4, 2024).

EPA. 2023c. *National rivers and streams assessment: The third collaborative survey*. https://riverstreamassessment.epa.gov/webreport/#per-and-polyfluoroalkyl-substances-pfas (accessed February 10, 2024).

Eriksen, M., W. Cowger, L. M. Erdle, S. Coffin, P. Villarrubia-Gómez, C. J. Moore, E. J. Carpenter, R. H. Day, M. Thiel, and C. Wilcox. 2023. A growing plastic smog, now estimated to be over 170 trillion plastic particles afloat in the world's oceans-urgent solutions required. *PLoS One* 18(3):e0281596.

FDA (U.S. Food and Drug Administration). 2011. *Mercury concentrations in fish from the FDA monitoring program (1990-2010)*. https://www.fda.gov/media/101237/download (accessed February 28, 2024).

FDA. 2014. *Quantitative assessment of the net effects on fetal neurodevelopment from eating commercial fish (as measured by IQ and also by early age verbal development in children)*. https://www.fda.gov/food/environmental-contaminants-food/quantitative-assessment-net-effects-fetal-neurodevelopment-eating-commercial-fish-measured-iq-and (accessed February 28, 2024).

FDA. 2021. *Appendix 5: FDA and EPA safety levels in regulations and guidance*. https://www.fda.gov/media/80400/download (accessed February 6, 2024).

FDA. 2022a. *Total diet study report*. https://www.fda.gov/food/reference-databases-and-monitoring-programs-food/fda-total-diet-study-tds (accessed February 4, 2024).

FDA. 2022b. *Technical information on development of FDA/EPA advice about eating fish for those who might become or are pregnant or breastfeeding and children ages 1–11 years.* https://www.fda.gov/food/environmental-contaminants-food/technical-information-development-fdaepa-advice-about-eating-fish-those-who-might-become-or-are (accessed January 1, 2024).

Ferriss, B. E., D. J. Marcinek, D. Ayres, J. Borchert, and K. A. Lefebvre. 2017. Acute and chronic dietary exposure to domoic acid in recreational harvesters: A survey of shellfish consumption behavior. *Environment International* 101:70-79.

Fisher, M., T. E. Arbuckle, C. L. Liang, A. LeBlanc, E. Gaudreau, W. G. Foster, D. Haines, K. Davis, and W. D. Fraser. 2016. Concentrations of persistent organic pollutants in maternal and cord blood from the maternal-infant research on environmental chemicals (MIREC) cohort study. *Environmental Health: A Global Access Science Source* 15(1):59.

Frank, J. J., A. G. Poulakos, R. Tornero-Velez, and J. Xue. 2019. Systematic review and meta-analyses of lead (Pb) concentrations in environmental media (soil, dust, water, food, and air) reported in the United States from 1996 to 2016. *Science of the Total Environment* 694:133489.

Fraser, A. J., T. F. Webster, and M. D. McClean. 2009. Diet contributes significantly to the body burden of PBDEs in the general U.S. population. *Environmental Health Perspectives* 117(10):1520-1525.

Gandhi, N., K. G. Drouillard, G. B. Arhonditsis, S. B. Gewurtz, and S. P. Bhavsar. 2017. Are fish consumption advisories for the Great Lakes adequately protective against chemical mixtures? *Environmental Health Perspectives* 125(4):586-593.

Gavelek, A., J. Spungen, D. Hoffman-Pennesi, B. Flannery, L. Dolan, S. Dennis, and S. Fitzpatrick. 2020. Lead exposures in older children (males and females 7–17 years), women of childbearing age (females 16–49 years) and adults (males and females 18+ years): FDA total diet study 2014–16. *Food Additives & Contaminants: Part A* 37(1):104-109.

Goyer, R. A., and T. W. Clarkson. 2001. Toxic effects of metals. In *Casarett and Doull's toxicology: The basic science of poisons*. Edited by C. D. Klassen. New York: McGraw-Hill. Pp. 811-867.

Grant, K. S., T. M. Burbacher, E. M. Faustman, and L. Gratttan. 2010. Domoic acid: Neurobehavioral consequences of exposure to a prevalent marine biotoxin. *Neurotoxicology and Teratology* 32(2):132-141.

Grieb, T. M., N. S. Fisher, R. Karimi, and L. Levin. 2020. An assessment of temporal trends in mercury concentrations in fish. *Ecotoxicology* 29(10):1739-1749.

Hamilton, K. A., A. Chen, E. de-Graft Johnson, A. Gitter, S. Kozak, C. Niquice, A. G. Zimmer-Faust, M. H. Weir, J. Mitchell, and P. Gurian. 2018. Salmonella risks due to consumption of aquaculture-produced shrimp. *Microbial Risk Analysis* 9:22-32.

Health Canada. 2007. *Human health risk assessment of mercury in fish and health benefits of fish consumption.* https://www.canada.ca/en/health-canada/services/food-nutrition/reports-publications/human-health-risk-assessment-mercury-fish-health-benefits-fish-consumption.html (accessed February 28, 2024).

Health Canada. 2019a. *Mercury–in fish - questions and answers.* https://www.canada.ca/en/health-canada/services/food-nutrition/food-safety/chemical-contaminants/environmental-contaminants/mercury/mercury-fish-questions-answers.html (accessed December 8, 2023).

Health Canada. 2019b. *Mercury in fish.* https://www.canada.ca/en/health-canada/services/food-nutrition/food-safety/chemical-contaminants/environmental-contaminants/mercury/mercury-fish.html (accessed February 4, 2024).

Health Canada. 2019c. *Fifth report on human biomonitoring of environmental chemicals in Canada.* Results of the Canadian Health Measures Survey cycle 5 (2016-2017). https://www.canada.ca/en/health-canada/services/environmental-workplace-health/reports-publications/environmental-contaminants/fifth-report-human-biomonitoring.html (accessed February 28, 2024).

Health Canada. 2021. *Mercury in Canadians.* https://www.canada.ca/en/health-canada/services/environmental-workplace-health/reports-publications/environmental-contaminants/human-biomonitoring-resources/mercury-canadians.html#a4 (accessed February 4, 2024).

Hight, S. C., and J. Cheng. 2006. Determination of methylmercury and estimation of total mercury in seafood using high performance liquid chromatography (HPLC) and inductively coupled plasma-mass spectrometry (ICP-MS): Method development and validation. *Analytica Chimica Acta* 567(2):160-172.

Hopf, N. B., A. M. Ruder, M. A. Waters, and P. Succop. 2013. Concentration-dependent half-lives of polychlorinated biphenyl in sera from an occupational cohort. *Chemosphere* 91(2):172-178.

Huang, Y., V. Ghate, L. Phua, and H. G. Yuk. 2012. Prevalence of *Salmonella* and *Vibrio* spp. in seafood products sold in Singapore. *Journal of Food Protection* 75(7):1320-1323.

Humphrey, H., J. C. Gardiner, J. R. Pandya, A. M. Sweeney, D. M. Gasior, R. J. McCaffrey, and S. L. Schantz. 2000. PCB congener profile in the serum of humans consuming Great Lakes fish. *Environmental Health Perspectives* 108(2):167-172.

IOM (Institute of Medicine). 2007. *Seafood choices: Balancing benefits and risks*. Washington, DC: The National Academies Press.

Jaishankar, M., T. Tseten, N. Anbalagan, B. B. Mathew, and K. N. Beeregowda. 2014. Toxicity, mechanism and health effects of some heavy metals. *Interdisciplinary Toxicology* 7(2):60-72.

Jankong, P., C. Chalhoub, N. Kienzl, W. Goessler, K. A. Francesconi, and P. Visoottiviseth. 2007. Arsenic accumulation and speciation in freshwater fish living in arsenic-contaminated waters. *Environmental Chemistry* 4(1):11-17.

Junqué, E., A. Tardón, A. Fernandez-Somoano, and J. O. Grimalt. 2022. Environmental and dietary determinants of metal exposure in four-year-old children from a cohort located in an industrial area (Asturias, northern Spain). *Environmental Research* 214:113862.

Kalloo, G., G. A. Wellenius, L. McCandless, A. M. Calafat, A. Sjodin, M. Karagas, A. Chen, K. Yolton, B. P. Lanphear, and J. M. Braun. 2018. Profiles and predictors of environmental chemical mixture exposure among pregnant women: The health outcomes and measures of the environment study. *Environmental Science & Technology* 52(17):10104-10113.

Karagas, M. R., A. L. Choi, E. Oken, M. Horvat, R. Schoeny, E. Kamai, W. Cowell, P. Grandjean, and S. Korrick. 2012. Evidence on the human health effects of low-level methylmercury exposure. *Environmental Health Perspectives* 120(6):799-806.

Karimi, R., T. P. Fitzgerald, and N. S. Fisher. 2012. A quantitative synthesis of mercury in commercial seafood and implications for exposure in the United States. *Environmental Health Perspectives* 120(11):1512-1519.

Kingsley, S. L., M. N. Eliot, K. T. Kelsey, A. M. Calafat, S. Ehrlich, B. P. Lanphear, A. Chen, and J. M. Braun. 2018. Variability and predictors of serum perfluoroalkyl substance concentrations during pregnancy and early childhood. *Environmental Research* 165:247-257.

Kroepfl, N., K. B. Jensen, K. A. Francesconi, and D. Kuehnelt. 2015. Human excretory products of selenium are natural constituents of marine fish muscle. *Analytical and Bioanalytical Chemistry* 407(25):7713-7719.

Lee, J.-W., H. Choi, U.-K. Hwang, J.-C. Kang, Y. J. Kang, K. I. Kim, and J.-H. Kim. 2019. Toxic effects of lead exposure on bioaccumulation, oxidative stress, neurotoxicity, and immune responses in fish: A review. *Environmental Toxicology and Pharmacology* 68:101-108.

Leng, F., S. Lin, W. Wu, J. Zhang, J. Song, and M. Zhong. 2019. Epidemiology, pathogenetic mechanism, clinical characteristics, and treatment of *Vibrio vulnificus* infection: A case report and literature review. *European Journal of Clinical Microbiology and Infectious Diseases* 38(11):1999-2004.

Lescord, G. L., T. A. Johnston, B. A. Branfireun, and J. M. Gunn. 2018. Percentage of methylmercury in the muscle tissue of freshwater fish varies with body size and age and among species. *Environmental Toxicology and Chemistry* 37(10):2682-2691.

Levin-Schwartz, Y., C. Gennings, B. Claus Henn, B. A. Coull, D. Placidi, R. Lucchini, D. R. Smith, and R. O. Wright. 2020. Multi-media biomarkers: Integrating information to improve lead exposure assessment. *Environmental Research* 183:109148.

Lischka, S., U. Arroyo-Abad, J. Mattusch, A. Kühn, and C. Piechotta. 2013. The high diversity of arsenolipids in herring fillet (*Clupea harengus*). *Talanta* 110:144-152.

Llop, S., M. Murcia, X. Aguinagalde, J. Vioque, M. Rebagliato, A. Cases, C. Iñiguez, M.-J. Lopez-Espinosa, A. Amurrio, and E. M. Navarrete-Muñoz. 2014. Exposure to mercury among Spanish preschool children: Trend from birth to age four. *Environmental Research* 132:83-92.

Lopez, M. C., R. F. Ungaro, H. V. Baker, L. L. Moldawer, A. Robertson, M. Abbott, S. M. Roberts, L. M. Grattan, and J. G. Morris, Jr. 2016. Gene expression patterns in peripheral blood leukocytes in patients with recurrent ciguatera fish poisoning: Preliminary studies. *Harmful Algae* 57(Pt B):35-38.

López-González, U., G. Riutort-Mayol, R. Soler-Blasco, M. Lozano, M. Murcia, J. Vioque, G. Iriarte, F. Ballester, and S. Llop. 2023. Exposure to mercury among Spanish adolescents: Eleven years of follow-up. *Environmental Research* 231:116204.

Lordan, R., and I. Zabetakis. 2022. Cadmium: A focus on the brown crab (*Cancer pagurus*) industry and potential human health risks. *Toxics* 10(10).

Luvonga, C., C. A. Rimmer, L. L. Yu, and S. B. Lee. 2020. Determination of total arsenic and hydrophilic arsenic species in seafood. *Journal of Food Composition and Analysis* 96(103729).

MacLeod, M., H. P. H. Arp, M. B. Tekman, and A. Jahnke. 2021. The global threat from plastic pollution. *Science* 373(6550):61-65.

Mahaffey, K. R., R. P. Clickner, and C. C. Bodurow. 2004. Blood organic mercury and dietary mercury intake: National Health and Nutrition Examination Survey, 1999 and 2000. *Environmental Health Perspectives* 112(5):562-570.

Mahaffey, K. R., R. P. Clickner, and R. A. Jeffries. 2009. Adult women's blood mercury concentrations vary regionally in the United States: Association with patterns of fish consumption (NHANES 1999–2004). *Environmental Health Perspectives* 117(1):47-53.

McAdam, J., and E. M. Bell. 2023. Determinants of maternal and neonatal PFAS concentrations: A review. *Environmental Health: A Global Access Science Source* 22(1):41.

Murphy, J., and K. D. Cashman. 2001. Selenium content of a range of Irish foods. *Food and Chemistry* 74:493-498.

Navarro-Alarcon, M., and C. Cabrera-Vique. 2008. Selenium in food and the human body: A review. *Science of the Total Environment* 400:115-141.

Notario-Barandiaran, L., S. Díaz-Coto, N. Jimenez-Redondo, M. Guxens, M. Vrijheid, A. Andiarena, A. Irizar, I. Riaño-Galan, A. Fernández-Somoano, and S. Llop. 2023. Latent childhood exposure to mixtures of metals and neurodevelopmental outcomes in 4–5-year-old children living in Spain. *Exposure and Health* 1-14.

OEHHA (California Office of Environmental Health Hazard Assessment). 2017. *Frequently asked questions about domoic acid in seafood.* https://oehha.ca.gov/fish/fact-sheet/frequently-asked-questions-about-domoic-acid-seafood (accessed February 4, 2024).

OHA (Oregon Health Authority). 2015. *Technical Report: Soft-shell clam advisory for the Oregon coast.* Salem, OR: Oregon Health Authority.

Olmedo, P., A. F. Hernández, A. Pla, P. Femia, A. Navas-Acien, and F. Gil. 2013. Determination of essential elements (copper, manganese, selenium and zinc) in fish and shellfish samples. Risk and nutritional assessment and mercury–selenium balance. *Food and Chemical Toxicology* 62:299-307.

Pacific Shellfish Institute. 2008. *Characterization of the cadmium health risk, concentrations and ways to minimize cadmium residues in shellfish: Sampling and analysis of cadmium in U.S. West coast bivalve shellfish.* Olympia, WA: Pacific Shellfish Institute.

Pennotti, R., E. Scallan, L. Backer, J. Thomas, and F. J. Angulo. 2013. Ciguatera and scombroid fish poisoning in the United States. *Foodborne Pathogens and Disease* 10(12):1059-1066.

Petersen, G. I., and P. Kristensen. 1998. Bioaccumulation of lipophilic substances in fish early life stages. *Environmental Toxicology and Chemistry* 17(7):1385-1395.

Petroff, R., T. Richards, B. Crouthamel, N. McKain, C. Stanley, K. S. Grant, S. Shum, J. Jing, N. Isoherranen, and T. M. Burbacher. 2019. Chronic, low-level oral exposure to marine toxin, domoic acid, alters whole brain morphometry in nonhuman primates. *Neurotoxicology* 72:114-124.

Pintó, R. M., M. I. Costafreda, and A. Bosch. 2009. Risk assessment in shellfish-borne outbreaks of hepatitis A. *Applied Environmental Microbiology* 75(23):7350-7355. https://doi.org/10.1128/AEM.01177-09. PMID: 19820160; PMCID: PMC2786421.

Radke, E. G., A. Reich, and J. G. Morris, Jr. 2015. Epidemiology of ciguatera in Florida. *American Journal of Tropical Medicine and Hygiene* 93(2):425-432.

Raml, R., G. Raber, A. Rumpler, T. Bauernhofer, W. Goessler, and K. A. Francesconi. 2009. Individual variability in the human metabolism of an arsenic-containing carbohydrate, 2′,3′-dihydroxypropyl 5-deoxy-5-dimethylarsinoyl-β-d-riboside, a naturally occurring arsenical in seafood. *Chemical Research in Toxicology* 22(9):1534-1540.

Rempelos, L., J. Wang, M. Barański, A. Watson, N. Volakakis, C. Hadall, G. Hasanaliyeva, E. Chatzidimitriou, A. Magistrali, H. Davis, V. Vigar, D. Średnicka-Tober, S. Rushton, K. S. Rosnes, P. O. Iversen, C. J. Seal, and C. Leifert. 2022. Diet, but not food type, significantly affects micronutrient and toxic metal profiles in urine and/or plasma; A randomized, controlled intervention trial. *American Journal of Clinical Nutrition* 116(5):1278-1290

Saktrakulkla, P., T. Lan, J. Hua, R. F. Marek, P. S. Thorne, and K. C. Hornbuckle. 2020. Polychlorinated biphenyls in food. *Environmental Science and Technology* 54(18):11443-11452.

Schaefer, A. M., M. Zoffer, L. Yrastorza, D. M. Pearlman, G. D. Bossart, R. Stoessel, and J. S. Reif. 2019. Mercury exposure, fish consumption, and perceived risk among pregnant women in coastal Florida. *International Journal of Environmental Research and Public Health* 16(24):4903.

Schartup, A. T., C. P. Thackray, A. Qureshi., C. Dassuncao, K. Gillespie, A. Hanke, and E. M. Sunderland. 2019. Climate change and overfishing increase neurotoxicant in marine predators. *Nature* 572:648-650.

Schecter, A., J. Colacino, K. Patel, K. Kannan, S. H. Yun, D. Haffner, T. R. Harris, and L. Birnbaum. 2010a. Polybrominated diphenyl ether levels in foodstuffs collected from three locations from the United States. *Toxicology and Applied Pharmacology* 243(2):217-224.

Schecter, A., D. Haffner, J. Colacino, K. Patel, O. Päpke, M. Opel, and L. Birnbaum. 2010b. Polybrominated diphenyl ethers (PBDEs) and hexabromocyclododecane (HBCD) in composite U.S. food samples. *Environmental Health Perspectives* 118(3):357-362.

Schmeisser, E., W. Goessler, and K. A. Francesconi. 2006. Human metabolism of arsenolipids present in cod liver. *Analytical and Bioanalytical Chemistry* 385:367-376.

Seshasayee, S. M., S. L. Rifas-Shiman, J. E. Chavarro, J. L. Carwile, P.-I. D. Lin, A. M. Calafat, S. K. Sagiv, E. Oken, and A. F. Fleisch. 2021. Dietary patterns and PFAS plasma concentrations in childhood: Project Viva, USA. *Environment International* 151:106415.

Shieh, Y. C., Y. E. Khudyakov, G. Xia, L. M. Ganova-Raeva, F. M. Khambaty, J. W. Woods, J. E. Veazey, M. L. Motes, M. B. Glatzer, S. R. Bialek, and A. E. Fiore. 2007. Molecular confirmation of oysters as the vector for hepatitis A in a 2005 multistate outbreak. *Journal of Food Protection* 70(1):145-150.

Signes-Pastor, A. J., E. Gutiérrez-González, M. García-Villarino, F. D. Rodríguez-Cabrera, J. J. López-Moreno, E. Varea-Jiménez, R. Pastor-Barriuso, M. Pollán, A. Navas-Acien, B. Pérez-Gómez, and M. R. Karagas. 2021. Toenails as a biomarker of exposure to arsenic: A review. *Environmental Research* 195:110286.

Sloth, J. J., V. Sele, and K. Julshamn. 2006. Of inorganic arsenic in blue mussel (*Mytilus edulis l.*) from the Norwegian coastline—Impact on seafood safety. Paper read at ISSEBETS, International Symposium on Speciation of Elements in Biological, Environmental and Toxicological Sciences.

Smith, J. L. 1999. Foodborne infections during pregnancy. *Journal of Food Protection* 62(7):818-829.

Soler-Blasco, R., M. Murcia, M. Lozano, X. Aguinagalde, G. Iriarte, M.-J. Lopez-Espinosa, J. Vioque, C. Iniguez, F. Ballester, and S. Llop. 2019. Exposure to mercury among 9-year-old Spanish children: Associated factors and trend throughout childhood. *Environment International* 130:104835.

Spungen, J. H. 2019. Children's exposures to lead and cadmium: FDA total diet study 2014-16. *Food Additives & Contaminants: Part A* 36(6):893-903.

Sunderland, E. M., M. Li, and K. Bullard. 2018. Decadal changes in the edible supply of seafood and methylmercury exposure in the United States. *Environmental Health Perspectives* 126(1):017006.

Taylor, V., B. Goodale, A. Raab, T. Schwerdtle, K. Reimer, S. Conklin, M. R. Karagas, and K. A. Francesconi. 2017. Human exposure to organic arsenic species from seafood. *Science of the Total Environment* 580:266-282.

Tee, P. G., A. M. Sweeney, E. Symanski, J. C. Gardiner, D. M. Gasior, and S. L. Schantz. 2003. A longitudinal examination of factors related to changes in serum polychlorinated biphenyl levels. *Environmental Health Perspectives* 111(5):702-707.

Tillett, T. 2008. Is arsenic "lactation intolerant"? *Environmental Health Perspectives* 116(7):A306.

Venkat, H., J. Matthews, P. Lumadao, B. Caballero, J. Collins, N. Fowle, M. Kellis, M. Tewell, S. White, R. Hassan, A. Classon, Y. Joung, K. Komatsu, J. Weiss, S. Zusy, and R. Sunenshine. 2018. *Salmonella enterica* serotype javiana infections linked to a seafood restaurant in Maricopa County, Arizona, 2016. *Journal of Food Protection* 81(8):1283-1292.

Vernon, R. E. 2013. Which elements are metalloids? *Journal of Chemical Education* 90(12):1703-1707.

Viganò, A., N. Pellissier, H. J. Hamad, S. A. Ame, and M. Pontello. 2007. Prevalence of *E. coli*, thermotolerant coliforms, *Salmonella* spp. and *Vibrio* spp. in ready-to-eat foods: Pemba Island, United Republic of Tanzania. *Annali di Igiene* 19(5):395-403.

von Stackelberg, K. 2011. PCBs. In *Encyclopedia of environmental health*. Edited by J. O. Nriagu. New York: Elsevier. Pp. 346-356.

Wagemann, R., W. Lockhart, H. Welch, and S. Innes. 1995. Arctic marine mammals as integrators and indicators of mercury in the arctic. *Water, Air, and Soil Pollution* 80:683-693.

Washington State Department of Health. 2024a. *PBDEs*. https://doh.wa.gov/community-and-environment/contaminants/pbdes (accessed February 4, 2024).

Washington State Department of Health. 2024b. *Paralytic shellfish poisoning (PSP)*. https://doh.wa.gov/community-and-environment/shellfish/recreational-shellfish/illnesses/biotoxins/paralytic-shellfish-poisoning (accessed February 4, 2024).

Wattigney, W. A., E. Irvin-Barnwell, Z. Li, and A. Ragin-Wilson. 2019. Biomonitoring of mercury and persistent organic pollutants in Michigan urban anglers and association with fish consumption. *International Journal of Hygiene and Environmental Health* 222(6):936-944.

Weitekamp, C. A., L. J. Phillips, L. M. Carlson, N. M. DeLuca, E. A. Cohen Hubal, and G. M. Lehmann. 2021. A state-of-the-science review of polychlorinated biphenyl exposures at background levels: Relative contributions of exposure routes. *Science of the Total Environment* 776:145912.

WHO (World Health Organization). 2010. *Persistent organic pollutants: Impact on child health*. https://iris.who.int/bitstream/handle/10665/44525/9789241501101 (accessed February 4, 2024).

Xiong, C., M. Stiboller, R. A. Glabonjat, L. Rieger, L. Paton, and K. A. Francesconi. 2020. Transport of arsenolipids to the milk of a nursing mother after consuming salmon fish. *Journal of Trace Elements in Medicine and Biology* 61:126502.

Xue, J., S. V. Liu, V. G. Zartarian, A. M. Geller, and B. D. Schultz. 2014. Analysis of NHANES measured blood PCBs in the general US population and application of SHEDS model to identify key exposure factors. *Journal of Exposure Science & Environmental Epidemiology* 24(6):615-621.

Yamashita, Y., H. Amlund, T. Suzuki, T. Hara, M. A. Hossain, T. Yabu, K. Touhata, and M. Yamashita. 2011. Selenoneine, total selenium, and total mercury content in the muscle of fishes. *Fisheries Science* 77:679-686.

Young, W., S. Wiggins, W. Limm, C. M. Fisher, L. DeJager, and S. Genualdi. 2022. Analysis of per-and poly (fluoroalkyl) substances (PFASs) in highly consumed seafood products from US markets. *Journal of Agricultural and Food Chemistry* 70(42):13545-13553.

Zafeiraki, E., W. A. Gebbink, R. L. Hoogenboom, M. Kotterman, C. Kwadijk, E. Dassenakis, and S. P. van Leeuwen. 2019. Occurrence of perfluoroalkyl substances (PFASs) in a large number of wild and farmed aquatic animals collected in the Netherlands. *Chemosphere* 232:415-423.

Zuri, G., A. Karanasiou, and S. Lacorte. 2023. Microplastics: Human exposure assessment through air, water, and food. *Environment International* 179: 108150.

6

Health Outcomes Associated with Seafood Consumption

Seafood provides an array of nutrients that are associated with beneficial health effects for those who are or may become pregnant or are lactating, and for infants, children, and adolescents. In particular, the long-chain omega-3 polyunsaturated fatty acids (n-3 LCPUFAs), as well as docosahexaenoic acid (DHA) and eicosapentaenoic acid, both synthesized from alpha-linolenic acid, have been shown to have a range of health benefits, including neurocognitive development.

As discussed earlier in this report, the average amount of seafood consumed by pregnant women is below recommended levels, and only about one in five U.S. women of childbearing age achieves an intake of seafood that is recommended for optimal maternal and child health. Furthermore, few children and adolescents in the United States and Canada consume the two or more servings of seafood per week recommended by the *Dietary Guidelines for Americans 2020–2025 (DGA)*. The *DGA*, however, acknowledges that robust research on specific health benefits associated with seafood consumption by children is limited, and further evidence is needed to clarify the contribution of seafood consumption to children's health (USDA and HHS, 2020).

This chapter considers seafood consumption patterns, dietary intake and nutrient composition of seafood, and exposure to contaminants associated with seafood consumption, and reviews the evidence on those relationships with child health outcomes. The committee determined that biomarkers of response to seafood consumption were outside the scope of its task.

SEAFOOD CONSUMPTION AND HEALTH OUTCOMES IN CHILDREN AND ADOLESCENTS

The discussion of evidence on seafood consumption and health outcomes in children and adolescents begins with results from systematic reviews commissioned by the committee (Appendix C). Additional evidence on outcomes not included in the commissioned systematic reviews was identified through a review of existing systematic reviews (Appendix D), as well as evidence submitted by the sponsor. Lastly, the committee obtained additional evidence through a narrative review of the published literature and technical reports. Examples of reports that the committee considered include the following:

- "Fish, Shellfish and Children's Health: An Assessment of Benefits, Risks and Sustainability" from the American Academy of Pediatrics Council on Environmental Health Committee on Nutrition (Bernstein et al., 2019)

- The U.S. Food and Drug Administration's (FDA's) *Quantitative Assessment of the Net Effects on Fetal Neurodevelopment from Eating Commercial Fish* (FDA, 2014)
- The *Report of the Joint FAO/WHO Expert Consultation on the Risks and Benefits of Fish Consumption* (FAO/WHO, 2011)
- The Summary and Conclusions from the second *Joint FAO/WHO Expert Consultation on Risks and Benefits of Fish Consumption* (FAO/WHO, 2023)
- The Norwegian Scientific Committee for Food and Environment (VKM) report *Benefit and Risk Assessment of Fish in the Norwegian Diet* (Andersen et al., 2022).

Updated Reviews

The committee commissioned the Texas A&M Agriculture, Food, and Nutrition Evidence Center to update three existing systematic reviews previously published by the U.S. Department of Agriculture's Nutrition Evidence Systematic Review team for the 2020 Dietary Guidelines Advisory Committee (DGAC). One review examined relationships between seafood consumption during pregnancy and lactation and neurocognitive development in the child, and another examined seafood consumption during childhood and adolescence and neurocognitive development. A third review examined seafood consumption during childhood and adolescence and cardiovascular disease. An analytic framework was developed to specify the interventions of interest (seafood consumption) during pregnancy and lactation and during childhood and adolescence and outcomes related to neurocognitive development or cardiovascular disease in children and adolescents (see Appendix D).

Summary of Key Systematic Reviews on Relationship Between Seafood Consumption During Pregnancy and Lactation and Neurocognitive Development in the Child

Two systematic reviews of seafood intake and neurocognitive outcomes conducted for the DGAC examined evidence on developmental outcomes, including:

- cognitive development,
- language and communication development,
- movement and physical development,
- social-emotional and behavioral development,
- attention deficit disorder (ADD)/attention deficit hyperactivity disorder (ADHD),
- autism spectrum disorder (ASD),
- academic performance, and
- anxiety and depression (Snetselaar et al., 2020a,b).

Snetselaar et al. (2020a) examined associations of seafood intake during pregnancy and lactation and a range of developmental outcomes. This systematic review found modest evidence that seafood intake during pregnancy is positively associated with measures of cognitive development in young children. The review also found limited evidence that seafood intake during pregnancy was associated with improved measures of language development in the child. There was insufficient evidence, however, to draw conclusions about other outcomes, and there were no studies of seafood intake during lactation that met their inclusion criteria.

Snetselaar et al. (2020b) described the results of the systematic review used by the 2020 DGAC to assess associations of seafood consumption with neurocognitive outcomes in children and adolescents. Based on 13 included studies, the review concluded that seafood intake during childhood and adolescence had either a beneficial or nonsignificant relationship across developmental domains, particularly in cognitive development, language and communication development, and movement and physical development. No conclusions were made regarding the relationships between seafood intake and developmental domains because of the inadequate number of studies, inconsistency in results, risk of bias in classification of exposures, and heterogeneity of outcome assessments.

Considerable variability was found across the instruments used to capture cognitive function; some authors used caregiver reporting and others used other tools to assess seafood consumption with outcomes.

Similarly, no conclusions were made regarding the relationships between seafood intake and academic performance, ADD/ADHD, anxiety and depression, or ASD, owing to an inadequate number of studies. It is important to note that neither review identified evidence of harm from maternal or child fish consumption in relation to child neurodevelopmental outcomes.

In the systematic review update commissioned by the committee, 11 additional studies were identified that met the review criteria. (Appendix C). Only one of the studies, a randomized controlled trial (RCT) conducted in a Norwegian population (Kvestad et al. 2021), found a significant beneficial effect of fish consumption during pregnancy and developmental outcomes in the child as measured by maternal reporting on developmental screening questionnaires. The study randomized 133 pregnant women (at 19 weeks of gestation or less) to receive 200 g cod fillet twice weekly (intervention) or to maintain their habitual diet (control) for 16 weeks. No difference was found between infants in the intervention and control groups on the total Ages and Stages Questionnaire, 2nd edition (ASQ-2), scores at 3, 6, and 11 months. A difference was found, however, on the ASQ: Social-Emotional scores in favor of the intervention group (P = 0.020). Thus, while there was no evidence for an effect of increased cod intake during pregnancy on overall child development in the first year of life, there was a positive effect on socioemotional development.

In contrast, two studies identified negative effects of fish (cod) consumption, one on gross motor development (Varsi et al., 2022) and one using the Bayley Scales of Infant Development cognitive composite scores (Markus et al., 2021). The remaining studies reported null findings and none of the studies found evidence of harm.

Summary of a Key Systematic Review on the Relationship Between Seafood Consumption During Childhood and Cardiovascular Disease

In the third review conducted for the 2020 DGAC, Snetselaar et al. (2020c) examined the relationship of seafood consumption during childhood and cardiovascular disease. The health outcomes included in this review were blood pressure, total cholesterol, low-density lipoprotein (LDL) cholesterol, high-density lipoprotein (HDL) cholesterol, HDL cholesterol, serum triglycerides, and overall cardiovascular disease. One RCT and one prospective cohort study reported no significant relationship between tuna or fish intake and blood pressure in children ages 10–12 years. One RCT reported lower total cholesterol with higher tuna consumption in girls, but not boys; two RCTs and one prospective cohort study reported lower triglyceride levels associated with higher fish consumption or no significant relationship. No studies on cardiovascular disease met the inclusion criteria for the systematic review. The authors could not derive any conclusions on these outcomes because of insufficient evidence, and a grade was not assignable.

Supplemental Reviews of Systematic Reviews

The committee's supplemental review (Appendix D) identified additional systematic reviews on associations of seafood consumption during pregnancy and lactation, and childhood, that included outcomes not covered by the commissioned systematic review update. The evidence from these reviews is summarized in the following sections.

Neurodevelopmental Outcomes

Hibbeln et al. (2019) conducted two systematic reviews on neurodevelopmental outcomes. The first review addressed the relationship between maternal seafood consumption during pregnancy and lactation and neurocognitive development of the infant. This review identified 29 studies representing 24 unique cohorts. Of the 29 studies, 24 reported beneficial outcomes associated with maternal seafood consumption and neurocognition on some or all the tests administered to children. Based on their analysis, the authors reported moderate and consistent evidence for an association of consumption of a broad range of amounts and types of commercially available seafood during pregnancy with improved neurocognitive development in the offspring as compared to not consuming seafood.

These studies suggested benefits to neurocognitive development occurred across the lowest (approximately 4 oz/week) to the highest (greater than 12 oz/week, including up to more than 100 oz/week) levels of intake. The authors further concluded that the evidence did not meet the criteria for "strong evidence" owing to a paucity of RCTs that may not be ethical or feasible to conduct during pregnancy.

The second review addressed the relationship between seafood consumption during childhood and adolescence (up to 18 years of age) and neurocognitive development. This review yielded 15 articles, comprising 25,031 children (six RCTs, four prospective cohorts, and nine case–control studies published between 2001 and 2019). They found moderate and consistent evidence indicating that seafood consumption of more than 4 oz/week and likely greater than 12 oz/week during childhood has beneficial associations with neurocognitive outcomes. No study in the review reported net adverse outcomes from seafood consumption in children; therefore, the authors concluded that it was unlikely that mercury exposure from seafood consumption by children was associated with substantive neurocognitive harms (Hibbeln et al., 2019).

Avella-Garcia and Julvez (2014) conducted a systematic review of primarily prospective cohort studies on seafood intake during pregnancy and childhood with a range of neurodevelopmental, behavioral, cognitive, and general developmental outcomes. Of the 16 publications identified in the review, 8 evaluated seafood exposure prenatally, 5 evaluated postnatal exposure, and 3 studies evaluated both pre- and postnatal exposure. All but two studies were prospective cohorts and most used food frequency questionnaires (FFQs) to assess seafood consumption.

Most of the studies found that seafood intake during pregnancy and postnatal periods appeared, overall, to be beneficial in connection with a wide range of neurodevelopmental outcomes, including neurological and cognitive functions, social competence, hyperactivity, and school performance, although potential risks such as inattention, hyperactivity, or impulsivity were identified at higher levels of intake. In general, prenatal exposure to seafood as part of the maternal diet was found to be associated with benefits in developmental outcomes in the child, including neurological, behavioral, and cognitive functioning. Seafood consumption was associated with improved neurological functions and lower disorder prevalence; better performances in cognitive functions related to verbal, memory, and visual-performance abilities; and improved behavioral outcomes such as hyperactivity, social competence, and school grades.

Some studies (de Groot et al., 2012; Freire et al., 2010; Mendez et al., 2009) observed an inverted U-shape pattern in the association between seafood intake and the neurodevelopment of children, which may be related to higher pollutant exposure in the heavy seafood consumers. Freire et al. (2010) suggested that consuming oily fish as a source of DHA concentrations counterbalanced some neurotoxic effects. Avella-Garcia and Julvez (2014) concluded from the review that public guidance should acknowledge the risk of contaminant exposure with large amounts of seafood, especially species with high mercury concentrations, while also noting the benefits of moderate intake.

Asthma and Allergic Outcomes

Yang et al. (2013) conducted a systematic review of studies on fish intake and risk of child asthma. A meta-analysis of three studies suggested that fish consumption in infants was associated with decreased risk of asthma during childhood. Two studies reported that higher levels of n-3 LCPUFAs in expressed breast milk were associated with lower incidence of asthma in their offspring. Maternal intake of fish during pregnancy was not reported to be related to development of asthma in their offspring.

A 2011 systematic review explored the associations between seafood intake and atopic or allergic outcomes in infants and children (Kremmyda et al., 2011). Positive associations were reported for maternal fish intake and atopic or allergic outcomes in their offspring, based on four cohort studies and one case–control study. When looking at associations between these outcomes and seafood intake by the infant or child, however, the results reported from five cohort, six cross-sectional, and three case-control studies were inconsistent. The authors concluded that more research is needed in this area before developing a conclusion.

Social-Emotional Outcomes

An RCT by Hysing et al. (2018) investigated associations between fish consumption and social/emotional development in Norway. Children ages 4–6 years were randomized to a fish lunch group (three lunches per week of fatty fish including herring and mackerel) or to a meat lunch group. No significant differences in social and/or emotional development were assessed using the Strengths and Difficulties Questionnaire (SDQ) for young children. In a second Norwegian RCT, teens (average age 14.6 years) were randomized to a high-fish lunch (three lunches of salmon, mackerel, or herring), a high-meat group, or a supplement group (fish oil supplement three times per week). Using the SDQ for older children, no significant differences were observed between groups (Skotheim, et al., 2017).

In a third RCT conducted in Denmark, children ages 9–10 years were randomized to a high-fish consumption group (compared with a high-poultry consumption group). Using the Behavior Rating Inventory of Executive Function, no significant differences were found in social and/or emotional developmental scores (Teisen et al., 2020).

Other Reports Related to Seafood Consumption and Child Health

The Food and Agriculture Organization of the United Nations (FAO) and World Health Organization (WHO) convened two Expert Consultations on the risks and benefits of fish consumption. The first, published in 2011, had the following three conclusions related to fish consumption by women and children:

1. When comparing the benefits of n-3 LCPUFAs with the risks of Hg among women of childbearing age, maternal fish consumption lowers the risk of suboptimal neurodevelopment in their offspring compared with the offspring of women not eating fish in most circumstances evaluated.
2. At levels of maternal exposure to dioxins (from fish and other dietary sources) that do not exceed the provisional tolerable monthly intake (PTMI) of 70 pg/kg body weight established by the Joint FAO/WHO Expert Committee on Food Additives (for polychlorinated dibenzodioxins [PCDDs], polychlorinated dibenzofurans [PCDFs], and coplanar PCBs), neurodevelopmental risk for the fetus is negligible. At levels of maternal exposure to dioxins (from fish and other dietary sources) that exceed the PTMI, neurodevelopmental risk for the fetus may no longer be negligible.
3. Among infants, young children, and adolescents, the available data are currently insufficient to derive a quantitative framework of the health risks and health benefits of eating fish. However, healthy dietary patterns that include fish consumption and are established early in life influence dietary habits and health during adult life (FAO/WHO, 2011, p. 33).

The most recent FAO/WHO Expert Consultation occurred in 2023, and while the full report has not yet been released, the published executive summary includes the following three conclusions relevant to this report:

1. Strong evidence exists for the benefits of total fish consumption during all life stages: pregnancy, childhood, and adulthood. For example, associations are found for maternal consumption during pregnancy with improved birth outcomes and for adult consumption with reduced risks for cardiovascular and neurological diseases. This evidence for health benefits of total fish consumption reflects the overall effects of nutrients and contaminants in fish on the studied outcomes, including nutrients and contaminants not specifically considered in the evidence review.
2. Benefits derived from general population studies and individual effects will vary depending on overall diet (e.g., selenium intake, exposure to other contaminants) and characteristics of consumers (e.g., n-3 [LC]PUFA status and individual susceptibility) and fish consumed (e.g., fish species and food preparation methods).
3. Risk–benefit assessments at regional, national, or subnational levels are needed to refine fish consumption recommendations considering local consumption habits, fish contamination levels, and nutrient content; nutritional status of the population of interest; cultural habits; and demographics (FAO/WHO, 2023, p. 3).

The VKM conducted a benefit and risk assessment of fish in the Norwegian diet (Andersen et al., 2022). This report consisted of a quantitative assessment of benefits and risks from fish consumption, a semiquantitative benefit assessment of nutrients in fish, and a semi-quantitative risk assessment of contaminants in fish. No associations were categorized as "convincing," but "probable" associations were found for a number of adult health outcomes, as well as for a benefit of fish consumption during pregnancy for preventing both preterm birth and low birth weight. The VKM found "limited, suggestive" evidence for a "protective association between maternal total fish consumption and child neurodevelopment" and also "limited, suggestive" evidence that "child fish consumption (total and fatty fish) benefits neurodevelopment" (Andersen et al., 2022, pp. 303, 320).

The committee notes that 62 percent of Norwegian women consume two or more meals of fish per week and mean intake was 238 grams (8 oz) per week. The overall conclusion of the Norwegian analysis was that low fish consumption is a potential health risk, and that optimal beneficial health effects of fish consumption are not obtained at current fish intake levels in Norway, which are substantially higher than those observed in the United States and Canada. The overall recommendation was for 300–450 g (about 10–16 oz) prepared fish per week for adults, of which at least 200 g should be fatty fish such as salmon, trout, mackerel, or herring. This recommendation is higher than the *DGA*, which recommends 8–12 oz of fish per week.

Summary on Evidence on Health Outcomes Associated with Consumption of Seafood in Pregnancy and Childhood

Taken together, the evidence reviewed by the committee indicates that higher fish consumption by women of childbearing age, including women who are pregnant and lactating, and by children, is not associated with any detectable adverse health outcomes, although one review found a neurocognitive benefit in 13 of 15 studies in the review. Moreover, there is evidence that greater fish consumption by women during pregnancy is likely associated with a number of health benefits, including improved birth outcomes. To date, available evidence for health benefits of child seafood consumption is overall not sufficient for conclusions to be drawn, but evidence does not suggest any harm from seafood consumption among children, in the studied populations, and potential benefits exist.

EXPOSURE TO TOXICANTS IN SEAFOOD AND CHILD GROWTH AND DEVELOPMENT

The Texas A&M Agriculture, Food, and Nutrition Evidence Center was commissioned to conduct a *de novo* systematic review to examine associations between seafood-related contaminants and health outcomes during pregnancy, lactation, childhood, and adolescence, and child growth and development.

An additional review of systematic reviews was carried out for mercury (Hg) exposure. An analytic framework was developed to specify the toxicant exposure to women during pregnancy or lactation and to children and adolescents, and the outcomes in infants, children, and adolescents (Appendix C).

De Novo Systematic Review

The *de novo* review began with a scoping review to determine the state of the current literature on specific exposure–outcome relationships. Some of these studies also reported associations of seafood consumption with the studied health outcomes; where such results are available, they are also summarized below.

Scoping Review

To determine the status of the evidence to support a *de novo* systematic review, a scoping review was conducted that included polychlorinated biphenyls (PCBs), dioxins, polybrominated diphenyl ethers, per- and polyfluoroalkyl substances (PFAS), arsenic, cadmium, lead, selenium, iron, magnesium, zinc, and dichlorodiphenyltrichloroethane (DDT) as exposures through fish consumption. Outcome measures included:

- cognition,
- language,
- motor skills,
- academic performance,
- neurological disorders (ASD, ADHD, seizures, tremors, and gait abnormalities),

- measures of growth and body composition,
- failure to thrive,
- malnutrition and protein deficiency,
- blood pressure, and
- allergy and immune response.

The scoping review was used to identify exposure–outcome pairs with at least three studies to justify a *de novo* systematic review. Of the 12 exposure categories only two exposure–outcome pairs had three or more articles. These were lead (Pb) exposure in pregnant and lactating women and child developmental domains (four studies) and PCB exposure in pregnant and lactating women and child growth-related outcomes (three studies).

Characteristics of Studies for Lead Exposure Through Seafood Consumption

Table 6-1 describes the characteristics of the identified studies for Pb exposure in pregnant and lactating women and child developmental domains.

Summary of Key Studies for Lead Exposure Through Seafood Consumption

Jeong et al. (2017) assessed associations of heavy metal concentrations in pregnant women with the concentrations in their offspring as part of the Mothers' and Children's Environmental Health study of 1,751 pregnant women in Korea. Metal concentrations included Pb, total Hg, and cadmium (Cd) in cord blood during early and

TABLE 6-1 Characteristics of Studies for Lead Exposure in Pregnant and Lactating Women and Child Developmental Domains

Study Characteristics: Name, Year, Study Design, Country, Cohort, Analytic sample (n)	Exposure Assessment		Outcomes			Results: Associations		ROBINS-E
	Fish/seafood exposure; timing	Pb exposure assessment; timing	Maternal seafood/fish intake and maternal Pb levels	Duration	Maternal seafood/fish intake and maternal Pb levels	Maternal Pb levels and child outcomes	Maternal seafood/fish and child outcomes	Overall risk of bias
Jeong, 2017 Prospective cohort Korea Mothers and Children's Environmental Health n= 553	Maternal fish intake Late pregnancy	Maternal blood Late pregnancy	Korean version of Wechsler Preschool and Primary Scale of Intelligence (K-WPPSI); Verbal, performance, and total IQ	60 months	NR	Maternal: NS Child: Beneficial	Maternal: NS Child: Direction NR	High
Rothenberg, 2016 Prospective Cohort China Daxin County n= 270	Maternal fish and shellfish intake Peripartum, during 3rd trimester	Maternal blood Peripartum	Bayley Scales of Infant Development (BSID)-II; Psychomotor Developmental Index (PDI); Mental Developmental Index (MDI)	12 months	NS, beneficial	Maternal: Significantly beneficial Child: NS, beneficial	Maternal: Significantly detrimental Child: NS, detrimental	High
Rothenberg, 2021 Prospective Cohort China Daxin County n= 190	Maternal fish and shellfish intake Peripartum, during 3rd trimester	Maternal blood Peripartum	Bayley Scales of Infant Development (BSID)-II; Psychomotor Developmental Index (PDI); Mental Developmental Index (MDI)	36 months	NR	Maternal: Significantly beneficial Child: NS, beneficial	Maternal and Child: NS, detrimental	High

NOTES: NR = not recorded; NS = nonsignificant; Pb = lead; ROBINS-E = Risk of Bias in Non-randomized Studies—of Exposure Tool.
SOURCE: Table created using data from Texas A&M Agriculture, Food, and Nutrition Evidence Center, 2023.

late pregnancy, and in children who were age 2, 3, and 5 years. Concentrations of Pb were lowest in cord blood, highest in children 2 years of age, and thereafter decreased with child age. Overall, the study found strong correlations between the Pb and total Hg levels during late pregnancy with the levels in cord blood. Correlations between the Pb and Hg levels in women during late pregnancy and cord blood with the levels in their children were weak.

Rothenberg et al. (2016) looked for associations of maternal consumption of seafood and Pb levels in rural China and found no significant correlation. All three studies (Jeong et al., 2017; Rothenberg et al., 2016, 2021) examined relationships between maternal Pb level and child development outcomes. Jeong et al. (2017) found no significant association, while Rothenberg et al. (2016) found a significant negative association between maternal Pb level and psychomotor index in the child at 12 months of age. Both Rothenberg studies found negative but nonsignificant associations between maternal Pb level and psychomotor index at 36 months of age. Taken together, the evidence from the three studies showed inconsistency in associations between Pb exposure through seafood consumption and health outcomes. As shown in Table 6-1, all the studies identified had a high risk of bias, which the committee considered when assessing the totality of the evidence on health outcomes related to exposure to metals.

Characteristics of Studies for PCB Exposure Through Seafood Consumption

Table 6-2 shows characteristics of the studies for PCB exposure during pregnancy and child development outcomes.

Summary of Key Studies for Exposure to PCBs

Using data from the Danish National Birth Cohort, Halldorsson et al. (2008) examined the associations between fatty fish intake and plasma PCB levels during pregnancy and the association of maternal PCB levels with fetal growth. The investigators obtained dietary intake data from a food frequency questionnaire and PCB concentrations from blood samples during pregnancy and at delivery. The study further found a positive correlation between total maternal lipid concentration and plasma PCB level, adjusting for plasma lipid concentrations. The study concluded that maternal exposure to PCBs through regular consumption of fatty fish was positively associated with PCB levels and inversely associated with both birth weight and placental weight.

In a study examining associations of maternal seafood consumption during pregnancy and small-for-gestational age (SGA) as a birth outcome, Mendez et al. (2009) obtained data from a population-based longitudinal study (*Infancia y Medio Ambiente*) in Spain with women enrolled in the first trimester of pregnancy. A food frequency questionnaire was used to obtain data on seafood consumption. Birth weight and lengths of infants and length of gestation were gathered at birth. The study found that higher maternal intake of crustaceans and tuna during pregnancy was associated with significantly greater risk of SGA, whereas there was no association among women who consumed lean fish or other shellfish. Associations of risk of SGA for infants of women who consumed fatty fish were not significant. The results of the study suggest that high maternal consumption of crustaceans and tuna may be associated with increased risk of SGA, although the causal chain that links fish consumption to SGA is unclear.

Miyashita et al. (2015) assessed the effects of in utero exposure to PCBs and methylmercury (MeHg) on birth size in the Japanese population. Levels of PCBs and n-3 LCPUFAs in maternal blood and the total Hg in hair were measured during pregnancy and at delivery. An FFQ, administered at delivery, was used to estimate maternal fish and shellfish consumption. This study found no association of PCB concentration and birth size. The study did find that risk of SGA decreased with increasing MeHg concentration when adjusted for n-3 LCPUFA intake.

Wohlfahrt-Veje et al. (2014) examined associations of dioxin and PCB exposure with insulin-like growth factor 1 (IGF1) levels and growth in early childhood. The investigation used data from the longitudinal Copenhagen Mother Child Cohort of Growth and Reproduction study of 2,098 mother–infant pairs recruited from 1997 to 2001. The study found associations of levels of exposure to environmental dioxin-like chemicals and accelerated infant height and weight gain as well as increased IGF1 concentrations at 3 months of age. Associations between dioxins and weight-for-length at birth were negative but not significant. The investigators concluded that early exposure to dioxins and dioxin-like compounds was associated with accelerated early childhood growth in height and weight, which is further associated with greater risk of adult obesity and associated chronic disease.

TABLE 6-2 Characteristics of Studies for PCB Exposure During Pregnancy and Child Development Outcomes

Study Characteristics: Name, Year, Study Design, Country, Cohort, Analytic sample (n)	Exposure Assessment		Outcomes		Results: Associations			ROBINS-E
	Fish/seafood exposure; timing	PCB exposure assessment; timing	Measured Outcomes	Age	Maternal seafood/fish intake and maternal PCB levels	Maternal seafood/ fish intake and child outcomes	Maternal PCB levels and child outcomes	Overall risk of bias
Halldorsson, 2008 Prospective cohort Denmark Danish National Birth Cohort n= 100	Maternal fatty fish 12, 25, and 30 weeks at gestation	Maternal blood plasma 8 and 25 weeks at gestation	Weight (g); length (cm); head circumference (cm); placental weight (g)	At birth	Significantly detrimental	NR	Maternal: NS Child: Direction NR	High
Mendez, 2009 Prospective Cohort Spain INfancia y Medio Ambiente (INMA) n= 592	Maternal seafood intake ~13 weeks at gestation	Maternal serum End of 1st trimester and beginning of 2nd trimester	Weight (g); small-for-gestational age (SGA) (cm); not clear if SGA measured by weight or length	At birth	Significantly detrimental	Maternal: Significantly detrimental Child: NS, mixed directions	NR	Some concerns
Miyashita, 2015 Prospective Cohort Japan Hokkaido on Environment and Children's Health n= 367	Maternal fish intake 3rd trimester	Maternal whole blood 3rd trimester or within 5 days postpartum if anemic	Weight (g); SGA by weight and length (cm); chest and head circumference (cm)	At birth	Significantly detrimental NS, detrimental	NS, mixed directions	NS, mixed directions	Very high
Wohlfahrt-Veje, 2014 Prospective Cohort Denmark Copenhagen Mother Child Cohort of Growth and Reproduction n= 417	Maternal fish intake During pregnancy	Breast milk Between 1-3 months post-natal	Weight and length	At birth, 3, 18, and 36 months	Significantly detrimental	NR	Maternal: Significantly, mixed directions Child: NS, mixed directions	High

NOTES: NR = not recorded; NS = nonsignificant; ROBINS-E = Risk of Bias in Non-randomized Studies—of Exposure Tool.
SOURCE: Texas A&M Agriculture, Food, and Nutrition Evidence Center, 2023.

Summary of Findings on Exposure to PCBs

Evidence from the four studies reviewed showed a significant positive association between seafood consumption during pregnancy and maternal PCB level. This finding was consistent irrespective of the PCB exposure indicator (i.e., maternal whole blood, plasma, serum, or human milk). Mendez et al. (2009) found a significant positive association between prenatal consumption of crustaceans and odds of an SGA infant. Other associations between seafood consumption by type and birth weight or SGA were nonsignificant. Miyashita et al. (2015), however, found no significant associations between seafood intake during pregnancy and growth outcomes. Among the three studies that examined an association of maternal PCB level and child growth outcomes, the findings were inconsistent (Halldorsson et al., 2008; Miyashita et al., 2015; Wohlfahrt-Veje et al., 2014).

As noted above for Pb exposure, the evidence from these studies also showed inconsistency in associations between PCB exposure through seafood consumption and health outcomes. Table 6-2 shows high risk of bias across all studies except Mendez, which was rated as "some concerns." The committee considered this inconsistency when assessing the totality of the evidence on health outcomes related to exposure to PCBs.

Review of Systematic Reviews on Maternal Exposure to Mercury

The Texas A&M Agriculture, Food, and Nutrition Evidence Center carried out a review of existing systematic reviews on maternal or childhood exposure to Hg and child growth to determine the state of current evidence on development outcomes not included in the *de novo* systematic review (see Appendix C). Eleven existing systematic reviews were identified that met the committee's criteria. No existing systematic reviews were identified for

TABLE 6-3 Systematic Reviews by Prioritized Outcomes and the Overall Quality of Evidence

Prioritized Outcome	Existing Review(s)	Overall Quality Assessment Rating
Developmental milestones (3 systematic reviews)	Dack et al., 2022	12 (Moderate–high)
	Ealo Tapia et al., 2023	10 (Moderate–high)
	Saavedra et al., 2022	9.5 (Moderate–high)
Neurological disorders: ASD (5 systematic reviews)	Ealo Tapia et al., 2023	10 (Moderate–high)
	Ding et al., 2023	9 (Moderate–high)
	Zhang et al., 2021	9 (Moderate–high)
	Amadi et al., 2022	9 (Moderate–high)
	Sulaiman et al., 2020	7 (Moderate–high)
Growth and body composition (3 systematic reviews)	Dack et al., 2022	12 (Moderate–high)
	Saavedra et al., 2022	9.5 (Moderate–high)
	Kumar et al., 2022	5 (Lower quality)

SOURCE: Texas A&M Agriculture, Food, and Nutrition Evidence Center, 2023.

academic performance or failure to thrive. Table 6-3 shows the studies identified in the initial scoping review by the committee's prioritized outcomes for exposure to Hg, and the overall quality of the evidence. Among these studies, three (Dack et al., 2022; Eola Tapia et al., 2023; Saavedra et al., 2022) were of moderate to high quality and covered the range of developmental domains included in the search.

Summary of Key Studies on Exposure to Mercury

Dack et al. (2022) conducted a systematic review of evidence for associations of prenatal Hg exposure and early neurodevelopment in children ages 3 days to 59 months. The investigators examined patterns of results by Hg biomarker (umbilical cord blood, whole blood, erythrocytes, and hair), the timing of measurement, and child age. Outcome groupings included cognition and language; attention, executive function, and memory; motor function; communication and language development; and composite measures of neurodevelopmental functioning. The analysis found that, at the levels of Hg recorded in studies reviewed, the evidence for an association of prenatal Hg exposure and neurodevelopmental functioning was weak.

The systematic review by Saavedra et al. (2022) examined the effects of maternal exposure to Hg during pregnancy on health outcomes in utero, and among newborns and children up to age 8 years. The review included studies from Europe, Asia, Africa, North America, and South America, and all were observational cohort studies. Levels of Hg were measured in cord blood, maternal venous blood, maternal hair, and umbilical cord tissue. Health outcomes included both cognitive and physical development. The age at assessment of health effects following in utero exposure ranged from birth to 7 years. The analysis suggested that maternal dietary exposure to Hg has a significant effect on the neurological and physical development of children, although the investigators noted wide heterogeneity among studies.

Ealo Tapia et al. (2023) conducted a systematic review to evaluate the scientific evidence on the effects of Hg exposure during the prenatal and postnatal periods and associations with neurodevelopmental disorders. Of 31 studies reviewed, 18 focused on the effects of Hg exposure on neurodevelopment and 13 on behavioral disorders. Of the 18 studies that assessed effects on neurodevelopment, 4 studies assessed the effect of pre- and postnatal exposure to Hg, 8 assessed prenatal exposure, and 6 assessed postnatal period exposure. The reported effects included association of Hg exposure with impaired cognitive and language functions and development of ASD and ADHD. The primary finding of the review indicates that the current scientific evidence on the effects of prenatal and postnatal Hg exposure and its incidence on neurodevelopmental and neurobehavioral disorders is limited.

Evidence from the Peer-Reviewed Published Literature and Technical Reports

Health Outcomes Related to Exposure to Metal and Metalloid Compounds Through Seafood

In 2014, FDA published an assessment of the overall net effects on the developing nervous system of the fetus from the consumption of commercial fish during pregnancy (FDA, 2014). The approach used was a quantitative risk assessment with the added component of calculating dose–response relationships for both adverse and beneficial effects. The assessment assumed that the beneficial and adverse effects act independently of one another but occur at the same time and included estimates of both population-level effects and individual effects.

The modeling component of the assessment included the net effects of consuming fish during pregnancy on three neurodevelopmental endpoints: (1) full IQ at age 9 years, (2) early age verbal development up to 18 months, and (3) later age verbal development through age 9 years. The model first estimated as a current baseline effect that on a population basis, the average neurodevelopment benefits were approximately 0.7 of an IQ point (95% confidence interval [CI] of 0.39–1.37 IQ points) in the United States from maternal consumption of fish during pregnancy. Because no IQ tests are sensitive to such a small difference, it is debatable whether a 0.7-point IQ difference is significant at the level of the individual. However, the assessment then estimated that optimum amounts of each of 47 individual species and market types sold in the United States could result in full-scale IQ gains in the vicinity of three IQ points depending on species and market type.

Optimum amounts always involved multiple IQ points although fish with lower levels of MeHg tended to produce greater gains than fish with higher levels. The assessment estimated somewhat greater gains for verbal IQ when optimum amounts are consumed and somewhat lesser gains for early age verbal development, again involving multiple IQ points. It further estimated that consumption beyond optimum amounts would result in gradual declines in the sizes of the gains, although the amounts necessary for the gains to dissipate completely or be replaced by net adverse effects were typically beyond what most people eat or could eat.

Collectively, these estimates are consistent with the current state of the evidence: higher fish consumption is associated with lower risk of IQ loss, and there is no evidence of increased risk of net adverse effects in the amounts that have been studied to date. At a population level, however, loss of a single IQ point may be meaningful. Furthermore, economic analyses have estimated each additional IQ point, at the population level, may result in 1.3 to 2.2 percent greater lifetime earnings (Grosse and Zhou, 2021).

The 2014 FDA report summarized the available literature on prenatal exposure to Hg from maternal fish consumption (primarily during pregnancy) and fetal neurodevelopment in children. It also examined postnatal exposure from the child's consumption of fish or breast milk that was consumed after the mother consumed fish. Whether the net effects of consuming fish were beneficial or harmful appears to depend on the amounts and types of fish consumed during pregnancy. In some studies, methylmercury (MeHg) likely reduced the size of beneficial effects and possibly caused the net effects to become adverse under some circumstances.

From the report's literature review, two studies from Poland examined exposure to MeHg from prenatal fish consumption and found an inverse association with the Bayley's Scale at 1 year but not at age 2 or 3 years. Three studies on prenatal fish consumption from the Avon Longitudinal Study of Parents and Children (ALSPAC) cohort in the United Kingdom found fatty fish consumption associated with development of stereoscopic vision (the perception of shape and distance of an object with binocular vision) at 3.5 years. Additionally, consumption of fish was shown to have a positive association with the Macarthur Communicative Development Inventory at age 15 months and with the Denver Developmental Screening Test at 18 months of age. Peak benefits were seen with 1–3 servings/week, with a waning or a plateau in benefits at higher intakes. No association was found with elemental Hg.

Four studies in the ALSPAC review from the United States showed positive associations between maternal fish consumption and multiple neurocognitive tests (including IQ) in children from age 6 months through 8 years. Each additional weekly serving of fish consumed by the mother was associated with a 4-point gain in IQ in the child, and each 1.0 ppm of Hg detected in maternal hair was associated with a loss of 7.5 points on visual recognition memory at age 5.5 to 8.4 months. Overall, fish consumption during pregnancy was associated with improvements in the Peabody Picture Vocabulary Test and the Wide Range Assessment of Visual Motor Abilities, and MeHg exposure was associated with reductions in those beneficial outcomes.

Among mothers who consumed two servings of fish per week, lower Hg exposure was associated with higher test scores than higher exposures—with both subgroups experiencing net benefits (compared with no fish consumption, with an overall plateau of effects at two servings/week). Maternal blood Hg levels were associated with reduced test scores and maternal fish consumption was associated with higher scores on the Bayley Scales at age 12, 24, and 36 months and with Wechsler Preschool and Primary Scale of Intelligence scores at age 48 months. In older children, higher maternal Hg and lower fish intake was associated with ADHD-related behaviors at age 8 years.

One study from Denmark did not directly measure exposure through maternal fish consumption, but assumed MeHg exposure was low in fish commonly consumed by the population. This study found that higher fish intake compared with no or lower intake during pregnancy resulted in better performance on developmental milestones including sitting unsupported at age 6 months and climbing stairs and drinking from a cup at age 18 months. Another study in Japan found beneficial outcomes with overall fish consumption, and adverse outcomes with higher Hg exposure in the "motor cluster" facet of the Neonatal Assessment Scale in infants at 3 days of age, but no evidence of a plateau associated with maternal fish consumption.

To determine the correlation of seafood intake and adverse cognitive outcomes associated with exposure to Hg through consumption of seafood, Golding et al. (2022) observed several groups of children across time in both a British and Seychelles cohort. From 1990 to 1992, the British Pre-Birth Cohort Study enrolled a geographic population of pregnant women and followed their pregnancies and their offspring throughout childhood, adolescence, and into adulthood. The results of the study found positive indicators of fish consumption among the children of this cohort.

Choi and Grandjean (2008) reviewed evidence for the effects of MeHg on developmental neurotoxicity and risk of heart disease. The review included two major prospective cohort studies from the Faroe Islands and the Seychelles. The primary sources of exposure were freshwater and marine fish. Biomarkers of exposure for MeHg included hair, cord blood, and cord tissue. The Faroe Island study associated prenatal exposure with decrements in attention, language, verbal memory, and motor speed at 7 and 14 years of follow-up. However, it did not find a protective effect of n-3 LCPUFA or selenium on neurocognitive outcomes. In the Seychelles study, no clear evidence was found for associations of prenatal exposure to MeHg and neurotoxicity, although decreased fine motor function was found among those with fetal exposure levels at or above 10 $\mu g/g$ in maternal hair by age 9 years.

Murcia et al. (2018) conducted a prospective cohort study of pregnant women in four Spanish regions between 2003 and 2008 and followed their children up to 4–5 years. The participants were recruited from the Spanish cohort study *Infancia y Medio Ambiente* (Environment and Childhood). The study found inverse associations between urinary iodine during pregnancy and both cognitive and motor function at ages 4–5 years, but no association with seafood intake was detected.

In a prospective cohort study conducted with a subset of the ALSPAC cohort, researchers examined the association between fish consumption (assessed via FFQ) among 3-year-olds. Using the SDQ, the authors reported no associations between fish consumption and problems reported on the conduct subscale. Collectively there was no evidence to support an association between fish consumption and social and/or emotional development (Ajmal et al., 2022).

The joint and interactive effects of prenatal exposure to Pb, manganese (Mn), Se, and MeHg on executive function behaviors were evaluated in 1,009 mother–child pairs from the Project Viva cohort in the United States (Fruh et al., 2021). An FFQ was used to assess food and beverage intake in early pregnancy and included questions on fish consumption. Parent and teacher evaluations of social, emotional, and self-regulatory behaviors were also included in the analysis. The elements of interest were measured in blood samples from women collected at the beginning of the second trimester of pregnancy. Executive function behaviors and behavioral difficulties were inferred from the Behavior Rating Inventory of Executive Function and the SDQ. The study did not find evidence of interaction between Pb, Mn, Hg, and Se. Overall, the study did not find strong evidence of adverse effects from exposure to the elements on neurobehavioral outcomes, but the investigators did observe a trend of worsening behavior associated with increasing concentrations of the mixture of elements.

As discussed above, exposure to metals and metalloids in early childhood can have adverse effects on neurodevelopment (Snetselaar et al., 2020a,b). A comprehensive study by Rahbar et al. (2020) examined a panel of metals (Pb, As, Mn, Hg, Cd, and aluminum [Al]) against the generalized Weighted Quantile Sum (gWQS) regression models algorithm developed by Lee et al. (2019) to compare exposure to the metals with each of three glutathione S-transferase (GST) genes (GSTP1, GSTT1, and GSTM1) and their possible interactions in relation to ASD. The analysis included an FFQ to collect information about the type and frequency of seafood consumed weekly by children. Specifically, data were collected on the consumption of sardine, mackerel, tuna, salt fish, shellfish, and shrimp. The investigators then compared their findings against a multivariable Conditional Regression Model. They also evaluated the overall mixture association of metals with ASD based on additive positive and negative gWQS models. Overall, the study found inverse associations of the mixture gWQS index score of the six metals. There were also marginally significant interactions identified between GSTP1 and Pb, Hg, and Mn in a mixture with regard to ASD status, although the interaction was no longer significant in the adjusted model.

Kim et al. (2020) investigated heavy metal exposure from domestic consumption of fishery products and proposed guidelines for the safe intake of seafood products to reduce consumer exposure. In this study, fishery products, including flounder, Pacific cutlass fish, chub mackerel, Pacific cod, Alaska pollock, Pacific saury, bastard halibut, Korean rockfish, Japanese Spanish mackerel, Okhotsk atka mackerel, shrimp, crab, croaker, alfonsino, monkfish, Filipino venous, mussel, squid, long arm octopus, and webfoot octopus were collected from local fish markets in Korea. Exposure assessment was conducted for children (age 1–11 years), adolescents (age 12–18 years), and adults (age 19+ years) by combining the heavy metal contamination values with the fishery product consumption data and dividing by body weight. Consumption data were obtained from the Korea National Health and Nutrition Examination Survey from 2010 to 2015. At the 95th percentile of consumption, squid was the leading Cd contributor, followed by Filipino venues, and chub mackerel was the leading contributor of Hg, followed by Alaska pollock. No species-specific differences were found for Pb exposure.

Chronic Disease Risk Associated with Exposure to Toxicants by Consumption of Seafood

An FAO/WHO (2011) risk–benefit analysis of fish consumption included a review of the evidence on the risk of chronic disease from seafood consumption. This study considered the effect of both nutrients and toxicants in seafood on health outcomes. Based on a review of previous reports and reviews, the authors concluded that seafood consumption lowers the risk of mortality from coronary heart disease in the adult population and little or no evidence exists for other health benefits including ischemic stroke or cancer. This report, however, did not include studies of fetal or childhood exposure.

Summary of Evidence on Health Outcomes Associated with Exposure to Toxicants by Consumption of Seafood

Taken as a whole, the evidence reviewed by the committee indicates that higher fish consumption is associated with lower risk of adverse health outcomes or no association with health outcomes. The evidence for increased risk of adverse health outcomes associated with seafood consumption was insufficient to draw a conclusion.

COMMON MECHANISMS OF ACTION OF CONTAMINANTS COMMONLY FOUND IN SEAFOOD

The committee was asked to consider evidence on how various compositions of a seafood matrix (i.e., the relative proportions and concentrations of nutrients or contaminants present) may function as exposures in the human body that have various mechanisms of action and interplay, including interactions between toxic and nutritive components. While there are many potential contaminants in seafood, the committee identified two common contaminants commonly found in seafood, MeHg and PCBs, for further consideration of seafood matrices.

Mechanism of Mercury-Mediated Toxicity

The mechanism of Hg toxicity is a complex chain of events. It has been postulated that co-exposure to selenium in seafood can modulate the effects of MeHg. For example, Moniruzzaman et al. (2021) conducted a study in mice to evaluate the effect of Se, vitamin C, and vitamin E on MeHg-toxified olive flounder fish muscle powder. The study assessed tissue Hg bioaccumulation, antioxidant enzyme activities, and oxidative stress. Mice were fed diets with three levels of Hg (0, 50, or 500 μg per kg) and two levels of Se in combination with vitamin C and vitamin E (Se: 0, 2 mg per kg; vitamin C: 0, 400 mg per kg; vitamin E: 0, 200 mg per kg). The findings included that dietary supplementation of antioxidants such as Se, vitamin C, and vitamin E had no effect on Hg bioaccumulation in mice. The antioxidants did, however, have a partial effect on reducing serum lipid peroxidation and a significant effect on the cumulative survival rate in the mice fed Hg-intoxicated diets.

Spiller (2018) described the role of selenium as follows.

Reduction of Hg toxicity depends in part on the form of Hg and may be multifaceted and may include:

- facilitating demethylation of organic Hg to inorganic Hg;
- redistribution of Hg to less sensitive target organs;
- binding to inorganic Hg and forming an insoluble, stable, and inert Hg:Se complex;
- reduction of Hg absorption from the gastrointestinal tract;
- repletion of Se stores (reverse Se deficiency); and
- restoration of target selenoprotein activity and restoring the intracellular redox environment (Fernandes et al., 2020).

The key interactions of Hg with Se identified are the sequestering of the chemical form and the counteracting of oxidative stress.

James et al. (2022) showed that for long-term low-level MeHg exposure from consuming fish, Hg speciation in human brain tissue demonstrates that MeHg coordinated to an aliphatic thiolate, resembling the coordinated environment observed in marine fish. The investigators also observed the presence of less bioavailable mercuric selenide deposits using high-energy resolution fluorescence detected X-ray absorption spectroscopy.

The selenoenzyme thioredoxin reductase (TrxR) is a critical component of the thioredoxin system. For example, selenoenzymes restore antioxidants such as vitamin C, thioredoxin, and glutathione to their functionally active forms. Branco and Carvalho (2019), Nogara et al. (2019), and Spiller (2018) reviewed the evidence about the interaction between Hg compounds, the thioredoxin system, and its implications for toxicity development due to co-exposure to selenium and Hg compounds. The TrxRs are a group of Se-containing pyridine nucleotide-disulphide oxidoreductases, whereby the mechanism of toxicity of Hg compounds involves a complex chain of events.

First, inhibition of TrxR, glutathione, and the glutaredoxin system (glutathione peroxidase) can result in the proliferation of intracellular reactive oxygen species. Next, glutamate excitosis, calcium dyshomeostasis, mitochondrial injury/loss, lipid peroxidation, compromised protein repair, and apoptosis can occur. Supplemental Se has been shown to have a protective effect on TrxR from the toxicity of inorganic Hg, but not from MeHg. The inhibition of TrxR can reduce thioredoxin by alternative mechanisms, which involve glutathione and glutaredoxin. If this pathway is compromised, apoptosis can occur. MeHg is a more potent inhibitor of the thioredoxin system, partially explaining its increased neurotoxicity. Whether the amount of selenium in seafood produces a similar response has not been established.

The current evidence shows that the MeHg and Se interaction is complex (Choi et al., 2008). The interactions can result in decreased Hg or Se toxicity, or an increase in Se deficiency. The nature or the interactions depends on several factors such as the form of Hg or Se, the affected organ, and the dose. Other factors have been shown to counteract the effects of Hg and other heavy metals. The nuclear factor erythroid 2 (Nrf-2) regulates cellular resistance to oxidants by controlling the expression of an array of genes dependent on the antioxidant response element. Glutathione (GSH) prevents damage to cellular components caused by reactive oxygen species and heavy metals.

In an investigation into the effect of zinc (Zn) on inorganic Hg-induced cytotoxicity in cultured cells, Hossain et al. (2021) used cellular toxicity assays to show that pretreatment was partially effective in reversing inorganic

Hg-induced toxicity. The mechanism of action was proposed to be through inhibiting formation of reactive oxygen species, GSH increase, and the Nrf-2-mediated pathway. In this model, Zn pretreatment was partially effective in protecting cells from inorganic Hg-induced cytotoxicity and intrinsic apoptosis through its antioxidant properties.

Mechanisms of PCB Toxicity

Yazdi et al. (2021) investigated the effects of PCBs found in food on hormone-responsive and nonresponsive cell lines. In this study, all cell lines were treated with serial concentrations of PCBs for 48 hours and tested for cell viability. The most effective PCB concentration was then applied and levels of paraoxonase-1—an HDL-associated protein that hydrolyzes LDL cholesterol with potential atheroprotective effects—were evaluated. In addition, a molecular modeling technique was used to determine the binding mechanism and predict the binding energies of PCB compounds to the aryl hydrocarbon receptor (AhR). The results showed that the hormone-responsive cell lines tested showed different concentrations of PCBs after treatment. Furthermore, the molecular modeling showed that PCBs had steric interaction with the AhR. The investigators concluded that PCBs have a significant effect on hormone-responsive cells.

Health Effects of Chemical Mixtures in Seafood

The traditional risk assessment approach relies on testing single chemicals across dosage concentrations in animal models or measuring selected biomarkers of exposure for selected chemicals in the studied populations and evaluating their associations with health outcomes (IOM, 2007). Therefore, the traditional risk assessment approach is only useful in considering selection of the nutrients and contaminants that are present in seafood. Moreover, as the relative proportions and concentrations of nutrients or contaminants in seafood vary, it is difficult to assess the cumulative effects or risks of the combined "chemical" exposure from seafood consumption using traditional approaches. There have been many recent efforts to enhance contaminant mixture modeling in epidemiological research (Yu et al., 2022) and efforts to enhance *in silico* prediction models (Gao et al., 2023). While a research priority, formal methods to assess risk from joint exposure to chemical mixtures have yet to be implemented (Nikolopoulou et al., 2023).

As reported in Liew and Guo (2022), six varying concentrations of an endocrine-disrupting chemicals (EDCs) mixture were identified in a cohort of Swedish mother–child pairs. These EDC mixtures were tested in multiple experimental models, including human cerebral organoids, *Xenopus laevis* tadpoles, and zebrafish larvae. Gene networks that were altered by the EDC mixture were identified in human cerebral organoids, and validated thyroid, estrogen, and peroxisome proliferator-activated receptor endocrine pathways as major convergent targets *in vivo*. The investigators estimated that about half of the children in the cohort had been prenatally exposed to EDC mixture concentrations that could cause biological effects, such as language development (Liew and Guo, 2022).

Summary of Evidence on Mechanisms of Action and Contaminants Found in Seafood

Some experimental evidence supports that the toxicity of mercury and PCBs can be modified by other factors (i.e., in antioxidant response pathways). This literature is complex, and the committee was not able to identify supportive evidence in humans.

FINDINGS AND CONCLUSIONS

Findings

Outcomes Associated with Seafood Consumption

1. Many of the studies reviewed by the committee reported outcomes correlated with seafood consumption generally and without differentiation as to species. One commonly accepted assumption has been that

omega-3 long-chain fatty acids in seafood, particularly DHA, contribute benefits, possibly in combination with other nutrients.
2. The evidence reviewed indicates that some gains in neurodevelopment may be achieved during childhood and are apparent in the children of women who consume greater quantities of seafood during pregnancy compared to those who consume lower quantities or no seafood.
3. Seafood consumption by women during pregnancy may also have a protective effect against adverse neurocognitive outcomes in their children that is linked to the nutrients in seafood, particularly the n-3 long-chain polyunsaturated fatty acids that are essential to brain development. Associations of health outcomes with seafood intake differ between the general populations and recreational and subsistence fishers.

Conclusions

1. *The results of the studies identified through the committee's evidence reviews did not support a beneficial association of seafood consumption during childhood and adolescence and reduced risk of cardiovascular disease.*
2. *No evidence was identified to determine whether seafood consumption among children or adolescents is associated with benefits to reducing risk of other diseases such as immune disease.*
3. *The evidence reviewed on health outcomes associated with seafood consumption for women of childbearing age, children, and adolescents is not adequate to support an accurate assessment of the health benefits and risks associated with meeting the recommended intakes of seafood for this population group.*

RESEARCH GAPS

- Additional research is needed to assess childhood health outcomes related to seafood consumption by children. This should include not only amounts and types consumed but also the age of introduction of seafood to infants and children.
- Additional research is needed to determine whether there are sensitive periods in child development during which seafood consumption or exposure to contaminants in seafood might have different effects on child health.
- Population studies that examine the effects of maternal and child seafood consumption on child health outcomes need to better characterize the seafood species (e.g., type of fish, source, and location) as well as nutrient composition and contaminant concentrations in the seafood consumed.
- Additional research is needed on the health effects of contaminant mixtures and varied exposure levels to determine applicability for these observations in seafood-consuming populations in the United States and Canada.
- Additional research is needed to assess how to effectively communicate seafood consumption recommendations to women of childbearing age, children, and adolescents.

REFERENCES

Ajmal, A., K. Watanabe, E. Tanaka, Y. Sawada, T. Watanabe, E. Tomisaki, S. Ito, R. Okumura, Y. Kawasaki, and T. Anme. 2022. Eating behaviour-consumption frequency of certain foods in early childhood as a predictor of behaviour problems: 6-year follow-up study. *Sultan Qaboos University Medical Journal* 22(2):225-232.

Amadi, C. N., C. N. Orish, C. Frazzoli, and O. E. Orisakwe. 2022. Association of autism with toxic metals: A systematic review of case-control studies. *Pharmacology Biochemistry and Behavior* 212:173313.

Andersen, L. F., P. Berstad, B. A. Bukhvalova, M. H. Carlsen, L. J. Dahl, A. Goksøyr, L. Sletting Jakobsen, H. K. Knutsen, I. Kvestad, and I. T. L. Lillegaard. 2022. *Benefit and risk assessment of fish in the Norwegian diet*. Oslo, Norway: Steering Committee of the Norwegian Scientific Committee for Food and Environment.

Avella-Garica, C. B., and J. Julvez. 2014. Seafood intake and neurodevelopment: A systematic review. *Current Environmental Health Reports* 1:46-77.

Bernstein, A. S., E. Oken, S. de Ferranti, Council On Environmental Health, and Committee on Nutrition. 2019. Fish, shellfish, and children's health: An assessment of benefits, risks, and sustainability. *Pediatrics* 143(6):e20190999. https://doi.org/10.1542/peds.2019-0999.

Branco, V., and C. Carvalho. 2019. The thioredoxin system as a target for mercury compounds. *Biochimica et Biophysica Acta* 1863(12):129255.

Choi, A. L., and P. Grandjean. 2008. Methylmercury exposure and health effects in humans. *Environmental Chemistry* 5(2):112-120.

Choi, A. L., E. Budtz-Jørgensen, P. J. Jørgensen, U. Steuerwald, F. Debes, P. Weihe, and P. Grandjean. 2008. Selenium as a potential protective factor against mercury developmental neurotoxicity. *Environmental Research* 107(1):45-52.

Dack, K., M. Fell, C. M. Taylor, A. Havdahl, and S. J. Lewis. 2022. Prenatal mercury exposure and neurodevelopment up to the age of 5 years: A systematic review. *International Journal of Environmental Research and Public Health* 19(4).

Ding, M., S. Shi, S. Qie, J. Li, and X. Xi. 2023. Association between heavy metals exposure (cadmium, lead, arsenic, mercury) and child autistic disorder: A systematic review and meta-analysis. *Frontiers in Pediatrics* 11:1169733.

de Groot, R. H., C. Ouwehand, and J. Jolles. 2012. Eating the right amount of fish: Inverted U-shape association between fish consumption and cognitive performance and academic achievement in Dutch adolescents. *Prostaglandins, Leukotrienes, and Essential Fatty Acids* 86(3):113-117.

Ealo Tapia, D., J. Torres Abad, M. Madera, and J. Márquez Lázaro. 2023. Mercury and neurodevelopmental disorders in children: A systematic review. *Archivos Argentinos de Pediatría* 121(5):e202202838.

FAO/WHO (Food and Agriculture Organization of the United Nations and World Health Organization). 2011. *Report of the joint FAO/WHO expert consultation on the risks and benefits of fish consumption, 25-29 January 2010, Rome, Italy.* Geneva, Switzerland: World Health Organization.

FAO/WHO. 2023. *Joint FAO/WHO expert consultation on the risks and benefits of fish consumption, 9-13 October 2023, Rome, Italy.* Geneva, Switzerland: World Health Organization.

FDA (U.S. Food and Drug Administration). 2014. *Quantitative assessment of the net effects on fetal neurodevelopment from eating commercial fish (as measured by IQ and also by early age verbal development in children).* https://www.fda.gov/media/88491/download (accessed February 29, 2024).

Fernandes, A., J. Falandysz, and I. Širič. 2020. The toxic reach of mercury and its compounds in human and animal food webs. *Chemosphere* 261:127765.

Freire, C., R. Ramos, M. J. Lopez-Espinosa, S. Díez, J. Vioque, F. Ballester, and M. F. Fernández. 2010. Hair mercury levels, fish consumption, and cognitive development in preschool children from Granada, Spain. *Environmental Research* 110(1):96-104.

Fruh, V., S. L. Rifas-Shiman, B. A. Coull, K. L. Devick, C. Amarasiriwardena, A. Cardenas, D. C. Bellinger, L. A. Wise, R. F. White, R. O. Wright, E. Oken, and B. Claus Henn. 2021. Prenatal exposure to a mixture of elements and neurobehavioral outcomes in mid-childhood: Results from Project Viva. *Environmental Research* 201:111540.

Gao, J., J. Zhao, X. Chen, and J. Wang. 2023. A review on in silico prediction of the environmental risks posed by pharmaceutical emerging contaminants. *Environmental Monitoring and Assessment* 195(12):1535.

Golding, J., C. Taylor, Y. Iles-Caven, and S. Gregory. 2022. The benefits of fish intake: Results concerning prenatal mercury exposure and child outcomes from the ALSPAC prebirth cohort. *Neurotoxicology* 91:22-30.

Grosse, S. D., and Y. Zhou. 2021. Monetary valuation of children's cognitive outcomes in economic evaluations from a societal perspective: A review. *Children (Basel)* 8(5):352.

Halldorsson, T. I., I. Thorsdottir, H. M. Meltzer, F. Nielsenn, and S. F. Olsen. 2008. Linking exposure to polychlorinated biphenyls with fatty fish consumption and reduced fetal growth among Danish pregnant women: A cause for concern? *American Journal of Epidemiology* 168:958-965.

Hibbeln, J. R., P. Spiller, J. T. Brenna, J. Golding, B. J. Holub, W. S. Harris, P. Kris-Etherton, B. Lands, S. L. Connor, G. Myers, J. J. Strain, M. A. Crawford, and S. E. Carlson. 2019. Relationships between seafood consumption during pregnancy and childhood and neurocognitive development: Two systematic reviews. *Prostaglandins, Leukotrienes, and Essential Fatty Acids* 151:14-36.

Hossain, K. F. B., T. Hosokawa, T. Saito, and M. Kurasaki. 2021. Zinc-pretreatment triggers glutathione and Nrf2-mediated protection against inorganic mercury-induced cytotoxicity and intrinsic apoptosis in pc12 cells. *Ecotoxicology and Environmental Safety* 207:111320.

Hysing, M., I. Kvestad, M. Kjellevold, L. Kolden Midtbø, I. E. Graff, Ø. Lie, H. Hurum, K. M. Stormark, and J. Øyen. 2018. Fatty fish intake and the effect on mental health and sleep in preschool children in Fins–KIDS, a randomized controlled trial. *Nutrients* 10(10).

IOM (Institute of Medicine). 2007. *Seafood choices: Balancing benefits and risks*. Washington, DC: The National Academies Press.
James, A. K., N. V. Dolgova, S. Nehzati, M. Korbas, J. J. H. Cotelesage, D. Sokaras, T. Kroll, J. L. O'Donoghue, G. E. Watson, G. J. Myers, I. J. Pickering, and G. N. George. 2022. Molecular fates of organometallic mercury in human brain. *ACS Chemical Neuroscience* 13(12):1756-1768.
Jeong, K. S., E. Ha, J. Y. Shin, H. Park, Y. C. Hong, M. Ha, S. Kim, S. J. Lee, K. Y. Lee, J. H. Kim, and Y. Kim. 2017. Blood heavy metal concentrations in pregnant Korean women and their children up to age 5 years—Mothers' and Children's Environmental Health (MOCEH) birth cohort study. *Science of the Total Environment* 605-606:784-791. https://doi.org/10.1016/j.scitotenv.2017.06.007.
Kim, T. H., J. H. Kim, M. D. Le Kim, W. D. Suh, J. E. Kim, H. J. Yeon, Y. S. Park, S. H. Kim, Y. H. Oh, and G. H. Jo. 2020. Exposure assessment and safe intake guidelines for heavy metals in consumed fishery products in the Republic of Korea. *Environmental Science and Pollution Research International* 27(26):33042-33051.
Kremmyda, L. S., M. Vlachava, P. S. Noakes, N. D. Diaper, E. A. Miles, and P. C. Calder. 2011. Atopy risk in infants and children in relation to early exposure to fish, oily fish, or long-chain omega-3 fatty acids: A systematic review. *Clinical Reviews in Allergy and Immunology* 41(1):36-66.
Kumar, S., A. Sharma, and S. Sedha. 2022. Occupational and environmental mercury exposure and human reproductive health-a review. *Journal of the Turkish German Gynecological Association* 23(3):199.
Kvestad, I., M. Hysing, M. Kjellevold, S. Næss, L. Dahl, and M. W. Markus. 2021. Maternal cod intake during pregnancy and infant development in the first year of life: Secondary analyses from a randomized controlled trial. *Journal of Nutrition* 151(7):1879-1885.
Lee, M., M. H. Rahbar, M. Samms-Vaughan, J. Bressler, M. A. Bach, M. Hessabi, M. L. Grove, S. Shakespeare-Pellington, C. Coore Desai, J. A. Reece, K. A. Loveland, and E. Boerwinkle. 2019. A generalized weighted quantile sum approach for analyzing correlated data in the presence of interactions. *Biometrical Journal* 61(4):934-954.
Liew, Z., and P. Guo. 2022. Human health effects of chemical mixtures. *Science* 375(6582):720-721.
Markus, M. W., M. Hysing, L. K. Midtbo, I. Nerhus, S. Naess, I. Aakre, I. Kvestad, L. Dahl, and M. Kjellevold. 2021. Effects of two weekly servings of cod for 16 weeks in pregnancy on maternal iodine status and infant neurodevelopment: Mommy's food, a randomized-controlled trial. *Thyroid* 31(2):288-298.
Mendez, M. A., E. Plana, M. Guxens, C. M. Foradada Morillo, R. Martorell Albareda, R. Garcia-Esteban, F. Goni, M. Kogevinas, and J. Sunyer. 2009. Seafood consumption in pregnancy and infant size at birth: Results from a prospective Spanish cohort. *Journal of Epidemiology and Community Health* 64(3):216-222.
Miyashita, C., S. Sasaki, T. Ikeno, A. Araki, S. Ito, J. Kajiwara, T. Todaka, N. Hachiya, A. Yasutake, K. Murata, T. Nakajima, and R. Kishi. 2015. Effects of in utero exposure to polychlorinated biphenyls, methylmercury, and polyunsaturated fatty acids on birth size. *Science of the Total Environment* 15(533):256-265.
Moniruzzaman, M., S. Lee, Y. Park, T. Min, and S. C. Bai. 2021. Evaluation of dietary selenium, vitamin C and E as the multi-antioxidants on the methylmercury intoxicated mice based on mercury bioaccumulation, antioxidant enzyme activity, lipid peroxidation and mitochondrial oxidative stress. *Chemosphere* 273:129673.
Murcia, M., M. Espada, J. Julvez, S. Llop, M. J. Lopez-Espinosa, J. Vioque, M. Basterrechea, I. Riaño, L. González, M. Alvarez-Pedrerol, A. Tardón, J. Ibarluzea, and M. Rebagliato. 2018. Iodine intake from supplements and diet during pregnancy and child cognitive and motor development: The INMA mother and child cohort study. *Journal of Epidemiology and Community Health* 72(3):216-222.
Nikolopoulou, D., E. Ntzani, K. Kyriakopoulou, C. Anagnostopoulos, and K. Machera. 2023. Priorities and challenges in methodology for human health risk assessment from combined exposure to multiple chemicals. *Toxics* 11(5):401.
Nogara, P. A., C. A. Oliveira, G. L. Schmitz, P. C. Piquini, M. Farina, M. Aschner, and J. B. T. Rocha. 2019. Methylmercury's chemistry: From the environment to the mammalian brain. *Biochimica et Biophysica Acta* 1863(12):129284.
Rahbar, M. H., M. Samms-Vaughan, M. Lee, J. Zhang, M. Hessabi, J. Bressler, M. A. Bach, M. L. Grove, S. Shakespeare-Pellington, C. Beecher, W. McLaughlin, and K. A. Loveland. 2020. Interaction between a mixture of heavy metals (lead, mercury, arsenic, cadmium, manganese, aluminum) and GSTP1, GSTT1, and GSTM1 in relation to autism spectrum disorder. *Research in Autism Spectrum Disorder* 79:101681.
Rothenberg, S. E., X. Yu, J. Liu, F. J. Biasini, C. Hong, X. Jiang, Y. Nong, Y. Cheng, and S. A. Korrick. 2016. Maternal methylmercury exposure through rice ingestion and offspring neurodevelopment: A prospective cohort study. *International Journal of Hygiene and Environmental Health* 219(8):832-842.
Rothenberg, S. E., S. A. Korrick, J. Liu, Y. Nong, H. Nong, C. Hong, E. P. Trinh, X. Jiang, F. J. Biasini, and F. Ouyang. 2021. Maternal methylmercury exposure through rice ingestion and child neurodevelopment in the first three years: A prospective cohort study in rural China. *Environmental Health: A Global Access Science Source* 20(1):50.

Saavedra, S., Á. Fernández-Recamales, A. Sayago, A. Cervera-Barajas, R. González-Domínguez, and J. D. Gonzalez-Sanz. 2022. Impact of dietary mercury intake during pregnancy on the health of neonates and children: A systematic review. *Nutrition Reviews* 80(2):317-328.

Skotheim, S., K. Handeland, M. Kjellevold, J. Øyen, L. Frøyland, Ø. Lie, I. Eide Graff, V. Baste, K. M. Stormark, and L. Dahl. 2017. The effect of school meals with fatty fish on adolescents' self-reported symptoms for mental health: FINS-teens—a randomized controlled intervention trial. *Food & Nutrition Research* 61(1):1383818.

Snetselaar, L., R. Bailey, J. Sabaté, L. Van Horn, B. Schneeman, J. Spahn, J. H. Kim, C. Bahnfleth, G. Butera, N. Terry, and J. Obbagy. 2020a. *Seafood consumption during pregnancy and lactation and neurocognitive development in the child: A systematic review.* Alexandria, VA: USDA Nutrition Evidence Systematic Review.

Snetselaar, L., R. Bailey, J. Sabaté, L. Van Horn, B. Schneeman, J. Spahn, J. H. Kim, C. Bahnfleth, G. Butera, N. Terry, and J. Obbagy. 2020b. *Seafood consumption during childhood and adolescence and neurocognitive development: A systematic review.* Alexandria, VA: USDA Nutrition Evidence Systematic Review.

Snetselaar, L., R. Bailey, J. Sabaté, L. Van Horn, B. Schneeman, J. H. Kim, J. Spahn, C. Bahnfleth, G. Butera, N. Terry, and J. Obbagy. 2020c. *Seafood consumption during childhood and adolescence and cardiovascular disease: A systematic review.* Alexandria, VA: USDA Nutrition Evidence Systematic Review.

Spiller, H. A. 2018. Rethinking mercury: The role of selenium in the pathophysiology of mercury toxicity. *Clinical Toxicology* 56(5):313-326.

Sulaiman, R., M. Wang, and X. Ren. 2020. Exposure to aluminum, cadmium, and mercury and autism spectrum disorder in children: A systematic review and meta-analysis. *Chemical Research in Toxicology* 33(11):2699-2718.

Teisen, M. N., S. Vuholm, J. Niclasen, J. J. Aristizabal-Henao, K. D. Stark, S. S. Geertsen, C. T. Damsgaard, and L. Lauritzen. 2020. Effects of oily fish intake on cognitive and socioemotional function in healthy 8-9-year-old children: The FiSK Junior randomized trial. *American Journal of Clinical Nutrition* 112(1):74-83.

USDA and HHS (U.S. Department of Agriculture and U.S. Department of Health and Human Services). 2020. *Dietary Guidelines for Americans, 2020-2025.* 9th ed. http://www.dietaryguidelines.gov/ (accessed August 17, 2023).

Varsi, K., I. K. Torsvik, S. Huber, M. Averina, J. Brox, and A. L. Bjorke-Monsen. 2022. Impaired gross motor development in infants with higher PFAS concentrations. *Environmental Research* 204(Pt D):112392.

Wohlfahrt-Veje, C., K. Audouze, S. Brunak, J. P. Antignac, B. le Bizec, A. Juul, N. E. Skakkebæk, and K. M. Main. 2014. Polychlorinated dibenzo-p-dioxins, furans, and biphenyls (PCDDs/PCDFs and PCBs) in breast milk and early childhood growth and IGF1. *Reproduction* 147(4):391-399.

Yang, H., P. Xun, and K. He. 2013. Fish and fish oil intake in relation to risk of asthma: A systematic review and meta-analysis. *PLoS One* 8(11):e80048.

Yazdi, F., S. Shoeibi, M. H. Yazdi, and A. Eidi. 2021. Effect of prevalent polychlorinated biphenyls (PCBs) food contaminant on the MCF7, LNCap and MDA-MB-231 cell lines viability and PON1 gene expression level: Proposed model of binding. *Daru* 29(1):159-170.

Yu, L., W. Liu, X. Wang, Z. Ye, Q. Tan, W. Qiu, X. Nie, M. Li, B. Wang, and W. Chen. 2022. A review of practical statistical methods used in epidemiological studies to estimate the health effects of multi-pollutant mixture. *Environmental Pollution* 306:119356.

Zhang, J., X. Li, L. Shen, N. U. Khan, X. Zhang, L. Chen, H. Zhao, and P. Luo. 2021. Trace elements in children with autism spectrum disorder: A meta-analysis based on case-control studies. *Journal of Trace Elements in Medicine and Biology* 67:126782.

7

Risk–Benefit Analysis

This chapter presents the committee's work to evaluate when or when not to conduct a risk–benefit analysis (RBA) relative to risk–benefit factors, including how to assess quality and uncertainty, evaluate confidence in the potential conclusions of an RBA, identify relevant factors that are additive to the findings of an RBA, and discuss any implications or applications that may inform policy decision making.

In this report, the RBA approach integrates relevant evidence from components, including nutrition, toxicology, microbiology, and epidemiology toward a comprehensive assessment of health outcomes related to seafood consumption. The goal is to facilitate evidence-based decision making and support policy development and public health advice.

APPROACH TO REVIEWING EVIDENCE ON CONDUCTING A RISK–BENEFIT ANALYSIS

The assessment of risks and benefits to human health associated with seafood consumed as a food product or part of a dietary pattern can be quantitative or semiquantitative. The steps in the process are identification of any chemical and/or microbiological hazards, assessment of intake response, assessment of the nature of the risk, and characterization of health outcomes (IOM, 2007). The balance of positive and negative health outcomes is used to inform policy decisions and develop guidelines for public health practitioners. The committee reviewed a range of evidence on how RBAs are conducted, which included an evidence scan provided by the sponsor as well as additional published literature identified in a supplementary literature review conducted by the committee (Appendix G).

ASSESSMENT OF THE STATE OF THE SCIENCE ON RISK–BENEFIT ANALYSIS

Evidence Scan on Risk–Benefit Analysis

The study sponsors provided to the committee an evidence scan on existing risk–benefit analyses related to seafood and health as an approach to exploring the current state of the evidence on seafood consumption and health outcomes and as a contribution to the committee's review of the state of the science of risk–benefit analyses. The committee notes that apart from the evidence scan there is a preponderance of "grey" literature on this topic.[1] In

---

[1] Grey literature is defined as literature that is not formally published in books or journal articles. Examples include government reports, conference proceedings, white papers, or dissertations.

consideration of its task, however, the committee used only peer-reviewed literature and published reports from the European Food Safety Authority (EFSA) and the Food and Agriculture Organization of the United Nations (FAO) as part of its evidence base.

The data sources for the sponsor-provided evidence scans included PubMed, Cumulative Index to Nursing and Allied Health Literature, Cochrane, and Embase. The final screening results identified 176 relevant publications for full-text review. The study types included in the evidence scan were randomized controlled trials, cohort studies (prospective and retrospective), case–control studies, cross-sectional studies, ecological studies, case–cohort studies, nested case–control studies, case series, and case studies. The interventions and exposures included the following: type, duration, placebo/control (if used); exposure level quantified; dietary assessment (with emphasis on seafoods and/or with high methylmercury [MeHg], such as food records and food frequency questionnaires, and other screeners; and biochemical assays or markers of exposure such as, urinalysis, blood, hair, nail, and fecal markers.

The evidence scan also included primary health outcomes and conditions that affect health outcomes, including neurodevelopment, reproductive biology, pregnancy, psychiatric or behavioral, allergy, cardiovascular, endocrine, cancer/tumor, genetic expression, growth, immune function, inflammation, and infections.

The evidence scan identified three types of risk–benefit analyses:

- Tier 1: Initial—A qualitative RBA that determines whether the health risks clearly outweigh the health benefits or vice versa;
- Tier 2: Refined—A semiquantitative or quantitative estimate of risks and benefits at relevant (toxicant, essential nutrient) exposure levels; and
- Tier 3: Composite Metric—A quantitative RBA that compares risks and benefits as a single net health effect value, such as disability-adjusted life year (DALY) or quality-adjusted life year (QALY).

Across the body of epidemiological evidence, the evidence scan showed differences in exposure levels and in exposure and outcome measurements and windows of time, questionable population representation, and generalizability of diverse and specialized study samples. From a biostatistical perspective, variation existed in the covariates, confounders, and effect modifiers that were considered. There were also a range of statistical methods and approaches to addressing biases during the conduct of a study and in assessing the risks and effects of bias in interpreting results.

The findings from the evidence scan suggest a need for sufficient planning, preparation, discussion, consensus building, and further innovation when applying evolving review methodologies, incorporating emerging findings from new studies, and exploring triangulation approaches for integrating and synthesizing evidence.

METHODOLOGIES AND FRAMEWORKS USED TO CONDUCT RISK–BENEFIT ANALYSES

In addition to the sponsor-provided evidence scan, the committee reviewed evidence gathered in its supplemental review of the literature. Relevant studies and reports from the literature review are discussed in the following sections.

Evidence from the European Food Safety Authority Scientific Committee

In response to a request for an RBA of risks of MeHg exposure and nutritional benefits associated with consuming seafood, the EFSA Scientific Committee used previous work performed by the EFSA Panel on Contaminants in the Food Chain and the EFSA Panel on Dietetic Products, Nutrition, and Allergies to create scenarios based on typical seafood consumption patterns among European population groups at risk of exceeding the tolerable weekly intake (TWI) for MeHg (EFSA, 2015). The number of servings of seafood per week were estimated that would reach both the TWI and the recommended intake (dietary reference value) for n-3 long-chain polyunsaturated fatty acids (LCPUFAs). Additional assumptions included that the form of mercury (Hg) was 100 percent MeHg in fish meat, fish products, fish offal, and seafood, and 80 percent in crustaceans, mollusks, and amphibians. All other foods were assumed to contain inorganic Hg.

Analysis of the scenarios showed that children, including those younger than age 3 years, exceeded the TWI for MeHg at the fewest number of seafood servings per week. The results were expressed as "total mercury" for the various product categories because Hg speciation is not performed routinely by national laboratories. The EFSA Scientific Committee identified wild-caught tuna as the source of the highest levels of MeHg exposure among all fish and seafood commonly consumed in the European Union. Inadequate data precluded full characterization of the benefits of seafood consumption from being performed. For the risk assessment of seafood consumption at the EU population level, no other representative longitudinal follow-up study was identified that could have simultaneously provided good quality data on seafood consumption and clinical/physiological endpoints in this population. The EU committee concluded that the estimated mean dietary exposures to MeHg across age groups did not exceed the TWI, except for children.

Models from the Peer-Reviewed Literature

A study by Hoekstra et al. (2013) that was identified in the evidence scan described a process for conducting a quantitative RBA of seafood consumption for the Dutch population. In their approach the researchers expressed risk and benefits using the DALY metric, and evaluated the data using a software tool, QALIBRA,[2] to compare the net effect of eating seafood on health outcomes. A potential impact fraction (PIF) was used to calculate the proportional change in average disease incidence following a change in exposure of a risk factor. Specifically, the factors considered in the PIF were a decrease in the risk of fatal coronary heart disease (CHD), increase in IQ in newborns, decrease in sperm count, decrease in the production of TT4 (thyroid) hormone, and increase in the incidence of diffuse fatty liver. The health outcome scenarios were based on a population intake model of consuming 200 and 500 g of seafood per week (equivalent to about 7 and 15 oz per week). The analytical finding was expressed as the relative risk of an adverse outcome. The results indicated a net benefit for populations consuming 200 g of seafood per week.

Overall, the study concluded that the beneficial effect associated with increased seafood consumption was attributable in large part to the balance of intake against the relative burden of disease from CHD and stroke, and a decrease in thyroid hormone and sperm count. Specifically, the alternative diet scenarios resulted in a decrease in DALYs and an average net annual health benefit. A loss of IQ points owing to Hg exposure from seafood consumption was compensated for by a gain in IQ points owing to the contribution of docosahexaenoic acid in fish.

Cohen et al. (2005) investigated the aggregate effect of hypothetical shifts in seafood consumption using a modeling approach. The level of risk versus benefit was modeled as the product of exposure to the active agent (MeHg or n-3 LCPUFAs) and the dose–response relationship for that agent (incremental risk per microgram per day of MeHg, or reduction in risk per gram per day of n-3 LCPUFAs, or number of seafood servings per week). The investigators then quantified the effect of changes in seafood consumption on MeHg exposure, n-3 LCPUFA intake, and the average number of servings consumed per week.

In the model, seafood consumption was estimated for 42 species from data collected in the U.S. Department of Agriculture's Continuing Survey of Food Intake by Individuals reporting years from 1989 to 1991 and the third National Health and Nutrition Evaluation Survey reporting years from 1988 to 1994. The authors modeled five scenarios of seafood consumption and measures to increase consumption. To aggregate disparate health effects across the population, the authors reexpressed the health effects in terms of QALYs. After accounting for uncertainties in the model, the investigators found that among women of childbearing age, a shift to consumption of low-MeHg seafood resulted in a substantial improvement in cognitive development in the offspring. Alternatively, the model showed that when women of childbearing age reduced seafood consumption, the aggregate effect on cognitive development remained positive but was substantially smaller than the women who modified their consumption choices.

---

[2] QALIBRA is a general model for food risk–benefit assessment that quantifies variability and uncertainty.

The authors concluded that risk managers should carefully and quantitatively evaluate how the population will react to changes in consumption advice and how such reactions will affect exposure to contaminants and intake of nutrients as well as how changes in contaminant exposure and nutrient intake will affect the probability of both adverse and beneficial health effects.

Boué et al. (2015), also identified in the evidence scan, conducted a systematic review of the published literature to synthesize RBA studies associated with food consumption and summarize the current methodological options and/or tendencies carried out in the field. The final review consisted of 126 articles focused on studies of RBAs and 34 on methodological frameworks. The recommended methodology for conducting RBAs followed a risk assessment framework similar to that used in science-based research, but with a risk–benefit comparison step added. Most of the studies in the review compared nutritional benefits and adverse health effects related to fish consumption based on safety reference values. The studies reviewed identified two categories of reference values, recommendations by food safety authorities, and process and formulation designs by manufacturers.

To help public health programs know which commercial or locally caught fish species may be eaten more frequently, considering only Hg and n-3 LCPUFAs, Ginsberg et al. (2015) updated a previous RBA methodology published in 2009. The previous model predicted a net risk for neurodevelopmental outcomes for many species when risk data were calibrated against benefit data and compared with risk–benefit models, including models from the World Health Organization (WHO) and the U.S. Food and Drug Administration (FDA). Among commonly eaten fish high in Hg, the calibrated model identified risks that are consistent with current fish advisories, although other models predicted greater net neurodevelopmental benefits.

The calibrated model was used to propose a three-step framework for setting consumption advisories:

1. Set an initial consumption level based on the Hg reference dose (RfD).
2. Adjust consumption estimates upward if the risk–benefit model indicates a net benefit.
3. Limit fish consumption based on the saturation of benefit from n-3 LCPUFAs.

To advise the public on the frequency of consuming those species that exceed the RfD requires confidence that there is a net benefit. Upper bound and lower bound slope estimates can be used to identify where a benefit is substantial relative to uncertainties in slope estimates. Borderline benefits may not warrant increasing consumption beyond relatively minor rounding to the next whole meal, and a net risk may warrant downgrading of consumption advice. Where a clear net benefit exists, the saturation of n-3 LCPUFA benefit as introduced by FAO/WHO (2011) appears to be a reasonable way to limit meal frequency and prevent excessive risk of Hg exposure.

Simple n-3 LCPUFA-to-Hg ratios in fish tissue have been proposed as a useful screen for estimating risk–benefit trade-offs associated with consuming a particular species. The simplicity of such an approach could encourage more species sampling. In this approach, an n-3 LCPUFA-to-Hg ratio of 30 or greater would represent a clear neurodevelopmental benefit (see Table 4 in Ginsberg et al., 2015). This approach could also help assessors determine when it may be appropriate to recommend that it is acceptable for consumers to exceed the RfD on a species-specific basis.

In a different approach, Ginsberg and Toal (2009) developed a method to quantitatively analyze the net risk–benefit of individual fish species based on MeHg and n-3 LCPUFA content, which was intended to allow a more nuanced approach to providing advice about risks of consuming seafood. This study identified dose–response relationships for MeHg and n-3 LCPUFA's effects on CHD in adults and neurodevelopment in infants. The investigators used the MeHg and n-3 LCPUFA content of 16 commonly consumed species to calculate the net risk–benefit for each species. The results indicated that the estimated benefits from n-3 LCPUFAs outweighed the risks from MeHg for some species (e.g., farmed salmon, herring, trout), while the opposite was true for others (e.g., swordfish, shark). Other species were associated with a small net benefit (e.g., flounder, pollack, canned light tuna) or a small net risk (e.g., canned white tuna, halibut). The results were used to place fish into one of four meal frequency categories. However, the advice was considered provisional owing to limitations in the underlying dose–response information.

The overall results of the study showed a framework for risk–benefit analysis that could be used to develop categories of consumption advice ranging from *do not eat* to *unlimited*, with the caveat that the term *unlimited* may need to be moderated for certain fish (e.g., farm-raised salmon) because of other contaminants and end points (e.g., cancer risk) that may be present. Furthermore, the authors proposed a tailored approach because of uncertainties in the underlying dose–response assessment. Although showing possible directions for species-specific advisories, the analysis also identifies key research areas—such as examining the adverse effects of MeHg on cardiovascular outcomes in adults—for improving RBAs for fish consumption.

Summary of Evidence on Methodologies Used to Conduct Risk–Benefit Analyses

The committee determined that a quantitative approach to fish type and specific toxicant health impact could be useful for assessing risk compared with benefits where one size does not fit all, and where the concentrations of MeHg by fish species provide more appropriate guidance for the public. However, this approach could benefit from identifying further directions needed for high consumers and providing specific calculations for updating current information on both nutrient and toxicant.

MODELING BENEFITS AND RISKS OF FISH CONSUMPTION

FDA's 2014 quantitative risk assessment (also discussed in Chapter 6) estimated the effects on the developing nervous system of the fetus from the consumption of commercial fish during pregnancy (FDA, 2014). The assessment also reviewed the evidence on the effects of fish consumption by young children on their own neurodevelopment. The methodology for this assessment included exposure modeling and dose–response modeling. Exposure modeling was based on previously published work by Carrington and Bolger (2002). The dose–response models were developed from results from selected observational research studies in humans. The preferences for selecting research results for input into the dose–response modeling included outcomes for neurodevelopment that were biologically plausible, sufficiently detailed, and reasonably consistent with effects seen in other studies.

The data and results from which the Hg dose–response relationship with IQ was derived established that IQ is a representative indicator of effect, and sufficient detail was available to conduct dose–response modeling. The results were biologically plausible and reasonably consistent with effects seen in other studies. Furthermore, the MeHg effects are not likely to have been substantially confounded as exposure levels were relatively high and the combined study population was relatively large.

The assessment estimates that for each of the endpoints modeled, consumption of commercial fish during pregnancy is beneficial for most children in the United States. On a population basis, average neurodevelopment is estimated to benefit by nearly 0.7 of an IQ point (95% confidence interval [CI] of 0.39–1.37 IQ points) from maternal consumption of commercial fish. For comparison purposes, the average population-level benefit for early-age verbal development is equivalent in size to 1.02 of an IQ point (95% CI of 0.44–2.01 IQ size equivalence). For a sensitive endpoint as estimated by tests of later age verbal development, the average population-level benefit from fish consumption is estimated to be 1.41 verbal IQ points (0.91, 2.00).

The assessment also estimates that a mean maximum improvement of about three IQ points is possible from fish consumption, depending on the types and amounts of fish consumed. Fish lower in MeHg generally produce greater benefits and have a lower likelihood of an adverse net effect than fish higher in MeHg. The amount of fish consumed that is needed to obtain the greatest benefit, meaning the greatest gain in IQ points, can vary depending on fish species, but in the hypothetical scenarios modeled, the largest benefits on a population-wide basis occurred when all pregnant women ate 12 oz of a variety of fish per week.

By contrast, an FDA survey of young women indicated that pregnant women on average ate slightly less than 2 oz of fish per week (FDA, 2017). The assessment modeled the net effects of maternal fish consumption on early-age verbal development as a representative indicator of the net effects from fish consumption on neurodevelopment generally. This updated assessment focused on IQ but retained the modeling approach for early-age verbal development for purposes of comparison. The estimated effects on both endpoints were not identical, but they were consistent and appear to provide a plausibly narrow range in which net effects are likely to fall. The assessment also included modeling based on scores of later-age verbal development because the scores appear to reflect a particular sensitivity to the effects of both MeHg and nutrients in fish. The results allow for a comparison between a particularly sensitive endpoint and more representative endpoints.

The FDA assessment also included species-by-species modeling for 47 selected species and market types of commercial fish. This included both population-level modeling, which estimates percentiles of the population experiencing various net effects, and individual-level modeling, which estimates the net effects of eating commercial fish during pregnancy on IQ measured through 9 years of age as indicative of how eating fish can affect neurodevelopment and verbal development. There is evidence that the neurodevelopmental test results for this endpoint are sensitive to both detrimental effects of MeHg exposure (e.g., the Boston Naming Test as administered in the Faroe Islands study) and beneficial nutrients in fish consumed by the mother.

Nauta et al. (2018) identified 10 key challenges to be addressed when developing an RBA, such as application of different definitions of *risk* or *benefit*. For example, the term *benefit* can be used for anything from the agent causing the health effect to the probability and magnitude of the effect. Another challenge is how to assess health effects in an RBA. The approach chosen usually depends on whether the health effects associated with food components are obtained from animal experiments or human observational studies. A top-down approach to human consumption data is presented as a more feasible approach, particularly if data have a large n value and the data needs are diverse.

Nauta et al. (2018) also discussed dose–response models as well as the modeling process, which is often based on relative risk, although the uncertainties can be large. The committee notes that the level of scientific evidence needed to identify a risk may be low because indication of a risk is sufficient for scientific validation. Lastly, the study concluded that risk communication is a key pillar in risk analysis and should be a part of RBAs applied to foods.

Future Work

With the availability of new evidence on the risks and benefits of fish consumption, FAO and WHO in October 2023 conducted an *Expert Consultation on the Risks and Benefits of Fish Consumption* to update the previous report (FAO/WHO, 2011) on this topic. Although the full report has not yet been published, the "Meeting Report" with executive summary was published on November 1, 2023.[3]

FAO and WHO commissioned a systematic literature review from the Norwegian Institute of Marine Research (IMR) that was used to generate a FAO/WHO background document on the risks and benefits of fish consumption to inform the expert consultation. The IMR review covered existing evidence scans, including the following:

- *Benefit and Risk Assessment of Fish in the Norwegian Diet* published by the Norwegian Scientific Committee for Food and Environment (Andersen et al., 2022);
- report from the World Cancer Research Fund (WCRF International, 2018);
- reports from the EFSA containing expert opinion on MeHg (EFSA Panel on Contaminants in the Food Chain, 2012) and dioxins (EFSA Panel on Contaminants in the Food Chain, 2018); and
- additional publications identified from a systematic literature search to identify publications not considered in these prior evidence scans.

After reviewing the background document on the risks and benefits of fish consumption, the 2023 Joint FAO-WHO Expert Consultation agreed on the following overall conclusions regarding human health benefits from fish consumption:

- Fish consumption provides energy, protein, and a range of other nutrients important for health.
- Fish consumption is part of the cultural traditions of many peoples. In some populations, fish are a major source of food, animal protein, and a range of other nutrients that are important for health.

---

[3] Available at https://cdn.who.int/media/docs/default-source/food-safety/jecfa/summary-and-conclusions/jecfa-summary-risks-and-benefits-of-fish-consumption.pdf?sfvrsn=af40f32c_5&download=true (accessed February 29, 2024).

- "Strong evidence exists for the benefits of total fish consumption during all life stages: pregnancy, childhood, and adulthood. For example, associations are found for maternal consumption during pregnancy with improved birth outcomes and for adult consumption with reduced risks for cardiovascular and neurological diseases. This evidence for health benefits of total fish consumption reflects the overall effects of nutrients and contaminants in fish on the studied outcomes, including nutrients and contaminants not specifically considered in the evidence review."
- "Benefits derived from general population studies and individual effects will vary depending on overall diet (e.g., selenium intake, exposure to other contaminants) and characteristics of consumers (e.g., n-3 LCPUFA status and individual susceptibility) and fish consumed (e.g., fish species and food preparation methods)."
- Risk–benefit assessments at regional, national, or subnational levels are needed to refine fish consumption recommendation, which should consider local consumption habits, contamination levels, and nutrient content of fish species present, as well as the population of interest's nutritional status, cultural habits, and demographics.

Summary of Evidence on Modeling Benefits and Risks of Fish Consumption

It is a reasonable hypothesis that fish consumption by young children can affect their neurodevelopment. They may be especially vulnerable to MeHg but could also be especially responsive to the beneficial nutrients in fish. Consistent evidence indicates that young children can benefit from fish consumption, but the evidence is not consistent with regard to whether young children are especially vulnerable to adverse effects from MeHg from postnatal exposure.

DEVELOPING A FRAMEWORK FOR CONDUCTING A RISK–BENEFIT ANALYSIS

The risk–benefit framework is based on three key elements: assessment of risks and benefits, management of risks and benefits, and communication of risks and benefits. Boué et al. (2022) proposed an approach to assessing the effect of diet on public health using RBA methods that simultaneously consider both beneficial and adverse health outcomes. Their aim was to develop a harmonized, transparent, and documented methodological framework for selecting nutritional, microbiological, and toxicological RBA components. The investigators used a stepwise approach to component selection that involved conducting a comprehensive literature search to first identify an initial, long list of components to consider for each of the three domains. To trim each domain's long list of components to a shorter list, they applied a series of predefined criteria that were established based on occurrence and severity of health outcomes related to these components. The final list of components was developed by refining the short list based on availability and quality of data for a feasible inclusion in the RBA model.

The final list included the components and health outcomes to be considered in the RBA to estimate the overall public health impact of using the DALY composite metric. The limitations of using DALYs as a composite metric to quantify health impact include that the criteria for occurrence and severity may not specifically distinguish between the general populations and the vulnerable populations nor identify potential allergic reactions. Additionally, the use of DALYs as a metric in analysis could limit the inclusion criteria because of data model gaps. The investigators thus concluded that the RBA should not be considered as a one-dimensional process, rather as a process that could benefit from the integration of environmental, economic, and sociological assessments. The committee's assessment of this study was that it presented an insufficient and complicated approach to using RBA as a means of harmonizing the findings.

Membré et al. (2021) also shows some of the complexity involved in attempting to conduct an accurate RBA that can reflect, to the extent possible, the net risks and benefits to a population. For example, complications can arise from the differences between specific population groups and the general population, from the challenges to obtaining the large amount of data often required for an RBA, and from the substantial time required to perform it. Additional factors influencing the conduct of an RBA include the availability of the food type, costs, personal preference, and food quality, among others. Separate studies often result in conflicting messages, and several examples were given. Although fish is one of the most widely studied foods in an RBA, it can be highly complicated and difficult to capture the overall effect of fish consumption on health among different populations. Often, large states of risk and benefit must be tailored for specific groups. Hence, clear communication of the results or findings is essential to ensure that consumers can make balanced and objective choices.

As stated by Membré et al. (2021), the first message component is often the most influential. An accurate and effective RBA is essential to supporting informed decision making by both the target population and specific subgroups within it. Transparency about the data and input incorporated into an RBA are important for public acceptance of the RBA and to help promote behaviors aligned with the RBA's results.

Scherer et al. (2008) conducted a comparative analysis of state websites to assess health messages accessible to vulnerable populations, including pregnant women and women of childbearing age. These advisories were issued by state, tribal, and local governments. The study demonstrated that of the 48 fish consumption-related state advisories that were examined, 90 percent targeted pregnant women and 58 percent targeted women of childbearing age. Six of the 48 advisories mentioned only one contaminant (Hg), and the other 42 mentioned anywhere from 2 to 12, most frequently mercury, polychlorinated biphenyls (PCBs), chlordane, dioxin, and dichlorodiphenyltrichloroethane. Beneficial health effects mentioned were limited to effects associated with n-3 fatty acids found in fish. The two states without advisories at the time of the analysis, Alaska and Wyoming, subsequently issued guidelines for fish consumption.

Scherer at al. (2008) attempted to answer the question, do advisories convey risk and benefit information about fish that is sufficient to provide context for the advice offered? Advisories provided numerous recommendations for consumption frequency across multiple groups. For children, the specific age ranges mentioned varied from children younger than 6 years to those children younger than 18 years. Thirty-eight percent of advisories were offered in non-English language, and that language was Spanish only. All advisory websites reviewed (except for Nebraska) offered meal frequency advice, although states varied by whether they issued such advice in units per week, per month, or per day. Some websites referenced the 2004 Environmental Protection Agency/FDA recommendations to consume up to 12 oz per week, while 75 percent provided meal size and 10 percent targeted sensitive populations. Some websites also provided advice about preparation and cooking.

In 2011, the Joint FAO/WHO Expert Committee on Food Additives (JECFA) issued a report and framework for the assessment of health benefits or risks of fish consumption to guide public health authorities and decision making (FAO/WHO, 2011). Although several potential contaminants can be present in fish, MeHg and dioxin are the major toxicants addressed in the JECFA report. The health benefits of fish consumption or dietary intake of n-3 LCPUFAs are often assessed using imprecise dietary estimates, whereas health risks of contaminants are often assessed using objective biomarkers. After reviewing the literature, JECFA compared the effects of prenatal exposure to n-3 LCPUFAs and MeHg on child IQ, and exposure to n-3 LCPUFAs and dioxins on mortality. Several meta-analyses have established linear dose–response relationships between dietary exposure to n-3 LCPUFAs and MeHg and child IQ.

The JECFA report concluded that convincing evidence exists for benefits of maternal fish consumption during pregnancy on neurodevelopment in their children. The JECFA further concluded that their differing quantitative analyses from different perspective cohorts, each employing different metrics and divergent assumptions, showed consistent dose–response relationships between maternal fish consumption and child IQ. Using a central estimate of MeHg risk, neurodevelopmental risks of not eating fish exceeded risks of eating fish for up to at least seven 100-g servings per week and MeHg levels up to at least 1 $\mu g/g$.

When comparing the benefits of n-3 LCPUFAs with the risks of MeHg among women of childbearing age, maternal fish consumption was found to lower the risk of suboptimal neurodevelopment in their offspring compared with the offspring of women not eating fish. At levels of maternal exposure to dioxins (from fish and other dietary sources) that do not exceed the provisional tolerable monthly intake of 70 pg/kg body weight established by JECFA for polychlorinated dibenzodioxins, polychlorinated dibenzofurans, and coplanar PCBs, neurodevelopmental risk for the fetus was negligible. From this study, the committee determined that among infants, young children, and adolescents, available data are currently insufficient to derive a quantitative framework of the health risks and health benefits of eating fish.

Summary of Evidence on Developing a Framework for Conducting a Risk–Benefit Analysis

The studies that the committee reviewed on addressing the risk and benefits of seafood consumption focused largely on pregnant women as one of the most vulnerable subpopulations. While some analyses included dioxins, most RBAs targeted MeHg as the contaminant of concern. From the benefit perspective, there was early recognition of the role of nutrition independently, and as a component of a broader public health approach. Together, the evidence from meta-analyses comparing dietary exposure of n-3 LCPUFAs and MeHg exposure with child IQ indicate that maternal fish consumption may be protective against potential toxic effects of MeHg exposure. However, in its framework for assessing health benefits or risks of fish consumption, the Joint FAO/WHO Expert Committee on Food Additives determined that there were insufficient data to develop an RBA for infants, children, and adolescents (FAO/WHO, 2011).

SCIENTIFIC PRINCIPLES UNDERPINNING A RISK–BENEFIT ANALYSIS

FAO/WHO (2023) identified principles for the analysis of risks versus benefits intended for application in the framework of the *Codex Alimentarius*. The objective was to provide guidance to the Codex Alimentarius Commission (CAC) and to JECFA to ensure that the food safety and health components of *Codex* standards and related texts are based on the analysis. Within the framework of CAC and its procedures, the responsibility for providing advice on risk management lies with CAC and its subsidiary bodies (risk managers), while the responsibility for risk assessment lies primarily with JECFA.

The general aspects of RBA used in the *Codex* report included consistent application, openness, transparency, and documentation. Analyses are conducted in accordance with both the statements of principle concerning the role of science in the *Codex* decision-making process and the extent to which other factors are considered and the statements of principle relating to the role of food safety risk assessment. Moreover, analyses are evaluated and reviewed as appropriate in light of newly generated scientific data. The RBA is intended to follow a structured approach comprising three distinct but closely linked components—risk assessment, risk management, and risk communication—with each component integral to the overall risk analysis.

Components of a Risk–Benefit Analysis

The three components of an RBA (risk assessment, risk management, and risk communication) should be documented fully, transparently, and systematically, and applied within an overarching framework for management of food-related risks to human health. While respecting legitimate concerns to preserve confidentiality, documentation should be accessible to all stakeholders. Furthermore, effective communication and consultation with stakeholders should be ensured throughout the analysis. There should also be a functional separation of risk assessment and risk management, to ensure the scientific integrity of the risk assessment, to avoid confusion over the functions to be performed by risk assessors and risk managers, and to reduce any conflict of interest. However, RBA is an iterative process, and interaction between risk managers and risk assessors is essential for practical application. When there is evidence that a risk to human health exists, but scientific data are insufficient or incomplete, CAC should not proceed with developing a standard, but should consider detailing a related text, such as a code of practice, provided that such a text would be supported by the available scientific evidence.

Uncertainty

As precaution is an inherent element of RBA, many sources of uncertainty exist in the process of risk assessment and risk management of food-related hazards to human health. The degree of uncertainty and variability in the available scientific information should be explicitly considered in the risk analysis. Where there is sufficient scientific evidence to allow *Codex* to proceed to elaborate a standard or related text, the assumptions used for the risk assessment, and the risk management options selected, should reflect the degree of uncertainty and the characteristics of the hazard. Lastly, the needs and situations of developing countries should be specifically identified and considered by the responsible bodies in the different stages of the risk analysis.

Risk Assessment Policy

The FAO/WHO (2023) Risk Assessment Policy posits that the determination of a risk assessment policy should be included as a specific component of risk management. It should be established by risk managers in advance of risk assessment in consultation with risk assessors and all other interested parties. The goal of this procedure is to ensure that the risk assessment is systematic, complete, unbiased, and transparent. The mandate given by risk managers to risk assessors should also be as clear as possible and, where necessary, risk managers should ask risk assessors to evaluate the potential changes in risk resulting from different risk management options.

Summary of Evidence on Scientific Principles Underpinning a Risk–Benefit Analysis

In their assessment of risk, FAO/WHO (2023) stated that the scope and purpose of the particular risk assessment being carried out should be clearly stated and in accordance with risk assessment policy. The committee's review of the evidence suggests that nutritional concerns may be prevalent in performing an RBA, as nutrients in themselves may pose both risks and benefits. Examples of risk include adverse effects of overconsumption, effects of adverse absorption of other nutrients, interaction among nutrients, and effect on other nutrients such as lowering their absorption or use.

APPROACH TO CONDUCTING A RISK–BENEFIT ANALYSIS

In 2010, the EFSA Scientific Committee designed a framework for performing an RBA with foods (EFSA, 2010). Its guidance acknowledges that sufficient evidence is lacking and proposes following a four-step risk assessment process. Once a problem has been formulated an initial assessment is performed; then a refined assessment and comparison of risks and benefits is made using a composite metric.

In a subsequent scientific opinion EFSA (2015) used a clear approach for establishing a risk overview and identifying data needed to assess fish consumption. This included work previously performed by the EFSA Panel on Contaminants in the Food Chain and the EFSA Panel on Dietetic Products, Nutrition, and Allergies to create scenarios based on typical seafood consumption patterns among European population groups at risk of exceeding the TWI for MeHg. The number of fish servings per week was estimated that would reach the TWI and the dietary reference value for n-3 LCPUFAs. The process and results of this activity were described earlier in the chapter, where it was reported that the estimated mean dietary exposures to MeHg across age groups did not exceed the TWI, except for children. No representative longitudinal follow-up data were available, however, that could have provided the information on seafood consumption and health outcomes that is needed for risk assessment (or for full characterization of benefits) of fish consumption at the level of the EU population.

Because of the variety of fish species consumed across the European Union, it is not possible to make general recommendations for fish consumption. The EFSA Scientific Committee therefore recommended "Each country needs to consider its own pattern of fish consumption and carefully assess the risk of exceeding the TWI of methylmercury while obtaining the health benefits from consumption of fish/seafood."

Summary of Evidence on an Approach to Conducting a Risk–Benefit Analysis

In its assessment of the EFSA (2015) report the committee identified inadequate data and uncertainties for fish species, season, location, diet, life stage, and age, as well as undefined regional differences as factors that had a major effect on both the nutrient and contaminant levels reported. Assessment of risks and benefits is further complicated by additional uncertainties in available epidemiological studies about actual serving sizes and actual contents of the potentially active positive and negative components in the seafood consumed.

STEPS IN EVALUATING WHEN OR WHEN NOT TO CONDUCT A RISK–BENEFIT ANALYSIS

The committee's review of the EFSA (2015) report along with additional evidence from peer-reviewed published literature led to the following interpretation of when or when not to conduct a risk–benefit analysis for seafood consumption by women of childbearing age, children, and adolescents.

Initial Assessment in Determining the Need for a Risk–Benefit Analysis

Because RBAs have an inherent requirement for concurrently evaluating both risks and benefits from seafood consumption, any evaluation should combine risks and benefits into a matrix that represents the overall assessment of a particular seafood. Risks are more likely to be included in an RBA leading to a potential bias in the RBA. The imbalance in the required level of scientific evidence for risks versus benefits demands a shift from the RBA as a sum of risks and benefit assessment to the RBA as a well-documented risk–benefit assessment.

Refining the Initial Assessment in Determining the Need for a Risk–Benefit Analysis

The EFSA Scientific Commission recommended that risk assessors consider risks and benefits independently and compare health outcomes to determine whether the benefits outweigh the risks or vice versa. If results demonstrate that neither a substantial risk nor benefit exists, the assessment is terminated. The first and second questions are derived from the model proposed by the EFSA Scientific Commission as it asks whether the scientific principles and evidence as well as the methodology supports assessment of both quality and uncertainty. The third question asks whether modifying factors and additional context are sufficient to establish confidence in the RBA. The final question asks whether the findings, conclusions, recommendations, and data gaps are sufficient to inform policy decision making (EFSA, 2017).

Figure 7-1 shows the committee's steps in the evaluating when or when not to conduct a formal risk–benefit analysis. The committee based its steps for refining risk–benefit decision making on the EFSA (2015) model. Step 1 of the model indicates the sources of evidence used to evaluate whether there is sufficient evidence to justify an RBA. Step 2 indicates the methodologies and framework for comparing risks and benefits as a single net health impact value. Step 3 identifies the factors that influence the decision of whether or not to conduct an RBA. Lastly, step 4 considers factors that the committee considered in developing a process for evaluating confidence and conclusions in the evaluation process.

Summary of Evidence Reviewed on Evaluating the Need for a Risk–Benefit Analysis

The committee notes that the EFSA guidance does not include critical factors such as socioeconomics, diversity, equity, inclusion, access to health care, and other considerations such as mechanisms of action and modifiers, which are essential components of the committee's charge. Therefore, the committee considered the following:

- inclusion of nutritional benefits;
- level of contaminant and microorganism exposure;
- mechanisms of action such as biomarkers, interactions, and intermediate variables;
- modifiers such as geography, access, dietary, and cultural practices;
- environmental stressors, including dimensions of community resilience;
- clinical outcomes relative to risk;
- presence of social determinants of health in the literature; and
- diversity, equity, and inclusion principles in demographic data, data gaps, and recommendations (see Chapters 4 and 5).

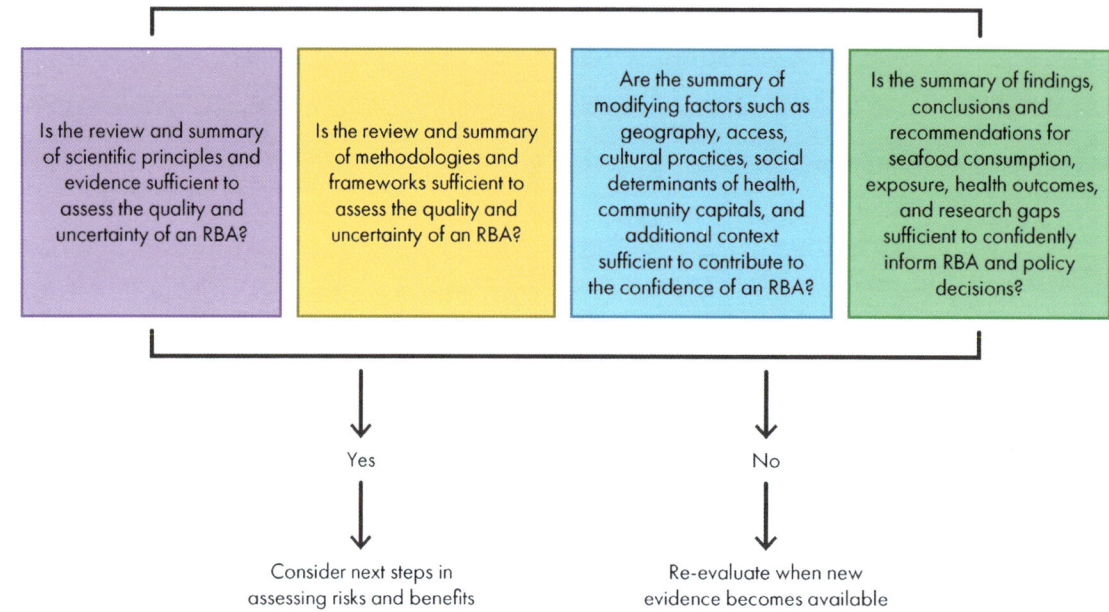

FIGURE 7-1 Steps in evaluating when or when not to conduct a formal risk–benefit analysis.

The committee reviewed the summary of evidence on health outcomes associated with potential risks factors identified in Chapter 6. Studies and reports on those factors that could potentially modify the decision-making process in evaluating whether to conduct an RBA were identified in a subsequent search and are summarized below. The committee considered exposure as it relates to consumption across the life stages of interest, meaning prenatal, infancy, and childhood as described in the analytical framework as important to understanding the interactions between nutrients consumed in seafood and health outcomes (Chapter 6).

A BASIS FOR DECISION MAKING

The committee's review of evidence on nutritional characteristics and potential toxicants in seafood, along with evidence on health outcomes associated with consumption, led to its overarching conclusion that seafood has the potential to exert both health benefits and health risks. Risk–benefit managers should have the ability to weigh those risks against the benefits based on either a qualitative or quantitative RBA. Implied in the decision-making process is that an imbalance exists between risks and benefits that would influence the need for an RBA. Important questions that risk managers should ask are the following:

1. What is the totality of the evidence on benefits and risks associated with seafood consumption?
   a. What are the implications of modifiers of benefit or risk, such as among populations with high vs. low seafood consumption?
2. How is the balance between the risks and benefits characterized?
   a. What is the balance between risks and benefits? Does the risk exceed any benefit or vice versa?
3. Can the benefit only be derived by exposure to seafood?
   a. For example, will a supplement of n-3 LCPUFA provide the same benefit as consumption of fish? That is, does the analysis need to consider the complexity of a food (nutrients, food components, food matrix, overall dietary pattern with or without seafood, etc.)?

4. What is contaminant exposure relative to the TWI?
    a. When can an existing RBA be adapted to the population of interest?
    b. Is there relevant evidence in the population of interest that should be factored into the decision-making process?

To be able to answer these questions requires both strength and adequacy of evidence to support an RBA. In this report the committee searched for new evidence published since the report *Seafood Choices: Balancing Benefits and Risks* (IOM, 2007) to understand the totality of evidence on both benefits and risk associated with consuming seafood and determined that the outcome of each step of an RBA must include a narrative of the strengths and weaknesses of the evidence base as well as the uncertainties.

The report *Guidance on the Use of the Weight of Evidence Approach in Scientific Assessments* (EFSA, 2017) states that the purpose of weighing evidence is to assess the relative support for potential answers to a scientific question, in this case, in support of an RBA. In some circumstances, the evidence supports only one answer with certainty. It is more often the case that multiple answers are possible, each with varying levels of support. Thus, a conclusion should state the range of answers that are possible rather than choose a single answer.

Assessing Quality and Uncertainty

The quantitative metric that is most often used in published RBAs involving food is the DALY. The DALY is increasingly used for risk ranking and in assessing the burden of disease. It is used as an aid to policy makers for decision making about where to spend available resources. When separate health effects need to be aggregated across populations, this analysis can also be expressed as QALYs, which are a measure of health impairment that takes into account changes in longevity and quality of life.

In considering seafood consumption, specifically in the United States and Canada, the committee's assessment was complicated by the finding that many pregnant women and young children do not consume large amounts of seafood (see Chapter 3). Furthermore, much of the data and many of the studies reviewed by the committee came from the European Union and countries outside of the United States and Canada.

Mapping the Decision-Making Process

The committee defined the parameters of risk by including toxins, toxicants, and micro-organisms and defined benefits by considering dietary intake, dietary patterns, and nutrients. In assessing the risks and the benefits, the committee included mechanisms of action such as biomarkers of susceptibility, interactions, and intermediate variables, as well as positive and negative modifiers such as geography, access, dietary patterns, cultural practices, social determinants of health, and community resilience. Lastly, the committee focused on the positive and negative health outcomes relative to growth and development, which includes neurodevelopment, cardiometabolic profiling, immune function, and disease, both chronic and acute. The committee developed a decision tree that takes a systematic approach to assessing when or when not to conduct a risk–benefit analysis for seafood consumption for the target population (Figure 7-2).

COMMUNITY RESILIENCE AND ACCESS TO HEALTH CARE

An example of community resilience is presented in the National Academies report *Advancing Health and Resilience in the Gulf of Mexico Region: A Roadmap for Progress* (NASEM, 2023). The goal of the report was to advance the development of sustainable systems that support activities focused on health and community resilience. The report identified four key roadblocks to achieving resiliency: (1) lack of a uniform systems approach to program development and service delivery; (2) incomplete, ineffective, and uncoordinated efforts to capture data; (3) insufficient resources reaching communities in need; and (4) an enduring failure of current systems to effectively account for the role and multiple dimensions of equity in rendering communities persistently vulnerable. The report then identified four overarching pillars corresponding to the four roadblocks: data, infrastructure, human capital, and governance.

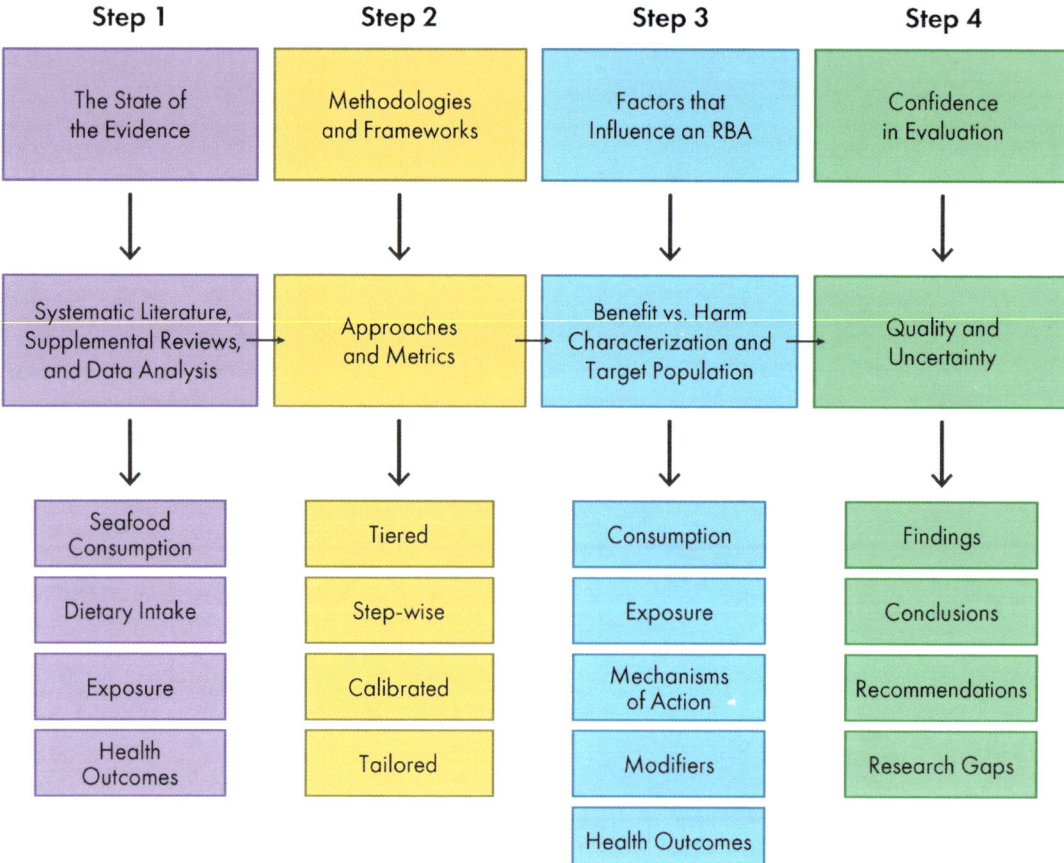

FIGURE 7-2 Decision process for evaluating when or when not to conduct a formal risk–benefit analysis.
NOTE: Steps 1–4 include hyperlinks to respective content in the report.

The report recommended that agencies within the U.S. Department of Health and Human Services- the Centers for Disease Control and Prevention, the National Institutes of Health, and the Federal Emergency Management Agency, as well as external partners, such as the U.S. Census Bureau, should be involved in developing the data pillar. The infrastructure and governance pillars included recommendations for active inclusion of state and legislative leadership with meaningful engagement of communities at state and local levels. The human capital and funding pillar recommendation included public participation to identify specific needs and priorities as well as supports that integrate with community resilience activities. Finally, the report recommended that both federal agencies and philanthropic funding be considered as a means to address issues identified in the report, and that funders should be explicit about their long-term research agendas, research gaps, and funding availability and sustainability expectations.

Social Determinants Influencing Seafood Consumption

Social determinants are defined as the conditions in environments where people are born, live, learn, work, play, worship, and age that affect a wide range of health, functioning, and quality-of-life outcomes and risks. Access to healthy foods is a potential determinant of nutritional health. A study by Guenther et al. (2009) used the Healthy Eating Index–2005 (HEI-2005) to compare food choices between higher-income and low-income individuals (family income less than 130 percent of poverty). The study found that, compared to higher-income individuals, lower-income individuals had significantly lower scores for vegetables, legumes, and whole grains, and higher scores for sodium (indicating a lower intake). However, there was no significant difference in total HEI-2005 scores among children ages 2–18 years by income level.

Among Indigenous female adolescents in Canada, aged 15–22 years, Hanemaayer et al. (2022) assessed the effects of determinants that included social environments (family and peer influence), physical environments (home, schools, and restaurants), and economic factors (income and socioeconomic status) on food choice behaviors. This study found that the built environment had an important influence on food choice, specifically the home and school settings. Family was found to be a facilitator of consistency and health choices, whereas the social environment, such as peers and community relationships, were barriers to healthy food choices. Cost had a detrimental influence on both food choice and regularity of meals. The ecological environment was not a consistent influence on food choice except seasonal consumption of traditional foods.

To understand the role of social factors, such as family structure, parental employment, and education level, as determinants of consumption of seafood and intake of n-3 LCPUFAs in children and adolescents Martínez-Martínez et al. (2020) administered a food frequency questionnaire to parents of school-age children to capture intake frequency and amount. This study identified dietary habit and food familiarity as well as ease of preparation as factors potentially contributing to low frequency of fish consumption. Additionally, the analysis found significantly lower consumption of fish high in n-3 LCPUFAs among children and adolescents whose mothers worked outside the home. An interesting finding was that children and adolescents whose mothers attained a secondary school education had lower intakes of n-3 LCPUFAs than those whose mothers had either a primary school or university education. The authors speculated that the difference could be caused by higher employment outside the home by these mothers.

Diversity, equity, and inclusion as contextual factors for consideration are discussed in Chapter 3 (seafood consumption); Chapter 4 (nutrient intake from seafood), and Chapter 5 (exposure to contaminants in seafood). A summary of contextual factors relevant to assessing risks and benefits associated with seafood consumption is shown in Figure 7-3.

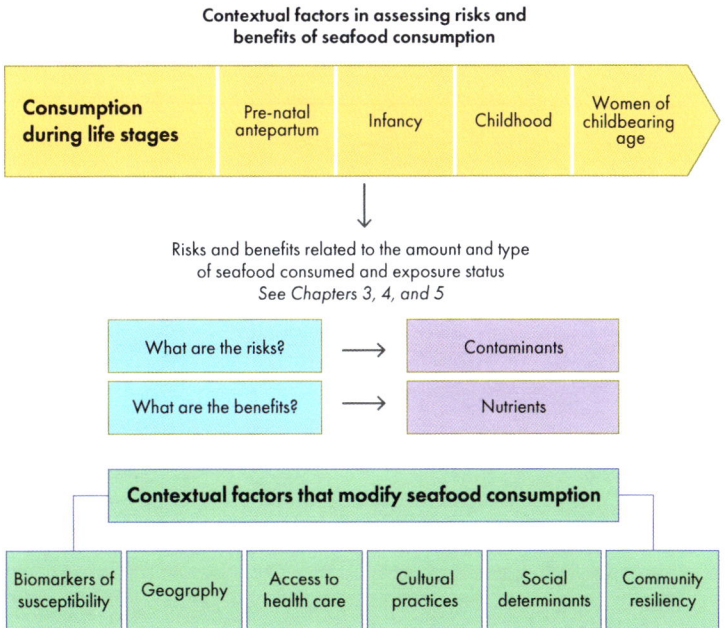

FIGURE 7-3 Contextual factors to consider in assessing risks and benefits associated with seafood consumption.

In summary, this chapter (1) discusses key gaps in the existing evidence, (2) proposes a three-step framework for conducting an RBA (Figures 7-1, 7-2, and 7-3), and (3) emphasizes the role of both individual- and community-level factors to consider when assessing risks and benefits associated with seafood consumption. The committee's comprehensive approach suggests a "big data" strategy that could be enabled by artificial intelligence and machine learning methodologies to allow for predictive modeling informing prevention and early intervention action.

FINDINGS AND CONCLUSIONS

Findings

Approach to Conducting a Risk–Benefit Analysis

1. The integration of diverse data sources and the heterogeneous nature of information available about risks and benefits presents a challenge when selecting metrics to adequately evaluate and compare these risks and benefits in a formal RBA. To date, many formal RBAs have focused on methylmercury as the contaminant and have not assessed contaminant mixtures and toxins. Many other contaminants present in mixtures showed gaps in evidence and hence were less suitable to conduct a formal RBA. Key factors influencing the conduct of RBAs include the social determinants of health at the individual level, such as poverty and health disparities, and cultural traditions and vulnerability at the community level.

Factors Influencing Risk–Benefit Analysis

2. All 50 U.S. states issue voluntary fish consumption advisories on potential contaminant exposure from consuming local fish. Advisories often include specific information about contaminants found in distinct fish species and waters. The evidence available showed variability in the information included in fish advisories for how these hazards are described, and even more variability in what (or if) nutritional information is included in these advisories, yet they are an information source for consumers. A key focus was observed on risks associated with the consumption of MeHg-contaminated fish by pregnant women. Most advisories do not adequately address the risk for specific vulnerable populations, especially subsistence fishers. The committee finds that this irregularity across advisories makes comparison of risks and benefits difficult for most consumers.

Conclusions

1. *A risk–benefit analysis can be an excellent tool to analyze, in a transparent matter, factors that affect both benefits and risks in an integrated approach, rather than as independent domains. This integrated approach toward assessing benefits and risks positions an RBA to effectively support decision-making processes regarding fish consumption. This tool can be applied at the population and individual levels and its scope extended beyond health concerns by including costs, environmental sustainability, and ethics.*
2. *The process for evaluating when or when not to conduct a formal RBA requires assessing the following four key areas: the state of evidence aided by systematic reviews of existing literature, the existence of validated approaches and metrics, an analysis of contextual factors affecting benefits or risk tailored to specific target populations, and the quality and uncertainty of the overall RBA evaluation.*
3. *Formal risk–benefit analyses of fish consumption are seldom conducted because no comprehensive source exists that provides necessary, available data on consumption, contextualization factors, and contamination.*
4. *Maximizing the usefulness of a risk–benefit analysis requires the integration of datasets addressing life stages, consumption patterns, information on nutrient status, exposure to contaminants, health outcomes, and contextual factors.*
5. *Communication about potential health benefits conferred by specific nutrients in seafood is varied. The advisories reviewed by the committee were voluntary and not subject to regulation.*

6. Strengthening the links between a formal risk–benefit analysis, management decisions, and dietary recommendations communicated to the public can improve transparency and advance public health outcomes by ensuring that the best science informs management decisions.

RECOMMENDATIONS

Recommendation 3: The U.S. Food and Drug Administration should consider conducting a risk–benefit analysis of maternal and child seafood intake and child growth and development, and, in doing so, routinely monitor data and scientific discoveries related to the underlying model and assumptions to ensure the assessment reflects the best available science.

Recommendation 4: In conducting a risk–benefit analysis, the U.S. Food and Drug Administration and the U.S. Environmental Protection Agency should include reviews of current evidence scans, systematic and supplemental reviews, approaches and metrics, benefit–harm characterization, and quality and assurance in evaluating the confidence in a risk–benefit analysis for policy decision making.

Recommendation 5: The U.S. Food and Drug Administration, in collaboration with the U.S. Environmental Protection Agency, should create an integrated database to support risk–benefit analyses for fish consumption, thoroughly considering implications of using a metric that reflects transparency and conflicts of interest for both risk and benefit.

Recommendation 6: To maximize the use of a formal risk–benefit analysis, the U.S. Food and Drug Administration in collaboration with the U.S. Environmental Protection Agency should present conclusions of a risk–benefit analysis, including a risk estimate, in a readily understandable and useful form to risk managers and be made available to other risk assessors and interested parties.

RESEARCH GAPS

- Research is needed to inform the use of emerging technologies, such as artificial intelligence and machine learning, to develop a comprehensive data integration framework to support the conduct of risk–benefit analyses.
- Research is needed to determine both the individual effect as well as the potential cumulative effects of factors that influence the conduct of a risk–benefit analysis.
- The science undergirding the conduct of a risk–benefit analysis should be periodically reviewed, such as every 3–5 years, and updated when needed.

REFERENCES

Andersen, L. F., P. Berstad, B. A. Bukhvalova, M. H. Carlsen, L. J. Dahl, A. Goksøyr, L. Sletting Jakobsen, H. K. Knutsen, I. Kvestad, and I. T. L. Lillegaard. 2022. Benefit and risk assessment of fish in the Norwegian diet—scientific opinion of the steering committee of the Norwegian Scientific Committee for Food and Environment.

Boué, G., S. Guillou, J.-P. Antignac, B. Le Bizec, and J.-M. Membré. 2015. Public health risk–benefit assessment associated with food consumption—A review. *European Journal of Food Research & Review* 5(1):32.

Boué, G., E. Ververis, A. Niforou, M. Federighi, S. M. Pires, M. Poulsen, S. T. Thomsen, and A. Naska. 2022. Risk–benefit assessment of foods: Development of a methodological framework for the harmonized selection of nutritional, microbiological, and toxicological components. *Frontiers in Nutrition* 9:951369.

Carrington, C. D., and M. P. Bolger. 2002. An exposure assessment for methylmercury from seafood for consumers in the United States. *Risk Analysis* 22(4):689-699.

Cohen, J. T., D. C. Bellinger, W. E. Connor, P. M. Kris-Etherton, R. S. Lawrence, D. A. Savitz, B. A. Shaywitz, S. M. Teutsch, and G. M. Gray. 2005. A quantitative risk–benefit analysis of changes in population fish consumption. *American Journal of Preventive Medicine* 29(4):325-334.

EFSA (European Food Safety Authority Scientific Committee). 2010. Guidance on human health risk–benefit assessment of food. *EFSA Journal* 8(7):1673.

EFSA. 2015. Statement on the benefits of fish/seafood consumption compared to the risks of methylmercury in fish/seafood. *EFSA Journal* 13(1):3982.

EFSA. 2017. Guidance on the use of the weight of evidence approach in scientific assessments. *EFSA Journal* 15(8).

EFSA Panel on Contaminants in the Food Chain. 2012. Scientific Opinion on the risk for public health related to the presence of mercury and methylmercury in food. *EFSA Journal* 10(12):2985.

EFSA Panel on Contaminants in the Food Chain. 2018. Risk for animal and human health related to the presence of dioxins and dioxin-like PCBs in feed and food. *EFSA Journal* 16(11: e05333.

FAO/WHO (Food and Agriculture Organization of the United Nation and World Health Organization). 2011. *Report of the joint FAO/WHO expert consultation on the risks and benefits of fish consumption.* Geneva, Switzerland: World Health Organization.

FAO/WHO. 2023. *Joint FAO/WHO expert consultation on the risks and benefits of fish consumption.* Geneva, Switzerland: World Health Organization.

FDA (U.S. Food and Drug Administration). 2014. *Quantitative assessment of the net effects on fetal neurodevelopment from eating commercial fish (as measured by IQ and also by early age verbal development in children).* https://www.fda.gov/food/environmental-contaminants-food/quantitative-assessment-net-effects-fetal-neurodevelopment-eating-commercial-fish-measured-iq-and (accessed February 29, 2024).

FDA. 2017. *FDA and EPA issue fish consumption advice.* https://www.fda.gov/food/cfsan-constituent-updates/fda-and-epa-issue-fish-consumption-advice (accessed December 5, 2023).

Ginsberg, G. L., and B. F. Toal. 2009. Quantitative approach for incorporating methylmercury risks and omega-3 fatty acid benefits in developing species-specific fish consumption advice. *Environmental Health Perspectives* 117(2):267-275.

Ginsberg, G., B. Toal, and P. McCann. 2015. Updated risk/benefit analysis of fish consumption effects on neurodevelopment: Implications for setting advisories. *Human and Ecological Risk Assessment: An International Journal* 21(7):1810-1839.

Guenther, P. M., W. Juan, M. Lino, H. A. Hiza, T. V. Fungwe, and R. Lucas. 2009. Diet quality of low-income and higher-income Americans in 2003-2004 as measured by the Healthy Eating Index-2005. *FASEB Journal* 23:540.545.

Hanemaayer, R., H. T. Neufeld, K. Anderson, J. Haines, K. Gordon, K. R. L. Lickers, A. Xavier, L. Peach, and M. Peeters. 2022. Exploring the environmental determinants of food choice among Haudenosaunee female youth. *BMC Public Health* 22(1):1156.

Hoekstra, J., A. Hart, H. Owen, M. Zeilmaker, B. Bokkers, B. Thorgilsson, and H. Gunnlaugsdottir. 2013. Fish, contaminants and human health: Quantifying and weighing benefits and risks. *Food and Chemical Toxicology* 54:18-29.

IOM (Institute of Medicine). 2007. *Seafood choices: Balancing benefits and risks.* Washington, DC: The National Academies Press.

Martínez-Martínez, M. I., A. Alegre-Martínez, and O. Cauli. 2020. Omega-3 long-chain polyunsaturated fatty acids intake in children: The role of family-related social determinants. *Nutrients* 12(11).

Membré, J. M., S. S. Farakos, and M. Nauta. 2021. Risk-benefit analysis in food safety and nutrition. *Current Opinion in Food Science* 39:76-82.

NASEM (National Academies of Sciences, Engineering and Medicine). 2023. *Advancing health and resilience in the Gulf of Mexico region: A roadmap for progress.* Washington, DC: The National Academies Press. https://doi.org/10.17226/27057.

Nauta, M. J., R. Andersen, K. Pilegaard, S. M. Pires, G. Ravn-Haren, I. Tetens, and M. Poulsen. 2018. Meeting the challenges in the development of risk-benefit assessment of foods. *Trends in Food Science & Technology* 76:90-100.

Scherer, A. C., A. Tsuchiya, L. R. Younglove, T. M. Burbacher, and E. M. Faustman. 2008. Comparative analysis of state fish consumption advisories targeting sensitive populations. *Environmental Health Perspectives* 116(12):1598-1606.

WCRF (World Cancer Research Fund) International. 2018. Meat, fish and dairy products and the risk of cancer. Continuous Update Project Expert Report. London, United Kingdom.

A

Committee Member Biosketches

Virginia A. Stallings, M.D. (*Chair*), is professor of pediatrics at the University of Pennsylvania Perelman School of Medicine, and director of the Nutrition Center and the Jean A. Cortner Endowed Chair in Gastroenterology and Nutrition at Children's Hospital of Philadelphia. Her research interests include pediatric nutrition, evaluation of dietary intake and energy expenditure, and nutrition-related chronic disease. Dr. Stallings has served on several National Academies of Sciences, Engineering, and Medicine Committees: the Committee on Food Allergies: Global Burden, Causes, Treatment, Prevention, and Public Policy; the Committee on Nutrition Standards for National School Lunch and Breakfast Programs; the Committee on Nutrition Services for Medicare Beneficiaries; the Committee on the Scientific Basis for Dietary Risk Eligibility Criteria for WIC (Women, Infants, and Children) Programs; the Committee to Review the WIC Food Packages (2003); the Committee to Review Child and Adult Care Food Program Meal Requirements; and the Committee to Review the Dietary Reference Intakes for Sodium and Potassium. She is a former member (1997–2000) and co-vice chair (2000–2002) of the Food and Nutrition Board. Dr. Stallings is board certified in pediatrics and clinical nutrition. She received the Fomon Nutrition Award from the American Academy of Pediatrics. Dr. Stallings is a member of the Board of Trustees of the Philadelphia College of Osteopathic Medicine and has served as a member of the Board of Directors for Danone. Dr. Stallings earned a B.S. in nutrition and foods from Auburn University, an M.S. in human nutrition and biochemistry from Cornell University, and an M.D. from the University of Alabama in Birmingham School of Medicine. She is a member of the National Academy of Medicine.

Laurie Hing Man Chan, Ph.D., has been a professor and Canada research chair (Tier 1) in toxicology and environmental health at the University of Ottawa since 2011. He was a founding member of the Centre for Indigenous Peoples Nutrition and Environment at McGill University and the holder of a BC Leadership Chair in Aboriginal Health at the University of Northern British Columbia. Professor Chan is a world-renowned expert in mercury toxicology and has worked with Indigenous populations for more than 30 years. Professor Chan's research in environmental and nutritional toxicology spans from the laboratory developing new techniques for contaminant analysis to participatory research in the community on the risk and benefits of traditional foods and the impact of environmental change on food security. He is the principal investigator of the First Nations Food, Nutrition and Environment Study and the Food, Environment, Health, and Nutrition of First Nations Children and Youth Study. Professor Chan has published more than 300 peer-reviewed scientific papers and supervised more than 90 graduate students. He has also served as an advisor for international and national governments and organizations and numerous Indigenous communities on environmental health issues. He was a member of Expert Consultation by the World Health Organization/Food Agriculture Organization on the Risks and Benefits of Fish Consumption in 2010. Professor Chan is a Fulbright Scholar and a Fellow of the Canadian Academy of Health Sciences.

Elaine M. Faustman, Ph.D., DABT, ATS, is professor and director, Institute for Risk Analysis and Risk Communications, School of Public Health, University of Washington, Seattle, Washington. Her previous service has included adjunct professorship in the Department of Engineering and Public Policy at Carnegie Mellon University, Pittsburgh, Pennsylvania, and she currently is adjunct professor, Daniel J. Evans School of Public Policy and Governance at the University of Washington. She is an elected fellow of the American Association for the Advancement of Science, the Society for Risk Analysis, and the Washington State Academy of Science. Her past service has included membership on the U.S. Environmental Protection Agency (EPA) Science Advisory Board, the National Institute of Environmental Health Sciences (NIEHS) National Advisory Environmental Health Sciences Council, and the National Toxicology Program Board of Scientific Counselors. She has served as the Secretary General for the International Union of Toxicology and as cochair of the steering committee of the International Science Council World Data Systems and the Health Professionals Advisory Board for the International Joint Commission (United States and Canada) for Boundary Waters. Her research expertise is on identifying molecular mechanisms of developmental, reproductive, and neurotoxicants; characterizing *in vitro* techniques for toxicology assessment; and developing the biological basis for dose–response and cost–benefit models. She has directed the National Science Foundation and NIEHS Center for Oceans and Human Health at the University of Washington. She has more than 250 peer-reviewed research publications and reports including co-editorship of a *Handbook for Life Course Health Studies*. Her service on National Academies committees includes chair of the Committee for Developmental Toxicology, chair of recent workshops for EPA (AI and Triangulation), and membership of the Upper Limits subcommittee, Food and Nutrition Board, National Academy of Medicine. Research efforts include her leadership as principal investigator for the EPA Predictive Toxicology Center and her work with NIEHS and the National Institute of Child Health and Human Development directing various children's cohort studies. Dr. Faustman received her B.A. degree from Hope College with a dual degree in chemistry and biology, Ph.D. from Michigan State University in pharmacology and toxicology, and her postdoctoral fellowship in pharmacology, pediatrics, and pathology.

Claude Earl Fox, M.D., M.P.H., is currently a professor emeritus of the University of Miami Miller School of Medicine, and he retired as a research professor of the Department of Epidemiology and Medicine there in 2006. He previously was the founding director of the Johns Hopkins Urban Health Institute and the Florida Institute for Health Innovations as well as founding chair of the editorial board of *Progress in Community Health Partnerships: Research, Education and Action*, Johns Hopkins University Press. Dr. Fox served on the Institute of Medicine committee that authored the 2007 report *Seafood Choices: Balancing Benefits and Risks* and was cochair of the Nutrition Policy Board for the Department of Health and Human Services (HHS). He also was cochair of the federal HHS Steering Committee Implementing the Children's Health Insurance Program passed by Congress and chairman of the Steering Committee for the HHS Healthy People 2000 plan. He was awarded the Alumnus of the Year from the University of North Carolina School of Public Health in 1999 and the John Farrell Prize for Outstanding Contributions to Preventive Medicine and Public Health, University of North Carolina, in 2001. Dr. Fox has served as the President of the Association of State and Territorial Health Officials and Chair of the Alabama Task Force on Prevention and Prenatal Care. In addition to his master's degree in public health in maternal and child health at the University of North Carolina, Dr. Fox is board certified in preventive medicine and public health, and he received pediatric clinical training at the University of Mississippi and the Johns Hopkins Hospital in Baltimore.

Delbert M. Gatlin III, Ph.D., is a regents professor in the Department of Ecology and Conservation Biology and member of the Intercollegiate Faculty of Nutrition at Texas A&M University. He has had an academic appointment with Texas A&M University since 1987. Dr. Gatlin's research program encompasses many different aspects of fish nutrition in support of aquaculture, including determination of requirements for, and metabolism of, various nutrients, as well as development and evaluation of diet additives, formulations, and feedstuffs for various fish species including channel catfish, hybrid striped bass, red drum, and tilapia. The targeted goal of his research program is improving sustainability and production efficiency in aquaculture and enhancing the health and well-being of cultured organisms. Gatlin was Vice Chair of the Committee on Nutrient Requirements of Fish and Shrimp of the National Academies from 2009 to 2010. He has coauthored over 300 peer-reviewed journal articles, 19 book chapters, and four books. Gatlin has been Nutrition Section Editor for the journal *Aquaculture* since 2009 and Editor-In-Chief since 2019. Dr. Gatlin earned a B.S. in fisheries/aquaculture from Texas A&M University in 1980 and a Ph.D. in nutritional biochemistry from Mississippi State University in 1983. He is also a Certified Fisheries Scientist and member of the American Fisheries Society, World Aquaculture Society, and American Society for Nutrition.

Julie Herbstman, Ph.D., is a professor in the Department of Environmental Health Sciences, Director of the Columbia Center for Children's Environmental Health, and Director of the Certificate Program in Molecular Epidemiology at the Columbia University Mailman School of Public Health. Her research evaluates the associations between prenatal and early life environmental exposures and childhood outcomes primarily using longitudinal birth cohort studies. She has studied effects of exposures including polybrominated diphenyl ethers, per- and polyfluoroalkyl substances, polychlorinated biphenyls, and polycyclic aromatic hydrocarbons on child growth and neurodevelopment. Her research also incorporates biomarkers, including epigenetic measures. Dr. Herbstman received a Ph.D. in environmental epidemiology from the Johns Hopkins University and completed postdoctoral training in environmental health sciences from Columbia University.

Margaret R. Karagas, Ph.D., is the James W. Squires Professor and founding chair of the Department of Epidemiology at the Geisel School of Medicine at Dartmouth College and Director of its Center for Molecular Epidemiology. Her research encompasses interdisciplinary studies to illuminate the etiology of human cancers as well as adverse pregnancy and children's health outcomes. Her work seeks to identify emerging environmental exposures, host factors, and mechanisms that affect health from infancy to adult life, and to apply novel methods and technologies to understand disease pathogenesis. Among her current investigations is a rural cohort study of pregnant women and their offspring in northern New England designed to identify the sources and effects of nutrient and toxicant elements on childhood infection, allergy/atopy, growth, and neurodevelopment. Her collaborative studies examine a broad range of exposure biomarkers, individual susceptibility, and biological response to environmental agents including the developing microbiome and immune response. Furthermore, she has participated in synthesis papers on mercury and arsenic in food. She has served on international consensus panels (e.g., International Agency for Research on Cancer Monograph Program, European Food Safety Authority Scientific Opinions), and on expert committees for the U.S. National Cancer Institute, U.S. Environmental Protection Agency, and National Academies of Sciences, Engineering, and Medicine. She received her Ph.D. in epidemiology from the University of Washington.

Sibylle Kranz, Ph.D., RDN, FTOS, is tenured associate professor with primary appointment in the Department of Kinesiology, School of Education and Human Development. She holds an adjunct associate professor appointment in the Department of Public Health Sciences, School of Medicine, at the University of Virginia (UVA). As a registered dietitian with a Ph.D. in nutrition epidemiology from the University of North Carolina at Chapel Hill, she is the Director of UVA's Diet and Nutrition laboratory, and her research focuses on the role of dietary intake in children and the relationship between diet and health as well as changing dietary intake behavior. She conducts clinical feeding trials in laboratory and community settings serving young children in addition to performing epidemiologic research on diet quality and intake patterns in the United States, the United Kingdom, and China. She was principal investigator (PI) or co-PI on several systematic literature reviews and metanalysis. Prior to arriving at UVA, she was senior lecturer at the University of Bristol, United Kingdom (2014–2016), associate professor and Director of the Coordinated Undergraduate Program in Dietetics at Purdue University (2009–2014), faculty at East Carolina University (2008–2009), and the Pennsylvania State University (2002–2008) in its Nutrition Department. Dr. Kranz taught multiple courses in introduction to nutrition, life-cycle nutrition, diet therapy, and nutrition counseling at the undergraduate and graduate levels. She is actively engaged in a number of professional organizations as a member of the Obesity Society (since 2002) where she was awarded Fellow status since 2007, the American Public Health Association where she served as Chair of the Food and Nutrition Section (2009), the

American Society of Nutrition (Chair of the Nutrition Education and Behavioral Sciences Research Interest Sections, 2021–2023), and member of the American College for Sport Medicine and the Academy of Nutrition and Dietetics. She also held appointed or elected leadership positions for the Accreditation Council for the Academy of Nutrition and Dietetics to help guide the education standards and performance standards for future registered dietitians.

Maureen Lichtveld, M.D., M.P.H., is the dean of the School of Public Health, the Jonas Salk Chair in Population Health, and professor of environmental and occupational health at the University of Pittsburgh with more than 35 years of expertise in environmental health. As dean, Dr. Lichtveld oversees seven academic departments, more than 900 students, 165 faculty, and 320 staff. Her research focuses on environmentally induced disease, health disparities, climate and health, environmental health policy, disaster preparedness, public health systems, and community resilience. Dean Lichtveld is a member of the National Academy of Medicine (NAM), the NAM Council, and a member of many NAM and National Academies boards, roundtables, and committees. She serves on the Advisory Committees for the National Academies' Climate Communications Initiative and the Division of Earth and Life Sciences. Dean Lichtveld is the Chair of the Consortium of Universities for Global Health. She coauthored the textbook *Environmental Policy and Public Health*. Honors include Johns Hopkins University Society of Scholars, and Woman of the Year for the City of New Orleans for her contributions to science.

Charles A. Nelson III, Ph.D., is currently professor of pediatrics and neuroscience and professor of psychology in the Department of Psychiatry at Harvard Medical School, and professor of education in the Harvard Graduate School of Education. He also holds the Richard David Scott Chair in Pediatric Developmental Medicine Research at Boston Children's Hospital and serves as Director of Research in the Division of Developmental Medicine. His research interests center on a variety of problems in developmental cognitive neuroscience, including the development of social perception, developmental trajectories to autism, and the effects of early adversity on brain and behavioral development. Among his many honors, he has received the Leon Eisenberg award from Harvard Medical School and an honorary doctorate from Bucharest University (Romania). He was a resident fellow at the Rockefeller Foundation Bellagio (Italy) Center, has been elected to the American Academy of Arts and Sciences, the National Academy of Medicine, the British Academy, and along with Professors Fox and Zeanah has received the Ruane Prize for Child and Adolescent Psychiatric Research from the Brain & Behavior Research Foundation. In 2021 he received the Klaus J. Jacobs Research Prize, and in 2023 he received the Society for Research in Child Development Distinguished Scientific Contributions to Child Development award. In 2023, Dr. Nelson was retained by the law firm representing the plaintiffs in a class action suit to specifically address whether the educational deprivation experienced by children residing in state-run or privately run residential care settings in New Hampshire caused long-term harm.

Emily Oken, M.D., M.P.H., is professor in the Department of Population Medicine at Harvard Medical School and Harvard Pilgrim Health Care Institute. She is also professor in the Department of Nutrition at the Harvard T.H. Chan School of Public Health. Dr. Oken directs the Division of Chronic Disease Research Across the Lifecourse within the Department of Population Medicine. Her research focuses on the influence of nutrition and other modifiable factors during pregnancy and early childhood on long-term maternal and child health, including growth, cardiometabolic health, asthma, atopy, and cognitive development. She has also led a number of studies examining women's health outcomes across the life course, from the peripartum period through midlife. Her work on the toxicant risks and nutrient benefits of prenatal fish consumption has influenced national and international guidelines for fish consumption during pregnancy, helping to shift the previous focus of risk-only or benefit-only studies to a broader emphasis on the overall health effects of fish consumption for mother and baby. She authors the chapter on fish consumption during pregnancy for UpToDate, an online medical textbook. She participated, in a nonaffiliate capacity, in an expert consensus group, with a focus on high-dose docosahexaenoic acid supplementation and recommendations for the prevention of preterm birth. Additionally, she chaired the 2023 Food and Agriculture Organization of the United Nations/World Health Organization Expert Consultation on Risks and Benefits of Fish Consumption. She has led longitudinal studies commencing in the peripartum period and following mothers and children throughout childhood including related original qualitative and quantitative research. She has served on committees to develop nutrition guidelines both nationally and internationally, authored reviews and perspectives, and has participated in U.S. Food and Drug Administration and U.S. Environmental Protection Agency–sponsored conferences. For the National Academy of Medicine, she has served on the Committee for Evaluating the Process to Develop the Dietary Guidelines for Americans, 2020–2025; as a Planning Committee Member for the 2020 workshop on Nutrition in Pregnancy; and as a Planning Committee Member for the Food Forum's 2023 workshop on Dietary Patterns and Diet-Related Chronic Diseases Across the Lifespan. She serves on the National Institute of Child Health and Human Development Board of Scientific Counselors. Dr. Oken received her M.D. from Harvard Medical School and her M.P.H. from the Harvard School of Public Health. She completed her internship and residency in internal medicine and pediatrics, and fellowship in general internal medicine and primary care, at Harvard Medical School.

Ian J. Saldanha, M.B.B.S., M.P.H., Ph.D., is an associate professor of epidemiology at the Johns Hopkins Bloomberg School of Public Health. He also holds a joint appointment as associate professor of health services, policy, and practice at the Brown University School of Public Health. When at Brown (2018–2022), he was assistant director of the Brown University Evidence-based Practice Center, which is one of nine such centers funded by the Agency for Healthcare Research and Quality (AHRQ). Dr. Saldanha has expertise conducting systematic reviews and meta-analyses, developing and advancing methods to improve them, and teaching methods for their conduct. He has also researched the use of outcomes in clinical research. Dr. Saldanha has served on two National Academies of Sciences, Engineering, and Medicine's committees: (1) Scanning New Evidence on Nutrient Content of Human Milk and (2) Scanning for New Evidence on Riboflavin to Support a Dietary Reference Intake Review. Dr. Saldanha was the co–principal investigator (PI) of a National Academies contract to conduct a systematic review of public health emergency preparedness activities. He has been the PI of four AHRQ-funded systematic reviews: (1) management of primary headaches during pregnancy, (2) breast reconstruction after mastectomy, (3) postpartum care up to 1 year after delivery, and (4) postpartum management of hypertensive disorders of pregnancy. Additionally, he has been the PI of multiple AHRQ contracts to develop, advance, maintain, and support the Systematic Review Data Repository. Dr. Saldanha is an elected member of the Society for Research Synthesis Methodology and currently serves as its treasurer. He has served as the associate editor for various journals (e.g., *Trials*, *Systematic Reviews*, *Journal of Glaucoma*) and for the AHRQ Effective Healthcare Program. Dr. Saldanha has taught multiple courses and workshops related to systematic reviews, meta-analysis, clinical trials, and epidemiology at the undergraduate, graduate, and professional levels at various universities and other venues, such as the Centers for Disease Control and Prevention. He received his M.B.B.S. (M.D. equivalent) from Grant Medical College in Mumbai, India, and his M.P.H. and Ph.D. in epidemiology from the Johns Hopkins Bloomberg School of Public Health.

B

Open Session Agendas

The Role of Seafood Consumption in Child Growth and Development
Open Session
Evidence Scans to Explore the Available Evidence on Seafood and Health
February 23, 2023
1:45–3:00 pm ET

Objectives: The goal of this session is to:
- Review and discuss evidence scans conducted to explore the available evidence on seafood and health to inform the scope and tasks for a systematic review

1:45 pm	Introductions and Chair's Opening Remarks *Virginia Stallings, Chair*
1:55	Introduction to Evidence Scan *Kellie Casavale, FDA*
2:00	Epidemiology *Cecile Punzalan, FDA*
2:10	Mechanisms of Action *Emanuel Hignutt, FDA*
2:20	Risk–Benefit Analysis *Sofia Santillana Farakos, FDA* *Jacqueline Heilman, FDA*
2:30	Questions from the Committee *Virginia Stallings*

2:45   Closing Remarks
        Virginia Stallings

3:00   Adjourn

The Role of Seafood Consumption in Child Growth and Development
April 6, 2023
9:50 am–3:30 pm EST

9:50 am   Welcome and Introductions
           Virginia Stallings, M.D., Committee Chair

10:00   Session 1—Interaction Between Nutrients and Contaminants in Fish and Seafood
           Contaminant Mixture Effects During Pregnancy
           Emily Oken, M.D., M.P.H., Professor, Departments of Nutrition and Population Medicine, Harvard Medical School

           Lessons Learned from the Seychelles Child Development Study
           Edwin van Wijngaarden, Ph.D., Professor, Public Health Sciences, Environmental Medicine, Pediatrics and Dentistry, University of Rochester

           Interaction of Selenium with Environmental Contaminants in Fish and Seafood
           Nicholas Ralston, Ph.D., Research Scientist, University of North Dakota

11:00   Q&A

11:30   Session 2—Health Outcomes Associated with Nutrient Intake and Contaminant Exposure in Fish and Seafood
           Impact of Nutrients and Contaminants in Seafood on Neurodevelopment
           Joseph R. Hibbeln, M.D., CAPT, USPHS (ret.), Benjamin Meaker Distinguished Visiting Professor, University of Bristol, UK

           Impact of Nutrients and Contaminants in Human Milk on Growth and Development
           Christine D. Garner, Ph.D., RD, CLC, Assistant Vice President of Research, Assistant Professor, Department of Pediatrics, InfantRisk Center, Texas Tech University Health Sciences Center

12:10 pm   Q&A

12:30   Break

1:15   Session 3—Panel Discussion: The Lived Experience from Underserved and Native Communities
           Jamie Donatuto, Ph.D., Swinomish Indian Tribal Community
           Lanor Curole, M.A., United Houma Tribal Nation

2:15   Session 4—Seafood and Sustainability
           Management of Marine Ecosystems
           Daniel Pauly, FRSC, UBC Killam Professor, Sea Around Us; Institute for the Oceans and Fisheries & Department of Zoology

Equitable Access to Sustainable Marine Resources
Martin D. Smith, Ph.D., George M. Woodwell Distinguished Professor of Environmental Economics, Duke University

2:55   Q&A

3:15   Closing Remarks
Virginia Stallings, Committee Chair

3:30   Adjourn

C

Commissioned Systematic Reviews

BACKGROUND

The Agriculture, Food, and Nutrition Evidence Center at Texas A&M University (Evidence Center) was contracted to perform three systematic reviews examining the associations between seafood nutrition and toxicant intake during pregnancy, lactation, and child growth and development. These reviews addressed three key questions:

1. What are the associations between seafood consumption *during pregnancy and lactation* and child growth and development?
2. What are the associations between seafood consumption *during childhood* and child growth and development?
3. What are the associations between seafood toxicant exposure during pregnancy, lactation, and childhood and child growth and development?

The Evidence Center was asked to update two existing systematic reviews previously published by the USDA Nutrition Evidence Systematic Review Center conducted to inform the *Dietary Guidelines for Americans 2020–2025 (DGA)* that examined the relationship between seafood nutrition and health outcomes among pregnant and lactating women, as well as children (USDA/HHS, 2020). These two reviews are collectively referred to as the "nutrition reviews." In addition, a third *de novo* systematic review was requested to examine associations of seafood-related contaminants (toxicological) with health outcomes during pregnancy, lactation, and childhood on child growth and development. This review is referred to as the "toxicology review." For the toxicology systematic review, a scoping review was conducted to prioritize exposure–outcome associations with sufficient evidence to warrant a full systematic review. Relevant data and information for the systematic reviews was provided to the Evidence Center by the committee. The searches were run by the National Academies Resource Center librarian, and search results were provided to the Evidence Center. The Evidence Center drafted the review protocol, including relevant methodology, based on the provided information. Protocols for the three reviews were registered in PROSPERO (CRD42023432844).[1] Supplemental online Appendix F provides the full search strategy for each systematic review. The full methodology report from the Evidence Center is available in online Appendix H. The

---

[1] See https://www.crd.york.ac.uk/prospero/.

data extraction tables and lists of articles retrieved and evaluated by the Evidence Center are also described in online Appendix H.[2]

METHODOLOGY

PECOD Analytic Framework and Inclusion and Exclusion Criteria for Nutrition Reviews

Analytic Frameworks for Nutrition Reviews

The Evidence Center developed an analytic framework for the nutrition reviews. Figure C-1 shows the framework used for examining the associations of seafood consumption during pregnancy and lactation and neurocognitive development in the child. A similar framework was devised to examine associations of seafood consumption during childhood and adolescence and neurocognitive development in children. A complete description of the review methodology is provided in online Appendix H.

Inclusion and Exclusion Criteria

Inclusion and exclusion terms were provided by the committee and a PECOD (population, exposures, comparators, outcomes, designs [of studies]) table constructed for each nutrition review. Table C-1 shows the criteria

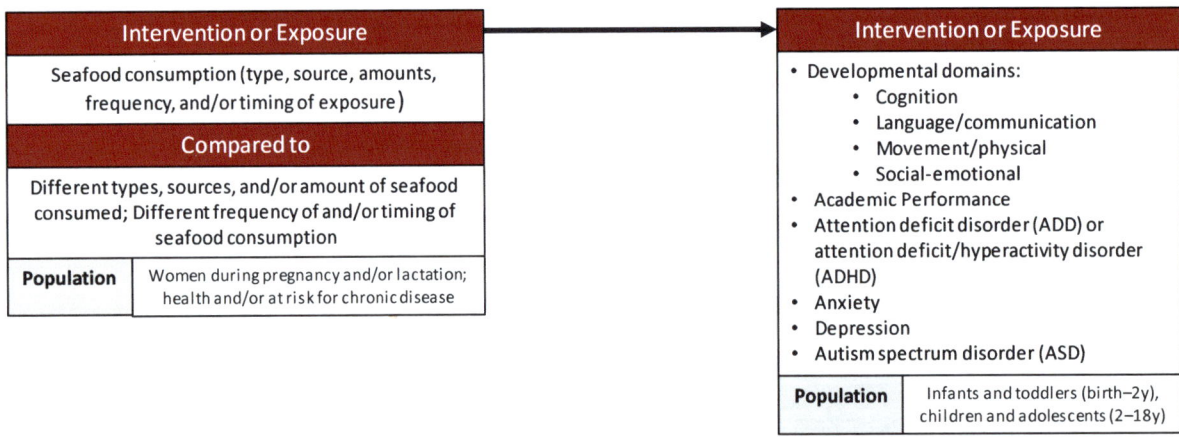

FIGURE C-1 Analytic framework for examining the associations of seafood consumption during pregnancy and lactation and neurocognitive development in the child.
SOURCE: Texas A&M Agriculture, Food, and Nutrition Evidence Center, 2023.

---

[2] Appendixes F through H can be found online at https://nap.nationalacademies.org/catalog/27623.

TABLE C-1 Inclusion and Exclusion Criteria for Associations of Seafood Consumption During Pregnancy and Lactation and Neurocognitive Development in the Child

Component	Inclusion Criteria	Exclusion Criteria

Populations	Individuals living in countries ranked as high or very high on the human development index during the study[a]
	• Exposed population: Individuals in the general population who are pregnant or lactating, infants, children, or adolescents up to age 18 years. Subgroups of interest:
	  ○ By race/ethnicity
	  ○ By income
	  ○ By cumulative exposure to nonchemical stressors (e.g., stress, depression)
	  ○ By cumulative exposure to environmental stressors (e.g., neighborhood or locale, food security)
	  ○ By preexisting disease burden
	• Outcome population: Children and adolescents (up to age 18 years). Subgroups of interest:
	  ○ Infants (ages 0–12 months)
	  ○ Toddlers (ages 1–3 years)
	  ○ Early childhood (ages 4–8 years)
	  ○ Puberty (ages 9–13 years)
	  ○ Adolescents (ages 14–18 years)
		• Studies exclusively of participants with a chronic condition, hospitalized with an illness or injury. Examples include:
		  ○ Diabetes (not including gestational diabetes)
		  ○ Cancer
		  ○ Cardiometabolic disorders
		  ○ Chronic kidney disease
		  ○ Malabsorption (any disorder that causes malabsorption from the gastrointestinal tract)
		  ○ Asthma

Exposures	• Seafood consumption:
	  ○ Types (e.g., salmon, tuna, bass)
	  ○ Sources (e.g., sea, freshwater, farmed, canned, wild)
	  ○ Amount (e.g., ounces per day, grams per meal)
	  ○ Frequency (e.g., daily, twice per week)
	  ○ Duration (e.g., length of time consuming seafood)
	  ○ Preparation (e.g., fried, baked)
	  ○ Timing (e.g., by trimester, age)
		• Supplements
		• Infant formula

Comparators:	• Different types, sources, amounts, frequencies, durations, preparations, or timings of seafood consumption • No seafood consumption	No comparator

Outcomes	Neurodevelopment and neurodevelopmental disorders
	  ○ Developmental domains: cognition, language/communication, movement/physical, social-emotional
	  ○ Social/emotional outcomes
	  ○ Academic performance
	  ○ Autism spectrum disorder (ASD)
	  ○ Anxiety
	  ○ Depression
	  ○ Attention deficit hyperactivity disorder (ADHD)	

Study Designs	• Randomized controlled trials • Controlled (nonrandomized) trials • Cohort (observational) studies, prospective or retrospective • Case–cohort studies	• Case reports • Studies reported in theses or conference abstracts only • Studies not reported in English • Studies without primary data, such as systematic reviews, narrative reviews, editorials, and commentaries

[a] https://worldpopulationreview.com/country-rankings/hdi-by-country.
SOURCE: Texas A&M Agriculture, Food, and Nutrition Evidence Center, 2023.

developed for associations of seafood consumption during pregnancy and lactation and neurocognitive development in the child.

Screening

All records captured in the search were screened independently by two reviewers. Screening occurred within a web-based program (DistillerSR) using screening forms developed based on the inclusion and exclusion criteria determined *a priori*. Each article was reviewed to determine if it met the inclusion criteria, in which case the article was included, or if any of the exclusion criteria were met, in which case the article was excluded.

Screening was conducted in three stages or levels following the methodology of the original existing review. In level 1, the title of the article was reviewed. Title screening was used to exclude clearly irrelevant studies. Potential reasons for exclusion at the title level included wrong study population or country. If there was not a clear reason for exclusion, the article was included and moved to level 2, abstract screening. If there was no reason to exclude the article based on information in the abstract, it was included and moved to level 3, full-text screening. When an article was excluded at level 2 (abstract) or level 3 (full text) the screener indicated at least one reason for exclusion. Any disagreements on whether to include or exclude an article were discussed and resolved by the two screeners. If necessary, a third party was consulted to resolve differences.

Piloting was done to ensure the screening forms were adequate and that screeners interpreted the eligibility criteria similarly. For the pilot, screeners reviewed a common set of references at each screening level. The screeners discussed their responses, any questions or uncertainties they had when making their decision, and any concerns regarding the screening form. If necessary, this was repeated with another common set of references.

Manual searching was performed on all articles included after full-text screening. If a reference was found to be relevant to the present review that was not identified in the electronic search, it went through the screening process as detailed above. If an article identified through manual searching was included in the review, the librarian was notified to determine why the article was not found through the electronic search. If necessary, the search strategy would be updated and rerun, and newly identified articles would go through the screening process.

Data Extraction

Data from all included articles were extracted by a trained analyst using a systematic approach. Only data relevant to the review were extracted. To ensure data were extracted in a consistent manner for all articles, standard data extraction forms were used. Data fields for extraction were based on information outlined in the protocol and included important characteristics of the study design, methodology, results, and limitations. Data extraction was piloted on two or three articles (varying in study design, when appropriate) by all reviewers to ensure all relevant information was recorded and done so in a consistent manner. For the nutrition reviews, data extraction forms included similar fields as the existing reviews (see online Appendix H for data extraction fields for the nutrition review update). A second analyst reviewed the extracted data for accuracy and completeness. Any suggested changes were discussed between the reviewers. If necessary, a third analyst was consulted.

Risk-of-Bias Assessment

Risk of bias was assessed independently by two analysts using standardized tools specific to each study's design for all included studies. If a study included multiple relevant results, the analysts assessed the risk of bias pertinent to each. If there were differences in risk of bias for the different results, more than one risk-of-bias assessment was reported for a paper. Cochrane risk-of-bias tools specific to the included study designs were used. These included ROB 2.0 for randomized controlled trials, Risk of Bias in Non-Randomized Studies–of Interventions (ROBINS-I), and Risk of Bias in Non-Randomized Studies–of Exposures (ROBINS-E) for nonrandomized studies of exposures. The analysts piloted the tools on two or three articles per study design to ensure a consistent approach and interpretation. Upon completion of the dual, independent risk-of-bias assessments, domain-level ratings and the overall rating were compared between the two reviewers to assess interrater reliability. If there were differences, the reviewers discussed and determined the appropriate rating. If necessary, a third reviewer was consulted.

Data Synthesis

Synthesis of the evidence was conducted by the committee. To prepare for synthesis, a description of the evidence was drafted to provide details on the body of evidence including but not limited to the number of included articles, the number of included studies, study designs, country of origin, participant characteristics, description of the exposure across studies, outcomes, and outcome assessment tools.

PECOD Analytic Framework and Inclusion and Exclusion Criteria for Toxicology Review

Prior to conducting systematic reviews on toxicants from seafood consumed during pregnancy, lactation, childhood, or adolescence on child development and health outcomes, the Evidence Center conducted a scoping review to identify (1) toxicant exposures with sufficient evidence to warrant a systematic review, and (2) gaps in the evidence. This allowed the committee to prioritize exposure–outcome relationships that warranted systematic review. The initial scoping review and subsequent *de novo* systematic review for the toxicology review followed the same protocol as described above for the nutrition reviews.

Using terms provided by the committee, the Evidence Center developed an analytic framework for examining associations of seafood toxicant exposure during pregnancy, lactation, and childhood and child growth and development (Figure C-2).

Inclusion and exclusion terms were provided by the committee and a PECOD table constructed for the toxicology scoping review. Table C-2 shows the criteria developed for associations of seafood toxicant exposure during pregnancy, lactation, and childhood and child growth and development.

The committee also expressed an interest in capturing and evaluating the evidence related specifically to mercury exposure. The inclusion criteria applied in the scoping review required that studies report both fish and seafood intake as an exposure and a toxicant exposure, with demonstration of the associations between fish and/or seafood exposure to the toxin and/or the outcome. However, given that the primary source of mercury exposure is through fish and seafood intake, the committee was interested in examining the association between mercury and child health outcomes using studies that did not explicitly report fish or seafood intake.

Grading the Strength of the Evidence

A rating of the certainty of the evidence was determined for each conclusion using the GRADE[3] approach. This includes an evaluation of the evidence by study design. For randomized controlled trials, the domains considered when determining the rating include risk of bias, indirectness, inconsistency, imprecision, and publication bias. Additional domains to be considered for other study designs included dose–response, magnitude of effect, and plausible confounding. Ratings were defined as high, moderate, low, or very low certainty.

RESULTS

Nutrition Systematic Reviews

The number of included articles from the combined nutrition updated systematic reviews are shown in Table C-3. Summary tables of the study characteristics, risk of bias, and outcomes for the nutrition reviews are provided in online Appendix H.

---

[3] GRADE = Grading of Recommendations, Assessment, Development and Evaluation.

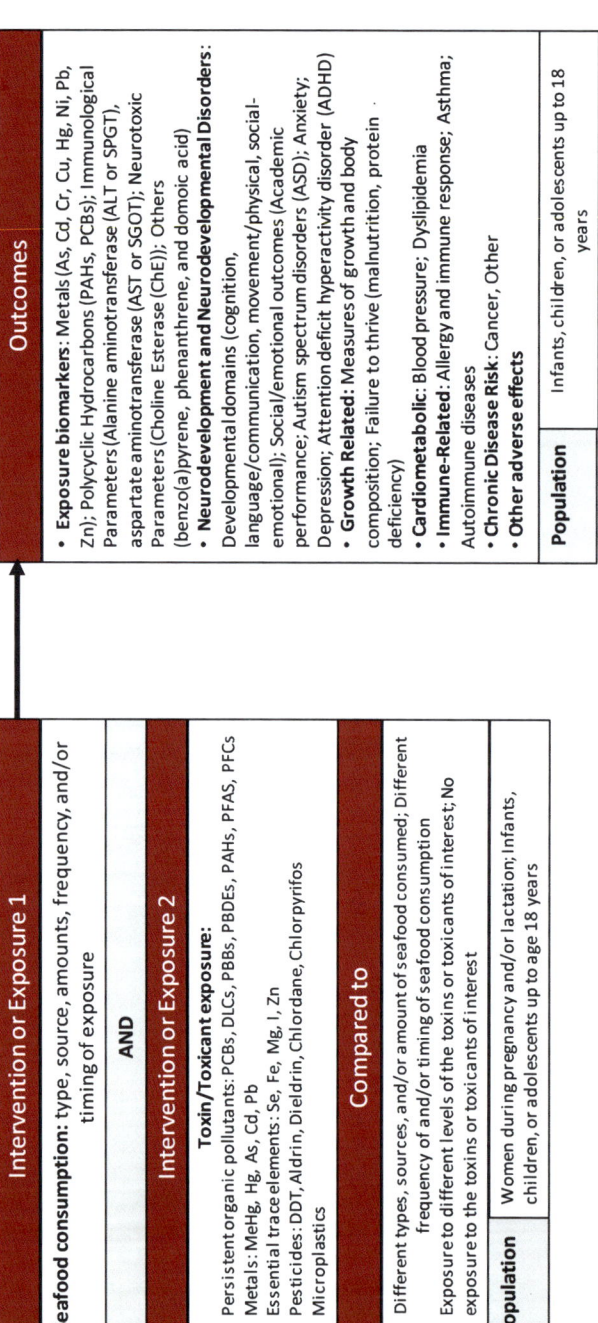

FIGURE C-2 Analytic framework for examining the relationship between seafood toxicant exposure during pregnancy, lactation, and childhood and child growth and development.
NOTE: As = arsenic; Cd = cadmium; Cr = chromium; Cu = copper; DDT = dichloro-diphenyl-trichloroethane; Fe = iron; Hg = mercury; I = iodine; MeHg = methyl-mercury; Mg = magnesium; Ni = nickel; PAHs = polycyclic aromatic hydrocarbons; Pb = lead; PBBs = polybrominated biphenyls; PBDEs = polybrominated diphenyl ethers; PCBs = polychlorinated biphenyls; PFAS = per- and polyfluoroalkyl substances; PFCs = perfluorochemicals; Se = selenium; Zn = zinc.
SOURCE: Texas A&M Agriculture, Food, and Nutrition Evidence Center, 2023.

TABLE C-2 PECOD Framework for Toxicology Review Inclusion and Exclusion Criteria

Component	Inclusion Criteria	Exclusion Criteria
Populations	Human individuals living in countries ranked as high or very high on the human development index during the study.[a] • Exposed population: Individuals in the general population who are pregnant or lactating, infants, children, or adolescents up to age 18 years. Subgroups of interest: 　○ By race/ethnicity 　○ By income 　○ By cumulative exposure to nonchemical stressors (e.g., stress, depression) 　○ By cumulative exposure to environmental stressors (e.g., neighborhood or locale, food security) 　○ By preexisting disease burden • Outcome population: Children and adolescents (up to age 18 years). Subgroups of interest: 　○ Infants (ages 0–12 months) 　○ Toddlers (ages 1–3 years) 　○ Early childhood (ages 4–8 years) 　○ Puberty (ages 9–13 years) 　○ Adolescents (ages 14–18 years)	• Studies exclusively of participants with a chronic condition, hospitalized with an illness or injury. Examples include: 　○ Diabetes (not including gestational diabetes) 　○ Cancer 　○ Cardiometabolic disorders 　○ Chronic kidney disease 　○ Malabsorption (any disorder that causes malabsorption from the gastrointestinal tract) 　○ Asthma • Nonhuman primates[b]
Exposures:	• Must contain Exposure 1 AND Exposure 2 *Exposure 1: Toxin or toxicants* • Persistent organic pollutants, e.g., 　○ Polychlorinated biphenyls (PCBs) e.g., dioxin and dioxin-like compounds (DLCs) 　○ Polybrominated biphenyls (PBBs) 　○ Polybrominated diphenyl ethers (PBDEs) 　○ Polycyclic aromatic hydrocarbons (PAHs) 　○ Per- and polyfluoroalkyl substances (PFAS) • Metals 　○ Methylmercury 　○ Mercury 　○ Arsenic 　○ Cadmium 　○ Lead • Essential trace elements 　○ Selenium 　○ Iron 　○ Magnesium 　○ Iodine 　○ Zinc • Pesticides 　○ DDT 　○ Aldrin 　○ Dieldrin 　○ Chlordane 　○ Chlorpyrifos • Microplastics *Exposure 2: Seafood consumption* • Types (e.g., salmon, tuna, bass) • Sources (e.g., sea, freshwater, farmed, canned, wild) • Amount (e.g., ounces per day, grams per meal) • Frequency (e.g., daily, twice per week) • Duration (e.g., length of time consuming seafood) • Preparation (e.g., fried, baked) • Timing (e.g., by trimester, age)	• Studies that do not report on any toxicant exposure in fish and seafood consumption • Supplements • Infant formula • Toxins from algal blooms:[b] 　○ Cyanobacteria 　○ Ciguatera 　○ Scombroid 　○ Domoic acid (red algae) • Microorganisms (hepatitis A, salmonella, *E. coli*)[b]

continued

TABLE C-2 Continued

Component	Inclusion Criteria	Exclusion Criteria
Comparators	• Exposure to different levels of the toxins or toxicants of interest; no exposure to the toxins or toxicants of interest • Different types, sources, amounts, frequencies, durations, preparations, or timings of seafood consumption; no seafood consumption	No comparator
Outcomes	Exposure biomarkers/indicators/levels (e.g., arsenobetaine) Neurodevelopment and Neurodevelopmental Disorders: • Developmental domains: cognition, language/communication, movement/physical, social-emotional • Social/emotional outcomes • Academic performance • Autism spectrum disorder (ASD) • Anxiety • Depression • Attention deficit hyperactivity disorder (ADHD) Growth-Related • Measures of growth and body composition • Failure to thrive (malnutrition, protein deficiency) Cardiometabolic • Blood pressure • Dyslipidemia Immune-Related • Allergy and immune response • Asthma • Autoimmune diseases Chronic Disease Risk • Cancer • Other Other adverse effects	
Study Designs	• Randomized controlled trials • Controlled (nonrandomized) trials • Cohort (observational) studies, prospective or retrospective • Case–cohort studies • Case–control studies • Before–after studies	• Case reports[c] • Studies reported in theses or conference abstracts only • Studies not reported in English • Studies without primary data, such as systematic reviews, narrative reviews, editorials, and commentaries • Cross-sectional studies[b]

[a] https://worldpopulationreview.com/country-rankings/hdi-by-country.

[b] A list of nonhuman primate and cross-sectional studies, as well as studies with algal toxin and microorganism exposures will be provided to the sponsor.

[c] Case reports will be excluded but will be reviewed on a case-by-case basis. If a case report meets the inclusion criteria, it will be included for further review.

SOURCE: Texas A&M Agriculture, Food, and Nutrition Evidence Center, 2023.

TABLE C-3 Nutrition Reviews: Number of Included Articles by Outcome Domains

Outcome	Exposure	
	Seafood Consumption During Childhood and Adolescence	Seafood Consumption During Pregnancy and Lactation
Developmental domains		
Cognition	10	28
Language/communication	0	13
Movement/physical	3	16
Social-emotional	3	10
Academic performance	1	0
Attention deficit disorder (ADD) or attention-deficit/hyperactivity disorder (ADHD)	1	4
Anxiety	0	0
Depression	2	0
Autism spectrum disorder (ASD)	0	4

SOURCE: Texas A&M Agriculture, Food, and Nutrition Evidence Center, 2023.

Toxicology Systematic Review

Toxicology Scoping Review

A risk-of-bias assessment was not carried out for the toxicology scoping review. After extraction of study characteristics of eligible articles, two toxicant exposure–prioritized outcome pairs were identified to proceed with *de novo* reviews. These were polychlorinated biphenyls (PCBs) and growth and body composition ($n = 4$); and lead and developmental domains ($n = 3$). Summary tables of the study characteristics, risk of bias, and outcomes for lead and PCBs are provided in online Appendix H.

Toxicology Systematic Reviews

The articles included in the scoping review were reorganized by toxicant and prioritized outcome for each of the two exposure populations (women who are pregnant or lactating and children and adolescents). Any toxicant exposure–prioritized outcome pair with three or more articles was determined to have sufficient data for conducting a *de novo* systematic review. For the full systematic review, screening, data extraction, risk-of-bias assessment, and evidence synthesis were carried out as described above for the nutrition reviews.

EVALUATION OF EXISTING SYSTEMATIC REVIEWS FOR MERCURY

In addition to the updated nutrition reviews and the *de novo* toxicology review, the committee expressed an interest in capturing and evaluating the evidence related specifically to mercury exposure. The inclusion criteria applied in the scoping review required that studies report both fish and/or seafood intake as an exposure and a toxicant exposure, with demonstration of the associations between fish and/or seafood exposure to the toxin and/or the outcome. However, given that the primary source of mercury exposure is through fish or seafood consumption, the committee was interested in examining the association between mercury and child health outcomes using studies that did not explicitly report fish/seafood intake.

To determine whether an existing systematic review could be used the relevancy, timeliness, and quality was assessed as follows:

- Relevancy is assessed by comparing PICO[4] elements of the existing review(s) to the desired review.
- Timeliness is based on the time of the literature search. What is considered "timely" will depend on the topic considering the volume of research being published and advancement in research methods.
- Quality of a systematic review is assessed using the AMSTAR 2 tool.

Given the large number of primary studies related to mercury exposure and child development, the committee's request to expand the inclusion criteria to include studies without measures of fish/seafood intake related to mercury exposure, and the likelihood of an existing relevant, recent systematic review, the decision was made to search the literature for relevant, timely, and good quality systematic reviews on mercury exposure during pregnancy, lactation, childhood, or adolescence on child health and development outcomes.

Methodology

The Evidence Center's information scientist conducted a search to identify existing recent relevant systematic reviews that examined the relationship between mercury exposure during pregnancy, lactation, childhood, or adolescence on child health and development outcomes including dates from 2020 to present. As described above, two reviewers screened all results from the search at the full-text level. Conflicts were resolved by a third reviewer.

The AMSTAR 2 quality assessment tool was used to assess the quality of included systematic reviews. The tool includes 16 items that were rated as "Yes," "Partial Yes," "No," or "No meta-analysis conducted." Some items were adapted for this review to account for the observational nature of the included studies. Two independent assessments were performed for each included review. Disagreements were discussed and resolved by the two reviewers. For the purposes of this review, an overall summary rating was determined for each systematic review by summing the item ratings (Yes = 1; Partial Yes = 0.5; No = 0; N/A = 1). Reviews that scored 8 or more (≥ 50 percent) were considered to be moderate-high quality; reviews that scored less than 8 (< 50 percent) were considered to be lower quality.

Results

A total of 53 articles were identified in the search for existing systematic reviews related to the association between mercury exposure during pregnancy, lactation, or childhood and child outcomes. After dual full-text screening, 12 articles were included. Existing systematic reviews were identified for all but two prioritized outcomes. No articles were identified in the search related to blood pressure; however, a review from 2019 was identified through manual searching and included. Table C-4 shows the identified systematic reviews by prioritized outcome for child health. The complete extracted data for mercury are provided in online Appendix H.

---

[4] PICO = Population, Intervention, Comparator, Outcome.

TABLE C-4 Systematic Reviews for Mercury: Number of Included Articles by Outcome Categories

Prioritized Outcome	Number of Systematic Reviews
Neurological disorders—ASD	5
Developmental domains	3
Growth—measures of growth or body composition	3
Biomarkers—gene expression	1
Neurological disorders—ADHD	1
Cardiometabolic—blood pressure	1
Immune-related—allergy, immune response	1
Academic performance	0
Growth—failure to thrive	0

SOURCE: Texas A&M Agriculture, Food, and Nutrition Evidence Center, 2023.

REFERENCE

USDA/HHS (U.S. Department of Agriculture and U.S. Department of Health and Human Services). 2020. *Dietary Guidelines for Americans, 2020–2025.* 9th ed. dietaryguidelines.gov.

D

Supplemental Review of Systematic Reviews

SUMMARY OF EVIDENCE

The committee was interested in exploring additional health outcomes and toxicity exposures related to fish and seafood consumption that were not included in the commissioned systematic reviews. To address these needs, the two supplemental reviews of systematic reviews were done. To identify relevant systematic reviews, two literature searches were conducted by the National Academies' Research Center. See Appendix G[1] for details on the literature search terms and search strategies. Figures D-1 and D-2 depict the PRISMA flow charts for each literature search. Summary details from the systematic reviews are provided in Table D-1 for additional health outcomes and in Table D-2 for toxicity exposures. Summary details from other reviewed literature are in Table D-3.

---

[1] Appendix G can be found online at https://nap.nationalacademies.org/catalog/27623.

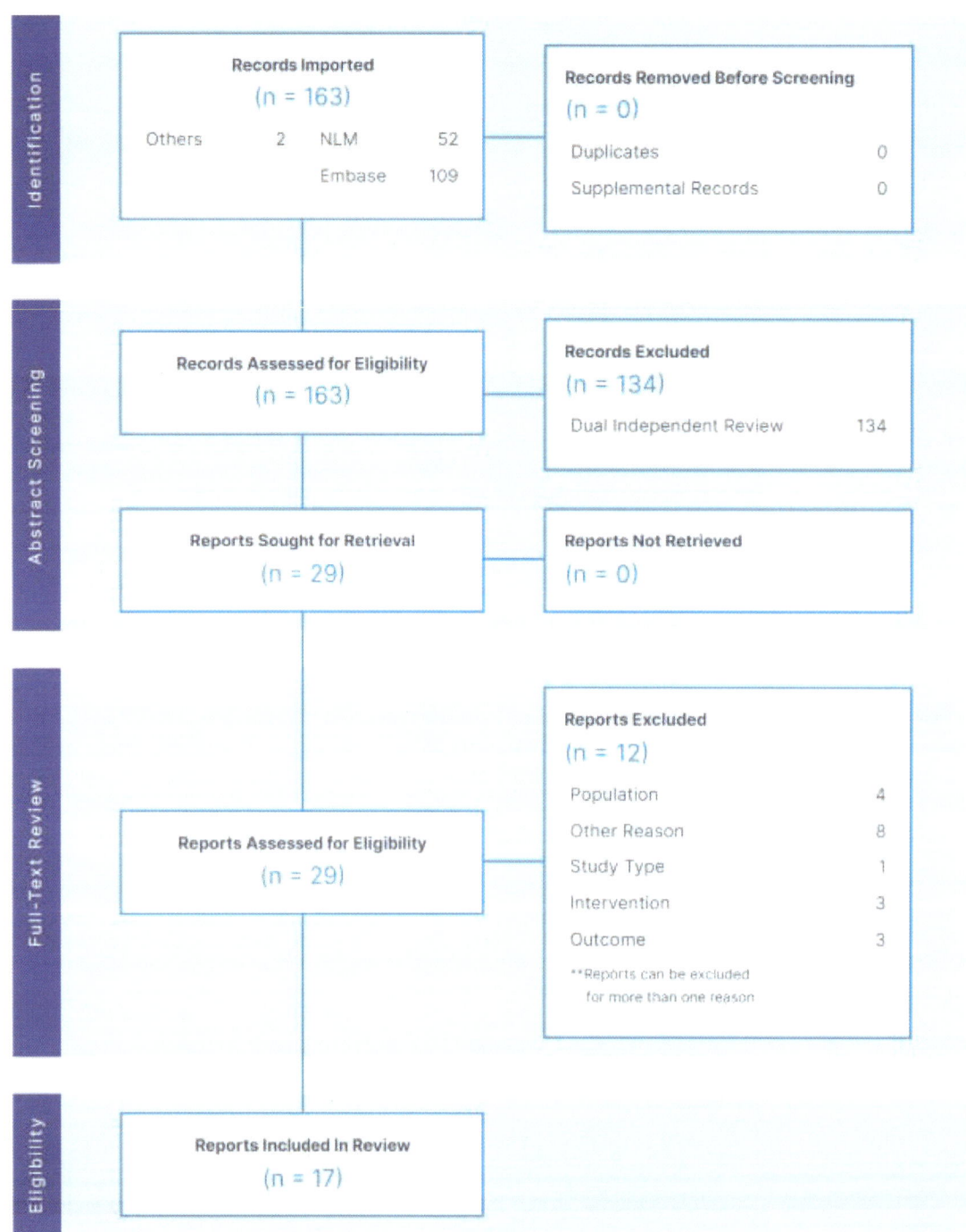

FIGURE D-1 PRISMA flow chart for literature review on additional health outcomes related to seafood consumption.
NOTE: NLM = National Library of Medicine.

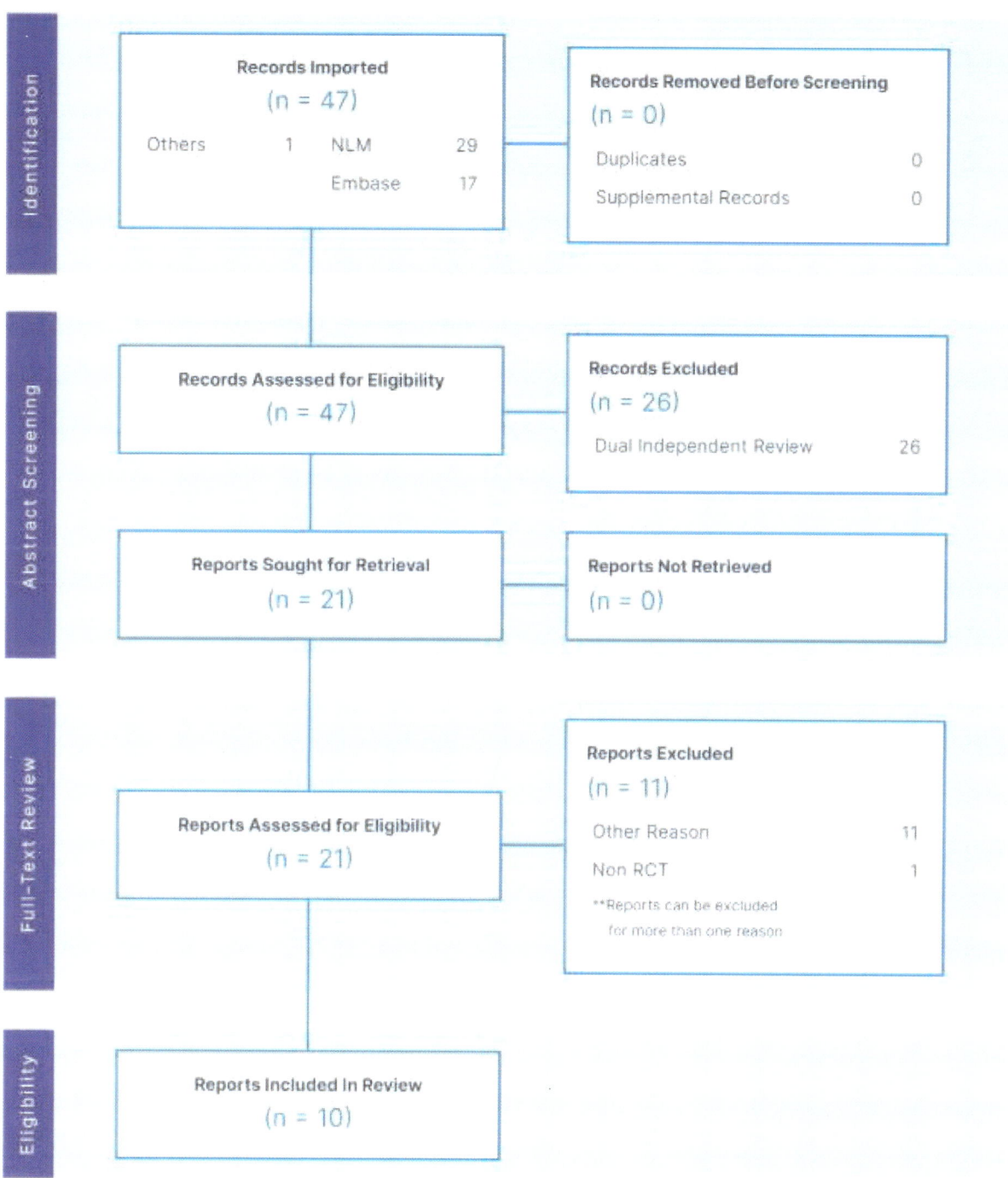

FIGURE D-2 PRISMA flow chart for literature review on additional toxicity exposures related to seafood consumption.
NOTE: NLM = National Library of Medicine.

TABLE D-1 Summary of Evidence from Systematic Reviews on Additional Health Outcomes Related to Fish and Seafood Consumption

Author, Year Country	Types of Studies Included	Population Measured	Exposure/ Intervention	Outcome and Results	Conclusion	AMSTAR2 Overall Quality
Cui and Mu, 2023 Multicountry (high-income countries)	27 cohort studies ranging from 2000 to 2021	Risk in early childhood (offspring) from exposure during pregnancy	Maternal fish consumption during pregnancy measured by food frequency questionnaire (FFQ)	Atopic dermatitis Based on 1 cohort study, higher maternal fatty fish consumption of around 35~69 g per week (1.17, 95% CI 1.00~1.38) is a dietary risk factor for atopic dermatitis	Higher maternal fatty fish consumption of around 35~69 g per week (1.17, 95% CI 1.00~1.38) is a potential dietary risk factor for atopic dermatitis	Partially well done/ reported
Prattico et al., 2023 Australia, United States, Europe, Chile, Japan	Majority were retrospective observational studies ($n = 26$); published 2012–2022	Children and adults	Fish as a food trigger (measurement method not reported)	Food-triggered food protein-induced enterocolitis syndrome (FPIES) Approximately 40% of the 42 studies reported that fish was a most frequently reported food trigger; in US-based studies ($n = 6$), cow's milk, grain, and soy were the most commonly reported triggers; fish was a commonly reported trigger in the Mediterranean region	Internationally, cow's milk was the most reported trigger; patterns of the most common triggers varied by country. Fish was one of the most common triggers in the Mediterranean region.	Not well done/ reported
Lampousi et al., 2021 Europe, North America, Asia, Australia, Africa, South America	42 cohort and 54 case–control studies	Children	Maternal fish consumption during pregnancy	Islet autoimmunity (IA) Reduced risk of IA in the offspring in relation to maternal fish intake during pregnancy (RR: 0.57, 95% CI 0.32–1.04, I2 = 0%), but no data on a potential association with type 1 diabetes	There was no association, or the evidence was of low certainty	Well done/ reported
Lampousi et al., 2021 Europe, North America, Asia, Australia, Africa, South America	42 cohort and 54 case–control studies	Children	Fish intake during childhood	Type 1 diabetes (T1D) No indication of a reduced risk of T1D in relation to childhood fish intake; fish intake (high vs. low/continuous) RR: 3.29, 95% CI 0.94–11.53, I2 = 0%)	There was no association, or the evidence was of low certainty	Well done/ reported

TABLE D-1 Continued

Author, Year Country	Types of Studies Included	Population Measured	Exposure/ Intervention	Outcome and Results	Conclusion	AMSTAR2 Overall Quality
Malmir et al., 2021 United States, Japan (Asia), Europe	31 studies in systematic review (2 cross-sectional; 2 case–control; 27 cohort) and 24 in meta-analysis (search time frame up to February 2020)	Children 10 years and younger	FFQs to assess dietary intake (N = 22)	Risk of allergic diseases (wheeze, food allergy, asthma, eczema, allergic rhinitis, inhalant allergy, dermatitis) (see article for results)	Greater fish consumption during pregnancy was associated with a 3% reduced risk of wheeze and 25% reduced risk of food allergy in the offspring. In addition, every additional 30 gram per week of maternal fish intake was associated with a 4% decreased risk of eczema in children.	Partially well done/ reported
Venter et al., 2020 Europe, North America, Asia, and Australia	17 RCTs and 78 observational (case–control, cross-sectional, and cohort) studies	Pregnant women and offspring	Maternal dietary intake during pregnancy measured via FFQs, unvalidated food questionnaires, and interviews	Wheeze/asthma, allergic rhinitis/rhino conjunctivitis/hay fever, food allergy, eczema, allergic sensitization (see article for results)	Insufficient evidence to provide guidance on diet diversity (no published reports), diet patterns, diet indices, or specific foods, food groups, and macro- or micronutrients that should be consumed or avoided during pregnancy for the prevention of allergic diseases	Partially well done/ reported
DGAC, 2020 United Kingdom Australia, United States, Portugal	4 prospective cohort studies	Children ages 2 years and older	Dietary pattern assessed by index or score analysis or factor and cluster analysis	Risk of cardiovascular disease later in life Limited evidence that dietary patterns consumed by children and adolescents reflecting higher intakes of vegetables, fruits, whole grains, fish, low-fat dairy, legumes, and lower intake of sugar-sweetened beverages, other sweets, and processed meat, are associated with lower blood pressure and blood lipid levels, including low-density lipoprotein cholesterol, high-density lipoprotein cholesterol, and triglycerides later in life	Limited evidence	Well done/ reported

continued

TABLE D-1 Continued

Author, Year Country	Types of Studies Included	Population Measured	Exposure/ Intervention	Outcome and Results	Conclusion	AMSTAR2 Overall Quality
Ferrante et al., 2019 European Atlantic coast and Mediterranean Sea	25 studies (type not specified)	Marine species (demersal fish, pelagic fish, and mollusks) for human consumption	Estimated average daily intake to inorganic arsenic from seafood	Cancer and carcinogenic risk (see article for results)	European populations more exposed to In-As from fish and mollusks are the French, Spanish, Italian, and Greek, with particular regards to children of 3–6 years old, which should minimize the consumption of mollusks to avoid carcinogenic and noncarcinogenic risks	Not well done/ reported
Middleton et al., 2018 Worldwide	70 RCTs	Pregnant women and offspring	Omega-3 supplementation during pregnancy	Preterm birth < 37 weeks; early preterm birth < 34 weeks; prolonged gestation > 42 weeks; perinatal death; neonatal care admissions; low birthweight; large-for-gestational age; small-for-gestational age or intrauterine growth restriction; induction postterm; maternal serious adverse events; maternal admission to intensive care; postnatal depression; gestational length; preeclampsia; cognition; IQ; vision; neurodevelopment and growth outcomes; language and behavior; body mass index at 19 years	Only 3/70 RCTs measured omega 3 food/dietary advice only vs. placebo/or no omega 3 fatty acids	Well done/ reported
Rahmani et al., 2018 Iran	23 studies (original observational, epidemiological, and/or cross-sectional studies)	Children and adults	Estimated daily intake (EDI)	Noncarcinogenic and carcinogenic risk Incremental lifetime cancer risk (ILCR) of arsenic (As) was 3.21E-5 in Adults and 4.18E-5 in children	Adults and children that consume canned tuna fish in Iran are not at noncarcinogenic risk but have a carcinogenic risk due to arsenic	Not well done/ reported

TABLE D-1 Continued

Author, Year Country	Types of Studies Included	Population Measured	Exposure/ Intervention	Outcome and Results	Conclusion	AMSTAR2 Overall Quality
Rahmani et al., 2018 Iran	23 studies (original observational, epidemiological, and/or cross-sectional studies)	Children and adults	Estimated daily intake (EDI)	Concentration of metals in canned tuna fish Ranking from high to low concentration of metals based on mean concentrations (μg/g wet weight) were Fe (13.17) > Zn (9.31) > Se (2.23) > Al (1.8) > Cr (1.63) > Cu (1.52) > As (0.38) > Ni (0.33) > Pb (0.24) > Cd (0.14) > Hg (0.11) > Sn (0.1)	Except for cadmium and selenium, concentrations were lower than the limits recommended by the U.S. Environmental Protection Agency, World Health Organization, Food and Agriculture Organization of the United Nations, and Iran National Standards Organization (INSO)	Not well done/ reported
Kibret et al., 2018 Worldwide	21 cohort and cross-sectional studies published between 2008 and 2016	Pregnant women	Adherence to a healthy dietary pattern (intake of vegetables, fruits, legumes, whole grains, and fish)	Hypertensive disorders of pregnancy; gestational diabetes mellitus; preterm birth; low birth weight (LBW); no studies included fish for LBW Preeclamsia: Healthy dietary pattern (high intake of fruits, vegetables, whole-grain foods, fish, and poultry) had significantly lower odds of preeclampsia (OR 0.78, 95% CI 0.70, 0.86; I2 39.0%) others Gestational diabetes mellitus (GDM): other studies found that women who had higher adherence to a healthy dietary pattern had lower odds of GDM (OR = 0.78; 95% CI 0.56, 0.99), with significant heterogeneity detected between studies (I 2 = 68.6%, P = 0.013) Preterm birth (PTB): women who had good adherence to a healthy dietary pattern were shown to have reduced odds of PTB (OR = 0.75; 95% CI 0.57, 0.93), although significant heterogeneity was observed (I2 = 89.6%, P = 0.0001)	Dietary patterns with a higher intake of fruits, vegetables, legumes, whole grains, and fish are associated with a decreased likelihood of adverse pregnancy and birth outcomes (preeclampsia and GDM); however, the evidence is inconsistent	Partially well done/ reported

continued

TABLE D-1 Continued

Author, Year Country	Types of Studies Included	Population Measured	Exposure/ Intervention	Outcome and Results	Conclusion	AMSTAR2 Overall Quality
Sioen et al., 2017 Europe (17 countries)	49 studies met study inclusion criteria	Pregnant women (10 studies), lactating women (4 studies), infants 6–12 months age (3 studies), children 1–3 years (6 studies), children 4–9 years (11 studies), adolescents 10–18 years (8 studies)	Polyunsaturated fatty acids (PUFAs) source (in children and adolescents) and PUFA content in human milk as a source Did not look at specific outcome	PUFAs source (in children and adolescents): In Belgian children (age 2.5–6.5 years), fats and oils were the major contributors to intakes of LA (23.6%) and ALA (33.1%), followed by cereal products with 17.6 and 13.5%, respectively. Meat, poultry, and eggs were the main contributors to ARA intake (72.0%), and fish and seafood were the main contributors to EPA (83.5%), DPA (57.8%) and DHA (75.7%) intake. In the multicountry HELENA study (adolescents age 12.5–17.5 years), the food group "meat, fish, eggs and meat alternatives" was the largest contributor to the intake of LA (31.7%), ALA (21.5), ARA (54.2%), EPA (92.3%), DPA (94.9%) and DHA (85.8%). PUFA content in human milk: DHA levels in human milk vary considerably among women and are strongly influenced by maternal diet, such as fish and seafood intake	Fish and seafood are main contributors to EPA, DPA, and DHA for Belgian children age 2.5–6.5 years. It is unclear (within the multiple countries of the HELENA study) how much PUFAs among adolescents (age 12.5–17.5) can be attributed to fish intake compared to other sources Inconsistent evidence for PUFA content in human milk	Not well done/ reported
Zhang et al., 2017 Multicountry	RCTs and prospective cohort studies	Women during pregnancy (1 RCT, 13 prospective cohorts)	Maternal and infant fish intake	Atopy, eczema, allergic rhinitis, wheeze, asthma, and food allergy See article for results	Maternal intake: no significant association with maternal intake of fish/seafood and any of the atopic outcomes Infant intake: There was a 39% reduction of eczema and 46% reduction of allergic rhinitis among infants who had a high intake of fish. There was no significant association of fish intake among infants and atopic outcomes of sensitization (food allergy), asthma, and wheeze	Partially well done/ reported

TABLE D-1 Continued

Author, Year Country	Types of Studies Included	Population Measured	Exposure/ Intervention	Outcome and Results	Conclusion	AMSTAR2 Overall Quality
Ierodiakonou et al., 2016 Worldwide	146 intervention trials and observational studies	Infants 0–12 months postpartum	Timing of fish introduction	Reduced allergic rhinitis and allergic sensitization Reduced allergic rhinitis: 3 of the cohort studies (13,472 participants) found that early fish introduction (before age 6–9 months) was associated with reduced allergic sensitization to any allergen or food allergens. Reduced allergic sensitization: 4 of the cohort studies (12,781 participants) found fish introduction before age 6–12 months was associated with reduced allergic rhinitis at age 4 years or younger (OR, 0.59; 95% CI, 0.40–0.87; high heterogeneity [I2 = 59%]) or at age 5–14 years (OR, 0.68; 95% CI, 0.47–0.98). In a sensitivity analysis excluding studies at high or unclear risk of bias, the association between early fish introduction and reduced allergic rhinitis at age 4 years or younger was not statistically significant.	No conclusion provided	Well done/ reported
Best et al., 2016 Various	13 publications from 10 prospective cohort studies	Maternal intake/child outcomes	Increased prenatal n-3 LCPUFA or fish intake	Incidence of 1 or more IgE-mediated allergic disease outcome in the child (eczema, rhino-conjunctivitis, asthma/ wheeze, sensitization) 8 of the studies found protective association between increased prenatal n-3 LCPUFA or fish intake and incidence of allergic disease symptoms in the child	No conclusion due to inconsistent results	Partially well done/ reported

continued

TABLE D-1 Continued

Author, Year Country	Types of Studies Included	Population Measured	Exposure/ Intervention	Outcome and Results	Conclusion	AMSTAR2 Overall Quality
Netting et al., 2014 Multicountry	43 studies (more than 40,000 children): 11 intervention studies (including 7 RCTs), 27 prospective cohort studies, 4 retrospective cohort studies and 1 case–control study	Children	Whole fish/ seafood intake	Eczema, asthma, hay fever, sensitization See article for results	No consistent association between mother's dietary intake and atopic outcomes in their children. Maternal consumption of Mediterranean dietary patterns, diets rich in fruits and vegetables, fish and vitamin D containing foods were suggestive of benefit. There were few studies that reported on the individual associations of maternal fish/ seafood intake and atopic outcomes.	Partially well done/ reported
Kremmyda et al., 2011 United States, Australia, Saudi Arabia, Taiwan, Japan, Europe	Cohort studies, case–control studies, cross-sectional studies	Children 2–16 years; pregnant women	Fish consumption during infancy or childhood	Atopic or allergic outcomes Maternal intake: positive associations between maternal fish intake during pregnancy and atopic or allergic outcomes in infants/ children (protective effect varied between 25% and 95%); 1 study of maternal fish intake during lactation did not observe any significant associations Infant and child intake: inconsistent results on association between infant/child intake of seafood and atopic outcomes; 9 (of 14) studies showed a protective effect; 2 studies found a negative effect; 3 studies found no effect	No conclusion on whether fish consumption during infancy or childhood can be protective; further studies needed	Not well done/ reported

APPENDIX D

TABLE D-1 Continued

Author, Year Country	Types of Studies Included	Population Measured	Exposure/ Intervention	Outcome and Results	Conclusion	AMSTAR2 Overall Quality
Shams et al., 2011 Country not reported	18 systematic reviews	Not reported	Maternal fish intake	Atopic eczema Results were unclear	Maternal intake of fish may be associated with a reduced risk of eczema in offspring, although further studies are needed	Not well done/ reported

TABLE D-2 Summary of Evidence from Systematic Reviews on Additional Toxicity Exposures Related to Fish and Seafood Consumption

Author, Year Country	Types of Studies Included	Population Measured	Exposure/ Intervention	Outcome and Results	Conclusion	AMSTAR2 Overall Quality
Raissy et al., 2022 Persian Gulf countries	30 studies	Children and adults	Concentration of potentially toxic elements in fish from the Persian Gulf (Hg, Pb, As, Cd)	Noncarcinogenic and carcinogenic risks Cancer risk factor of Cd was above 10^{-4}, which is the unsafe limit for Iranian and global consumers	Persian Gulf fish was safe for human consumption concerning Cd (THQ value < 1). In addition, except for Hg in global children consumers, the THQ for other elements was within the safe range (< 1). The total THQ for all consumers was > 1, except for Iranian and global adult consumers. The ELCR for Cd was more than Pb. Findings conservatively indicated that the risk of cancer caused by Pb exposure was within the USEPA safe limit. In the case of Cd, the ELCR for all consumers was higher than the range advised by USEPA.	Not well done/reported
Fakhri et al., 2021 Global	42 articles	Children and adults	Concentration of potentially harmful elements (PHEs) in fillet trout	Carcinogenic risks Adult consumers in China are at the threshold carcinogenic risk, and adult consumers in the other countries investigated are at the acceptable level for carcinogenic risk	Adult consumers in all countries studied were in the acceptable range of noncarcinogenic risk; however, children in Turkey were not in the acceptable range of noncarcinogenic risk. The carcinogenic risk of inorganic As revealed that adult consumers in China were in the threshold carcinogenic risk.	Not well done/reported

continued

TABLE D-2 Continued

Author, Year Country	Types of Studies Included	Population Measured	Exposure/ Intervention	Outcome and Results	Conclusion	AMSTAR2 Overall Quality
Fakhri et al., 2021 Global	42 articles	Children and adults	Concentration of PHEs in fillet trout	Noncarcinogenic risks Adult consumers in all the countries are at the acceptable range of noncarcinogenic risk; children in Turkey were at the not acceptable level for noncarcinogenic risk	Adult consumers in all countries studied were in the acceptable range of noncarcinogenic risk; however, children in Turkey were not in the acceptable range of noncarcinogenic risk. The carcinogenic risk of inorganic As revealed that adult consumers in China were in the threshold carcinogenic risk.	Not well done/reported
Kato et al., 2020 Global	64 articles	Shellfish	Bioaccumulation of arsenic in shellfish	No health outcomes reported	None	Partially well done/reported
Ferrante et al., 2019 Europe	7 articles	Fresh fish and mollusks caught in European waters; European populations of all ages	Arsenic in fresh fish and mollusks caught in the Mediterranean sea and the European coast of the Atlantic Ocean	Cancer risk THQ values above the level of risk for high frequency consumers of mollusks (7 meals per week) among adults and children (THQ: 1.056 and 2.320, respectively) from the Mediterranean area, and for medium-frequency consumers (4 meals per week) among children (THQ: 1.332) of the Mediterranean area. Based on In-As concentrations reviewed along European coasts, only children with a high frequency consumption of mollusks have a THQ above the level of risk (1.1)	No conclusion made on carcinogenic or noncarcinogenic risks	Not well done/reported

TABLE D-2 Continued

Author, Year Country	Types of Studies Included	Population Measured	Exposure/ Intervention	Outcome and Results	Conclusion	AMSTAR2 Overall Quality
Rahmani et al., 2018 Iran	23 observational, epidemiological, or cross-sectional studies	Children and adults	Concentration of 11 metals in canned tuna and estimated consumption per capita	Estimate of noncarcinogenic risk, total target hazard quotient, and estimate of carcinogenic risk	Concentration of Cd and Se were higher than the standard limits; risk assessment showed that the noncarcinogenic risk from Cd and Se in canned tuna in Iran does not represent a threat to adult and children consumers (THQ < 1). The carcinogenic risk assessment showed that adults and children are at threshold cancer risk due to the As content in canned tuna fish in Iran	Not well done/reported
Fakhri et al., 2018 Persian Gulf countries	9 articles (14 studies) cross-sectional studies	Persian Gulf shrimp	Arsenic and lead levels in shrimp	Cancer risk Overall arsenic levels in shrimp was significantly higher than WHO/FAO guidelines	Consumers are at considerable cancer risk due to arsenic from consumption of Persian Gulf shrimp	Partially well done/reported
Vilcins et al., 2018 Country not reported	69 observational and 2 experimental studies (2 observational studies on seafood)	Infants 0–2 y	Mercury in seafood	Stunting Neither study reported a statistically significant relationship between stunting and mercury, although one did show a nonsignificant trend between mercury level and reduced height for age Z-score	Inconclusive evidence	Not well done/reported

NOTE: FFQ = food frequency questionnaire; RCT = randomized control trial.

TABLE D-3 Summary of Evidence from Other Reviewed Literature on Additional Toxicity Exposures Related to Fish and Seafood Consumption

Author, Year Country	Types of Studies Included	Population Measured	Exposure/ Intervention	Outcome and Results	Conclusion
Amerizadeh et al., 2023 Azerbaijan, Russian Federation, Iran, Kazakhstan, and Turkmenistan (bordering countries of Caspian Sea)	14 studies with 30 different sets of results	Muscles of commercial fish	Commercial fish exposure to PTEs, including lead, chromium, arsenic, cadmium, and mercury	None	None
Chiocchetti et al., 2017 Africa, Europe and Asia	Research studies	Seafood products	Total and inorganic arsenic, cadmium, total mercury, methlymercury, lead, in seafood products	Adverse outcomes from toxicity of exposure elements	n/a
Collado-López et al., 2022 Global	152 studies including cross-sectional and longitudinal	Fish and shellfish	Heavy metal content of fish and shellfish	None	None

REFERENCES

Amerizadeh, A., M. Gholizadeh, and R. Karimi. 2023. Meta-analysis and health risk assessment of toxic heavy metals in muscles of commercial fishes in Caspian Sea. *Environmental Monitoring and Assessment* 195(4):457.

Best, K. P., M. Gold, D. Kennedy, J. Martin, and M. Makrides. 2016. Omega-3 long-chain PUFA intake during pregnancy and allergic disease outcomes in the offspring: A systematic review and meta-analysis of observational studies and randomized controlled trials. *American Journal of Clinical Nutrition* 103(1):128-143.

Chiocchetti, G., C. Jadan-Piedra, D. Velez, and V. Devesa. 2017. Metal(loid) contamination in seafood products. *Critical Reviews in Food Science and Nutrition* 57(17):3715-3728.

Collado-Lopez, S., L. Betanzos-Robledo, M. M. Tellez-Rojo, H. Lamadrid-Figueroa, M. Reyes, C. Rios, and A. Cantoral. 2022. Heavy metals in unprocessed or minimally processed foods consumed by humans worldwide: A scoping review. *International Journal of Environmental Research and Public Health* 19(14).

Cui, H., and Z. Mu. 2023. Prenatal maternal risk factors contributing to atopic dermatitis: A systematic review and meta-analysis of cohort studies. *Annals of Dermatology* 35(1):11-22.

DGAC (Dietary Guidelines Advisory Committee). 2020. USDA nutrition evidence systematic reviews. In *Dietary patterns and risk of cardiovascular disease: A systematic review*, Alexandria, VA: USDA Nutrition Evidence Systematic Review.

Fakhri, Y., A. Mohseni-Bandpei, G. Oliveri Conti, M. Ferrante, A. Cristaldi, A. K. Jeihooni, M. Karimi Dehkordi, A. Alinejad, H. Rasoulzadeh, S. M. Mohseni, M. Sarkhosh, H. Keramati, B. Moradi, N. Amanidaz, and Z. Baninameh. 2018. Systematic review and health risk assessment of arsenic and lead in the fished shrimps from the Persian Gulf. *Food and Chemical Toxicology* 113:278-286.

Fakhri, Y., A. Nematollahi, Z. Abdi-Moghadam, H. Daraei, S. M. Ghasemi, and V. N. Thai. 2021. Concentration of potentially harmful elements (PHES) in trout fillet (rainbow and brown) fish: A global systematic review and meta-analysis and health risk assessment. *Biological Trace Element Research* 199(8):3089-3101.

Ferrante, M., S. Napoli, A. Grasso, P. Zuccarello, A. Cristaldi, and C. Copat. 2019. Systematic review of arsenic in fresh seafood from the Mediterranean Sea and European Atlantic coasts: A health risk assessment. *Food and Chemical Toxicology* 126:322-331.

Ierodiakonou, D., V. Garcia-Larsen, A. Logan, A. Groome, S. Cunha, J. Chivinge, Z. Robinson, N. Geoghegan, K. Jarrold, T. Reeves, N. Tagiyeva-Milne, U. Nurmatov, M. Trivella, J. Leonardi-Bee, and R. J. Boyle. 2016. Timing of allergenic food introduction to the infant diet and risk of allergic or autoimmune disease: A systematic review and meta-analysis. *JAMA* 316(11):1181-1192.

Kato, L. S., R. G. Ferrari, J. V. M. Leite, and C. A. Conte-Junior. 2020. Arsenic in shellfish: A systematic review of its dynamics and potential health risks. *Marine Pollution Bulletin* 161(Pt A):111693.

Kibret, K. T., C. Chojenta, E. Gresham, T. K. Tegegne, and D. Loxton. 2018. Maternal dietary patterns and risk of adverse pregnancy (hypertensive disorders of pregnancy and gestational diabetes mellitus) and birth (preterm birth and low birth weight) outcomes: A systematic review and meta-analysis. *Public Health Nutrition* 22(3):1-15.

Kremmyda, L. S., M. Vlachava, P. S. Noakes, N. D. Diaper, E. A. Miles, and P. C. Calder. 2011. Atopy risk in infants and children in relation to early exposure to fish, oily fish, or long-chain omega-3 fatty acids: A systematic review. *Clinical Reviews in Allergy & Immunology* 41(1):36-66.

Lampousi, A. M., S. Carlsson, and J. E. Lofvenborg. 2021. Dietary factors and risk of islet autoimmunity and type 1 diabetes: A systematic review and meta-analysis. *EBioMedicine* 72:103633.

Malmir, H., B. Larijani, and A. Esmaillzadeh. 2022. Fish consumption during pregnancy and risk of allergic diseases in the offspring: A systematic review and meta-analysis. *Critical Reviews in Food Science and Nutrition* 62(27):7449-7459.

Middleton, P., J. C. Gomersall, J. F. Gould, E. Shepherd, S. F. Olsen, and M. Makrides. 2018. Omega-3 fatty acid addition during pregnancy. *Cochrane Database of Systematic Reviews* 11(11):CD003402.

Netting, M. J., P. F. Middleton, and M. Makrides. 2014. Does maternal diet during pregnancy and lactation affect outcomes in offspring? A systematic review of food-based approaches. *Nutrition* 30(11-12):1225-1241.

Prattico, C., P. Mule, and M. Ben-Shoshan. 2023. A systematic review of food protein-induced enterocolitis syndrome. *International Archives of Allergy and Immunology* 184(6):567-575.

Rahmani, J., Y. Fakhri, A. Shahsavani, Z. Bahmani, M. A. Urbina, S. Chirumbolo, H. Keramati, B. Moradi, A. Bay, and G. Bjorklund. 2018. A systematic review and meta-analysis of metal concentrations in canned tuna fish in Iran and human health risk assessment. *Food and Chemical Toxicology* 118:753-765.

Raissy, M., M. Ansari, R. S. Chaleshtori, V. Mahdavi, Z. Hadian, J. M. Lorenzo, G. Oliveri Conti, E. Huseyn, and A. Mousavi Khaneghah. 2022. A systematic review of the concentration of potentially toxic elements in fish from the Persian Gulf: A health risk assessment study. *Food and Chemical Toxicology* 163:112968.

Shams, K., D. J. Grindlay, and H. C. Williams. 2011. What's new in atopic eczema? An analysis of systematic reviews published in 2009-2010. *Clinical and Experimental Dermatology* 36(6):573-577; quiz 577-578.

Sioen, I., L. van Lieshout, A. Eilander, M. Fleith, S. Lohner, A. Szommer, C. Petisca, S. Eussen, S. Forsyth, P. C. Calder, C. Campoy, and R. P. Mensink. 2017. Systematic review on n-3 and n-6 polyunsaturated fatty acid intake in European countries in light of the current recommendations - focus on specific population groups. *Annals of Nutrition & Metabolism* 70(1):39-50.

Venter, C., C. Agostoni, S. H. Arshad, M. Ben-Abdallah, G. Du Toit, D. M. Fleischer, M. Greenhawt, D. H. Glueck, M. Groetch, N. Lunjani, K. Maslin, A. Maiorella, R. Meyer, M. Antonella, M. J. Netting, B. Ibeabughichi Nwaru, D. J. Palmer, M. P. Palumbo, G. Roberts, C. Roduit, P. Smith, E. Untersmayr, L. A. Vanderlinden, and L. O'Mahony. 2020. Dietary factors during pregnancy and atopic outcomes in childhood: A systematic review from the European Academy of Allergy and Clinical Immunology. *Pediatric Allergy and Immunology* 31(8):889-912.

Vilcins, D., P. D. Sly, and P. Jagals. 2018. Environmental risk factors associated with child stunting: A systematic review of the literature. *Annals of Global Health* 84(4):551-562.

Zhang, G. Q., B. Liu, J. Li, C. Q. Luo, Q. Zhang, J. L. Chen, A. Sinha, and Z. Y. Li. 2017. Fish intake during pregnancy or infancy and allergic outcomes in children: A systematic review and meta-analysis. *Pediatric Allergy and Immunology* 28(2):152-161.

E

NHANES Data Analysis Methodology

DESCRIPTION OF THE NHANES DATASET

Introduction

The National Health and Nutrition Examination Survey (NHANES) is a set of studies conducted since the 1970s that regularly collects dietary data from a representative sample of the American population. The primary source of dietary intake data in NHANES comes from two 24-hour recalls administered to participants, with the first recall administered in person at a mobile examination center and the second administered by phone 3–10 days later. The design of NHANES involves data collection across all days of the week and seasons of the year. The collection of data over 2 days instead of a single day allows for the minimization of measurement error associated with day-to-day variation in individual diets using methods described below.

NHANES also includes a food frequency questionnaire (FFQ) with questions about recalled consumption of 31 seafood items in the previous 30 days. This questionnaire does not ask about quantities consumed, only about the number of meals that were consumed that included each food item of interest. Since this module collects consumption data on commonly consumed seafood items over a longer recall period (30 days) than the 24-hour recalls, it can be integrated into models to estimate usual intake as described below.

General Overview of the Approach

Seafood is known to be an episodically consumed food in the United States, presenting a challenge for the use of 24-hour recall methods to estimate usual consumption because a large proportion of the population does not consume it regularly. The National Cancer Institute (NCI) has developed a two-step method that enables the use of multiple 24-hour recalls on nonconsecutive days to estimate usual intake of foods or nutrients, implemented through statistical analysis systems (SAS) macros (Tooze et al., 2006, 2010). The NCI SAS macros have been used to analyze NHANES 24-hour recall data to help inform the *Dietary Guidelines for Americans* and in various research studies (HHS/USDA, 2020; Krebs-Smith et al., 2010; Shan et al., 2019). The models use mixed-effects models, containing both random and fixed effects to estimate usual intake by separating and removing the within-person variation from between-person variation (Herrick et al., 2018).

For episodically consumed foods and nutrients, first a two-part model is fit to describe the relationship between usual intake and a set of covariates to partition the variance attributable to within and between individuals (Tooze et al., 2006). This two-part model estimates (1) usual intake as the probability of consuming a food on a given day and (2) the usual consumption day amount. Omega-3 fatty acids and certain other nutrients such as vitamin A are also known to be episodically consumed and require a two-part model. Other nutrients, such as total protein, are consumed daily and can be estimated with a one-part model. Further details about the NCI approach are available (Herrick et al., 2018; Luo et al., 2022).

DATASET PREPARATION AND ANALYSIS

The What We Eat in America (NHANES) day-1 and day-2 dietary recall dataset was analyzed for children (2–19 years old, $n = 13{,}171$) and women of childbearing age (16–50 years old, $n = 7{,}355$) in year cycles 2011–2012 to 2017–March 2020. Dietary intake and food pattern equivalent data were joined with the 30-day FFQ about seafood species meals consumed. Child age groups were defined as 2–5, 6–11, and 12–19 years old; three income-to-poverty ratio groups were used (less than 130 percent, between 130 and 499 percent, greater than 500 percent); and four race/ethnicity groups used (Hispanic, non-Hispanic Asian, non-Hispanic Black, and non-Hispanic White).

The per capita consumption of total seafood, seafood groups high and low in long-chain n-3 polyunsaturated fatty acids, total protein foods (e.g., red meat, processed meat, poultry, eggs, nuts and seeds, legumes, soy), seafood species, fatty acids, and micronutrients were calculated for the overall population of 2–19-year-old children and women and stratified by age, sex, race/ethnicity, and income. A two-part model was used for foods and nutrients consumed episodically, defined using the conventional approaches as more than 95 percent of the population having nonzero intake on the 24-hour recalls for the given food or nutrient (Herrick et al., 2018). In this model a correlation between the probability of consumption and the amount consumed was specified. All analyses of usual consumption also accounted for differences in weekend (defined as Friday–Sunday) versus weekday consumption. Covariates included in the prediction of both probabilities and amounts of seafood, protein types, and omega-3 fatty acids for children included sex, age groups, race, income quartiles, season, and consumption of any seafood meals in the seafood FFQ.

Separate modeling was conducted for each subgroup allowing for the estimation of distributions for subgroups. The same covariates were used for women's consumption, omitting sex. Percentiles of usual total fish consumption and total omega-3 fatty acid consumption were estimated using the Distrib SAS macro, which uses pseudo-populations derived from Markov chain Monte Carlo simulation modeling to estimate the percentile of usual consumption. A default of 100 pseudo-persons was used to create this dataset.

A one-part "amount" model was used for ubiquitously consumed foods or nutrients (those consumed by nearly everyone in the sample). Covariates used in the prediction of this model included sex, race, and income quartiles.

The frequency of seafood intake by food source (retail, restaurant, etc.), meal type (breakfast, lunch, dinner), and by the top 10 species (shrimp, tuna, salmon, etc.) by age, sex, race/ethnicity, and income groups was also performed. The top 10 species' frequencies were developed using the 30-day FFQ counts multiplied by the average seafood meal size among age-sex groups modeled using splines, and weighted by meal type (breakfast, lunch, dinner).

Separate analyses were conducted using data collected from children ($n = 1{,}750$) aged 6 months to 2 years for this same time period to examine patterns related to the timing of introduction of seafood. These analyses were primarily conducted using the 30-day FFQ data, although portion size analysis by age group used the 24-hour recall data. As seafood intake was found to be extremely infrequent in this age group the analyses were not intended to be representative, and therefore were reported as weight and unweighted estimates.

INCLUSIONS AND EXCLUSIONS

Analyses of women's intake included all women aged 16–50 years, including pregnant and lactating women. Analyses of children's (2–19 years) and women's intakes relied on participants with complete covariate data.

WEIGHTING

All NHANES analyses accounted for the complex sampling design using primary sampling units, strata, and survey weights to construct nationally representative estimates of food consumption.

Sample weights were constructed for multiple year cycles using methods described by the National Center for Health Statistics (NCHS, 2021). In brief, this involved taking the original weighting variables for each round of data collection and multiplying by the share each round contributes to the total years of the study period (2011–March 2020). The 2020–2021 round was stopped in March 2020 because of the COVID-19 pandemic. NHANES merged the 2019–March 2020 round with the 2017–2018 round for a 3.2-year combined dataset, while all other rounds lasted 2 years. Day 1 sample weights were used when working with 1 day of dietary recall, and day 2 sample weights were used when working with 2 days of dietary recall.

The NCI macro requires the use of balanced repeated replication (BRR) weights to account for both the complex survey design of NHANES and differential weighting in the nonlinear mixed-effects models. This approach is described in detail elsewhere (Herrick et al., 2018). Seventy-two BRR weights were calculated for each individual in the sample following this guidance for the 9.3 years of NHANES included in our sample, using a perturbation factor of 70 percent ($F = 0.3$), the standard factor used in the analyses of NHANES dietary intake data (Herrick et al., 2018; Moshfegh et al., 2009; NCI, 2019).

REFERENCES

Herrick, K. A., L. M. Rossen, R. Parsons, and K. W. Dodd. 2018. Estimating usual dietary intake from National Health and Nutrition Examination Survey data using the National Cancer Institute method. *Vital Health Statistics, Series 2* Feb(178):1-63.

HHS/USDA (U.S. Department of Health and Human Services and U.S. Department of Agriculture). 2020. *Dietary Guidelines for Americans, 2020–2025*. https://www.dietaryguidelines.gov/sites/default/files/2020-12/Dietary_Guidelines_for_Americans_2020-2025.pdf (accessed February 26, 2024).

Krebs-Smith, S. M., P. M. Guenther, A. F. Subar, S. I. Kirkpatrick, and K. W. Dodd. 2010. Americans do not meet federal dietary recommendations. *Journal of Nutrition* 140(10):1832-1838.

Luo, H., K. W. Dodd, C. D. Arnold, and R. Engle-Stone. 2022. Advanced dietary analysis and modeling: A deep dive into the National Cancer Institute method. *Journal of Nutrition* 152(11):2615-2625.

Moshfegh, A. J., J. D. Goldman, J. K. Ahuja, D. G. Rhodes, and R. P. Lacomb. 2009. *What We Eat in America, NHANES 2005-2006, usual nutrient intakes from food and water compared to 1997 dietary reference intakes for vitamin D, calcium, phosphorus, and magnesium*. http://www.ars.usda.gov/ba/bhnrc/fsrg (accessed February 26, 2024).

NCHS (National Center for Health Statistics). 2021. *NHANES analytic guidance and brief overview for the 2017-March 2020 pre-pandemic data files, 2021*. https://wwwn.cdc.gov/nchs/nhanes/continuousnhanes/overviewbrief.aspx?Cycle=2017-2020 (accessed November 7, 2023).

NCI (National Cancer Institute). 2019. *Usual dietary intakes: Food intakes, U.S. population, 2007-2010*. Epidemiology and Genomics Research Program. https://epi.grants.cancer.gov/diet/usualintakes/national-data-usual-dietary-intakes-2007-to-2010.pdf (accessed February 26, 2024).

Shan, Z. L., C. D. Rehm, G. Rogers, M. Y. Ruan, D. D. Wang, F. B. Hu, D. Mozaffarian, F. F. Zhang, and S. N. Bhupathiraju. 2019. Trends in dietary carbohydrate, protein, and fat intake and diet quality among US adults, 1999-2016. *JAMA* 322(12):1178-1187.

Tooze, J. A., D. Midthune, K. W. Dodd, L. S. Freedman, S. M. Krebs-Smith, A. F. Subar, P. M. Guenther, R. J. Carroll, and V. Kipnis. 2006. A new statistical method for estimating the usual intake of episodically consumed foods with application to their distribution. *Journal of the American Dietetic Association* 106(10):1575-1587.

Tooze, J. A., V. Kipnis, D. W. Buckman, R. J. Carroll, L. S. Freedman, P. M. Guenther, S. M. Krebs-Smith, A. F. Subar, and K. W. Dodd. 2010. A mixed-effects model approach for estimating the distribution of usual intake of nutrients: The NCI method. *Statistics in Medicine* 29(27):2857-2868.